X-RAY EQUIPMENT FOR STUDENT RADIOGRAPHERS

To R.W.A.
*who was first to take us
inside an X-ray set,
to show us by his articulate example
the value of saying what we mean
and to encourage us to believe that
we could teach as well as learn
about diagnostic X-ray equipment.*

X-ray Equipment for Student Radiographers

D. NOREEN CHESNEY
FCR, TE
Group Superintendent Radiographer
Coventry and Warwickshire Hospital

AND

MURIEL O. CHESNEY
FCR, TE
Principal, The Central Birmingham
School of Radiography
Central Birmingham Health Authority

THIRD EDITION

BLACKWELL SCIENTIFIC PUBLICATIONS
OXFORD LONDON EDINBURGH
BOSTON MELBOURNE

© 1971, 1975, 1984 by Blackwell Scientific
Publications
Editorial offices;
Osney Mead, Oxford, OX2 oEL
8 John Street, London, WC1N 2ES
9 Forrest Road, Edinburgh, EH1 2QH
52 Beacon Street, Boston
Massachusetts 02108, USA
99 Barry Street, Carlton
Victoria 3053, Australia

First published 1971
Second edition 1975
Reprinted 1978, 1981
Third edition 1984

Printed and bound in Great Britain by
William Clowes Limited, Beccles and London

DISTRIBUTORS

USA
  Blackwell Mosby Book Distributors
  11830 Westline Industrial Drive
  St Louis, Missouri 63141

Canada
  Blackwell Mosby Book Distributors
  120 Melford Drive, Scarborough
  Ontario, M1B 2X4

Australia
  Blackwell Scientific Book Distributors
  31 Advantage Road, Highett
  Victoria 3190

British Library Cataloguing in Publication
Data

Chesney, D. Noreen
  X-ray equipment for student
  radiographers.—3rd ed.
  1. X-rays—Apparatus and supplies
  I. Title   II. Chesney, Muriel O.
  616.07′57′028   RC78
  ISBN 0-632-01226-9

Contents

Preface to
Third Edition

In introducing this new edition to its readers—whom we naturally hope to find in the plural!—perhaps our first concern should be less to describe what the book includes than to explain what it omits. During the years which followed publication of the second edition, certainly two major diagnostic tools have established such firm places for themselves within the specialty that their presences are to be expected in a radiological department. One of these is medical ultrasound and the other is computed tomography. Now there is a third coming within our grasp: nuclear magnetic resonance or NMR as most of us know it. Readers may ask themselves—and wish to ask us—why this book attempts to explain only one of these three: perhaps our colleagues may even reprove us for what they regard as serious omissions.

Certain it is that, had we included medical ultrasound and NMR, production of this new edition would have been even longer delayed than now. Certain it is that we were not thoughtless of these matters. In the event, we decided to adhere to our title *X-ray Equipment for Student Radiographers* at least for the present book and so to exclude diagnostic usages which do not derive from an X-ray generator and an X-ray tube. Thus computed tomography—alone of the three methods—qualifies for inclusion and makes its appearance in Chapter 13.

For the rest, we have concerned ourselves with needed up-datings which have resulted in the introduction of certain generators, a review of available choices of generator and the application of each to diagnostic radiology. We have further reviewed automatic exposure control and have included some account of cassetteless radiography. In some control systems we have simplified the discussion of circuitry.

Chapter 11 (on image intensifiers) has been subject to hard pruning and to growth in order that it shall accord with present radiodiagnostic practice. The section in Chapter 12 on telecommand fluoroscopic/radiographic tables has been expanded, since these are now more widely used than they were; and the current availability of radiographic systems for trauma justifies another new section in Chapter 16. In Chapter 17 the section on functional tests of equipment has been expanded to include some of the test tools which are currently available for use by radiographers.

This book, like its predecessors, has been produced by the efforts not of its authors only. It is a pleasure now to have an opportunity to express our gratitude to others whom variously we have involved. Of each of them we have made demands of one kind or another and their unstinted responses have energized the realization of this book.

Mr Peter McAtamney of International General Electric Company of New York Ltd gave a number of hours—including the beginning of a Christmas holiday—to educating one of us in computed tomography: as also—fortunately at an earlier date—did Mr Alistair McIntosh, Head of the Department of Medical Physics and Bio-engineering at Walsgrave Hospital, Coventry. We are sincerely grateful for a generous gift of time from two fully occupied people.

Similar appreciation is due to Mr R. Basterfield of Siemens Ltd whose teaching on modern image intensifiers let light into previously dark places and who put references at our disposal. We are happy to say *Thank you* to Mr Ernest Orme of the same company who made this possible and provided always ready help and advice.

Mr C. W. Mead has shown continued interest in the book and has again sustained our efforts. We are grateful to him for reading a section of the manuscript and providing illustrations for others. Some of our illustrative needs have also been expeditiously met by Mr Mike Walker and his staff of the Department of Medical Illustration at Birmingham Dental Hospital and we much appreciate their work on our behalf.

We gladly recognize the courtesy of several companies in permitting us to use photographic material which they publish. In this respect, we offer our thanks to Siemens Elema AB, Shimadzu Medical X Ray and Picker International Ltd. We are grateful not least to Mr David Workman of International General Electric Co. for introducing us to his company's expertise in the first instance.

The efforts of all of us would have been invalidated if the authors had not been able to avail themselves—as always through a long association—of the skills and capabilities of their publishers. So we wish again to express our especial thanks to Mr Per Saugman and Mr John Robson of Blackwell Scientific Publications Ltd.

Finally, our wish for this book is that it may as unfailingly assist its readers as have the protagonists of this preface its authors.

1983

D.N.C.
M.O.C.

Preface to
First Edition

This is not the book we planned to write. When we began it the idea was to produce a book about diagnostic X-ray equipment which would be simple, primarily concerned with practicalities and reassuringly short. Instead we have a book which—we believe—should be reasonably easy to understand; we are encouraged in this respect by a physicist friend who is half-inclined to think it is too simple. It *is* very much concerned with the actual use of X-ray equipment. It is not, however, short.

Modern diagnostic apparatus is not a small subject, and perhaps we were foolish to believe that a brief manual on it could be written at a level likely to be useful to those who are presently preparing for the diploma examinations of the Society of Radiographers and always required to put to good use the expensive toys in their departments. We have tried to make every word in this book count, and we hope that student readers will not be intimidated by its appearance of length.

So far as we know this is the first book to be written about the subject called Diagnostic X-ray Equipment in the Society of Radiographers' syllabus for its qualifying diploma. True, X-ray equipment is included in other works but it is mixed with physics or radiographic technique. Because we enjoy using and understanding—if we can—properly designed apparatus, and because too few radiographers teach this subject in their schools, we have believed there is a place for a book that will concentrate on what X-ray equipment does, and provide basic explanations that may be helpful not only to students but perhaps also to the radiographers who teach them. We recognize that some of the topics in this book have been adequately covered elsewhere, for example the X-ray tube, but we would submit also that others have not appeared before in a formal textbook for radiographers, at least in the English language.

Because we wished to make the book one from which it is easy to learn, we have tried to avoid complexity in its many diagrams, especially in the circuit diagrams. This means that in various instances the drawings do not represent complete working arrangements and we make no apology for this, since their aim is to provide understanding and not to facilitate an X-ray installation.

Some references to physics have been essential, but we have generally assumed in our readers a certain knowledge of these matters and have limited our own probings as much as we can. Such subjects as electronoptics have been treated in relation to their application to a specific piece of equipment rather than in an academic context. This we believe to be the right approach because we are sure that the study of diagnostic X-ray equipment—if it is to be useful to radiographers—should be practical, its place the X-ray room as much as the classroom.

While the Society of Radiographers' syllabus for its qualifying diploma has established guide lines for the writing of this book, there are nevertheless matters here which do not appear in the present syllabus, though they are much in evidence in X-ray departments. It is therefore necessary to teach them to students and for post-diploma radiographers to have some understanding of them. We hope that both these groups of people will be helped by our small forays into television, electronics and other present advances in radiological equipment.

Perhaps the best part of writing the preface to a textbook is being able to say 'Thank you' to those from whom we have freely drawn assistance. That we have confidence in this book is due to the help of our friends among physicists and manufacturers of X-ray equipment who not only have given us much of their expensive time and unfailingly answered all our questions, but have not seemed to mind doing so. Our expert team of readers were Mr R. F. Farr, Chief Physicist at the United Birmingham Hospitals; Mr C. W. Mead of Watson and Sons (Electro-Medical) Ltd (G. E. C. Medical Equipment Ltd); Mr J. E. Steadman, who was then working with A. E. Dean and Co. (G. E. C. Medical Equipment Ltd); Mr G. Waters of Machlett X-ray Tubes (Great Britain) Ltd (G. E. C. Medical Equipment Ltd). Mr C. J. Hills, also of Watson and Sons, was let off lightly and kindly read Chapter 9. We hope that he did not regard his subsequent departure from the United Kingdom as an escape. Chapter 11 profited from the advice of Mr L. A. Newman of Philips Electrical Ltd. We are immeasurably grateful to them all. Their knowledge has provided this book with its sinews and their kindness has given to the writing of it a special reward.

We are grateful for the use of illustrative material supplied to us by several organizations. In particular we appreciate the energy displayed in our cause by Mr David Scott when he was Publicity Manager of Watson & Sons (Electro-Medical) Ltd, and by Mr Malcolm Holmes, Publicity Manager of G. E. C. Medical Equipment Ltd. The following have permitted us to publish photographs and diagrams belonging to them and it is a pleasure here to record our appreciation of this assistance: Barr and Stroud Ltd; Blackwell Scientific Publications Ltd; Mr D. Bourne; A. E. Dean and Co. Ltd (G. E. C. Medical Equipment Ltd); Elema-Schonander; Mr R. F.

Farr; Mr W. Herstel; International General Electric Co. of New York; Machlett X-ray Tubes (Great Britain) Ltd (G. E. C. Medical Equipment Ltd); Marconi Instruments Ltd; Mr G. Mountain; N. V. Optische Industrie; *Radiography*, the Journal of the Society of Radiographers; Sierex Ltd; The Technical Press Ltd; Watson and Sons (Electro-Medical) Ltd (G. E. C Medical Equipment Ltd).

Our colleague Mr D. S. Wilkinson took the photograph (Plate 12.2) of the handswitch of an AOT film changer, and we are grateful for his practical help.

Extracts in Chapter 5 from the British Standard Specifications for Composite Units of Switches and Fuses (British Standard 2510:1954) and for Heavy Duty Composite Units of Air-Break Switches and Fuses (British Standard 3185:1959) are reproduced by kind permission of the British Standards Institution, 2 Park Street, London W1Y 4AA, from whom copies of the complete Standard may be obtained.

Finally we would like once more to thank Mr Per Saugman of Blackwell Scientific Publications who, in telling us that he would publish this book, allowed us the self-indulgence of writing it.

1970

D.N.C.
M.O.C.

Chapter 1
The Electrical System and the Mains Supply

A true story is told of a radiologist and a radiographer who took a portable X-ray set to a patient's house in order to carry out a radiographic examination requested by the patient's doctor. When the two arrived with their equipment they found that the house, which was in a country district, was without any electrical supply.

The starting point in operating any X-ray equipment is the availability of electrical energy to make it work. This electrical energy is in most cases taken from the mains supply. Characteristics of the supply influence the operation of the equipment. So this book about X-ray equipment for diagnostic radiography may fairly begin with some account of the system by which electrical energy is generated and distributed in the United Kingdom. The account will be a very simple one, as there is no need for elaboration, which in any case the authors are not qualified to provide.

THE ELECTRICAL SYSTEM

One of the most advantageous features of electrical energy as a source of power is that it can be generated and easily transmitted over great distances to the places where it is going to be used. The generation and distribution of electrical energy are matters which most radiographers do not very easily understand. This lack of comprehension is not helped by the fact that it is not possible to *see* electricity; we can see only some of the effects of electricity. It is not easy to realize just how a process which starts in a power station can be used to make electrons flow along the wire filament of one's bedside lamp many miles distant from the generator. However, it is not necessary for radiographers fully to understand all of this. Provided we have certain knowledge concerning the electrical system as it relates to the operation of X-ray equipment, it may not matter if we continue to be slightly mystified by the processes which light our bedside lights.

It is clear that the electrical system we use embraces the three separate elements of (i) generation of the electrical energy in a power station, (ii) distribution and transmission of the electrical energy by means of copper cables or lines, and (iii) use of the electrical energy in various pieces of equipment for the provision of light and heat, and for doing countless other forms of work—one of which is the production of radiographic images.

GENERATION OF ELECTRICAL ENERGY

Direct and alternating currents

There is more than one kind of electrical current. The simplest division to make first of all is to consider that there are two kinds: (i) direct or continuous current, and (ii) alternating current.

Direct current is the simplest sort and is the type provided by a battery. It is a flow of electricity in one direction along conductors which carry it in complete circuits. A sketch (as in Fig. 1.1) can be made depicting a battery and a complete circuit, and a graph can be set beside it to show the current against a time-scale; such a graph is simply a picture of what is happening to the current as time goes by.

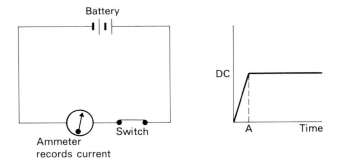

Fig. 1.1

It can be seen that the current once it reaches its full value at the point A in time is continuous and unvarying—i.e. it is *not* going up and down the vertical axis of the graph as in Fig. 1.2. It is not changing in direction—i.e. it does *not* come to the other side of the horizontal time-axis as in Fig. 1.3. The graph in Fig. 1.1 is the picture of direct current (d.c.).

Alternating current is quite different; it *does* vary and it *does* change its direction of flow in conductors which carry it in a complete circuit. Electricity is swinging back and forth in such a circuit. Alternating current can be produced by rotating a coil of wire in a magnetic field. The coil has induced in it an electromotive force (electrical pressure which tries to make

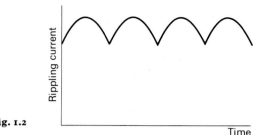

Fig. 1.2

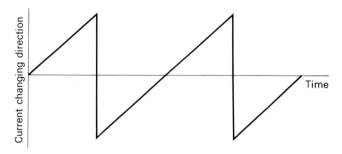

Fig. 1.3

electricity move) and this electromotive force can be used to make current flow in a complete circuit.

Again a sketch can be made depicting the coil which rotates at a uniform rate in its magnetic field, and the external circuit in which current can be made to flow by means of the electromotive force generated in the coil (Fig. 1.4). Beside it is a graph to show the current against a time-scale.

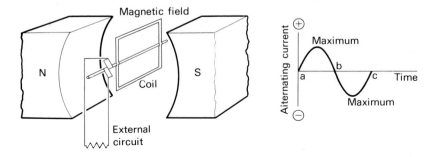

Fig. 1.4   Generating alternating current by rotating a coil in a magnetic field.

This is the picture of current which is varying in value (it is moving up and down the vertical axis of the graph) and is changing direction (it appears on both sides of the time-axis). During the period *ab* on the time-axis when the current is moving in one direction and a wave is shown above the horizontal axis, it is said to be *positive*. During the period *bc* when the current has reversed its direction and a wave is shown below the horizontal axis, it is said to be *negative*.

This form of alternating current, which is obtained by rotating a coil of wire at a uniform rate in a magnetic field and on the graph looks (if you have an active imagination!) like a wave of the sea, is called alternating current (a.c.) of sine wave form.

We should now consider how it comes to be that form of wave and why it is called a sine wave.

The sine wave of alternating current

The current flows in the complete circuit depicted in Fig. 1.4 because the coil of wire has generated in it an electromotive force which causes the current to flow. This electromotive force arises in the coil by reason of its *movement* in relation to the magnetic field in which it rotates at a uniform rate. Both the electromotive force which makes the current flow and the current itself have the same sort of pattern—this wave-like shape shown in the graph in Fig. 1.4. So we can stop talking about current for the purpose of this explanation and consider the electromotive force (e.m.f.). What is happening to it as time goes by?

It grows from zero up to a maximum value (considered a positive maximum); falls to zero again; changes direction and grows to a maximum value in this new direction (considered a negative maximum); then falls to zero again and the pattern repeats itself.

The reader may care to consider one edge of the coil—the one designated AB in Fig. 1.5(a). This describes a full circle as the coil rotates. In our imaginations we can replace this edge of the coil by a skipping-rope held by a girl who stands (for some reason or another) skipping in a magnetic field. She is seen in Fig. 1.5(b). Now let us imagine an observer watching her from one of the magnetic poles: his eye can be seen in Fig. 1.5(b) in front of the south pole.

The rope is rotating through a complete circle (360 degrees) but the observer will see this rotary motion as a vertical rise and fall of the rope— downwards in front of the skipper and upwards behind her if it is going clockwise. The rate of motion of the rope in its circular path is uniform (the coil rotates at a uniform rate); its rate of motion in an up and down direction is *not* uniform.

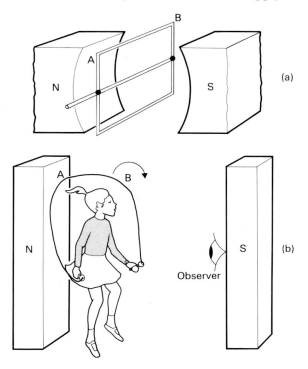

Fig. 1.5

This can be seen in Fig. 1.6 where xy is the edge of the coil (or the skipping-rope) in cross-section. xy_1, xy_2, xy_3, xy_4, xy_5 represent the positions of the coil as it moves through its first 15 degrees, its second 15 degrees, its third 15 degrees, its fourth 15 degrees and its fifth 15 degrees of rotation—equal amounts of rotary movement in equal periods of time. Its downward progress in a vertical direction is indicated by the spacing between the figures 1, 2, 3, 4, 5 on the vertical line in front of the observer's eye. It can be seen that the coil is moving through a bigger vertical distance with these successive degrees of rotation. As it is covering bigger vertical distances in the same periods of time, its vertical rate of motion must be increasing. It will continue to increase in the first quarter turn of the coil.

In the second quarter turn of the coil the vertical rate of motion will decrease again to a zero point (when the skipping-rope is swinging along the ground and for some instants is not moving vertically at all). Then the vertical rate of motion will increase again in the third quarter turn, but in a new direction (the rope is now rising vertically upwards and not moving vertically downwards). In the last quarter turn the vertical rate of motion again falls to zero (the rope, reaching the top of its circle, now travels parallel to the ground and for some instants is not moving vertically at all).

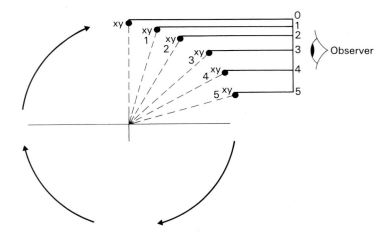

Fig. 1.6

This *vertical rate of motion* is the rate at which the coil is cutting the lines of magnetic force between the poles of the magnet. The electromotive force induced in the coil depends for its magnitude on the rate at which the coil cuts these magnetic lines, and for its direction on the direction the coil moves through them. Therefore the electromotive force increases from zero to maximum in the first quarter turn of the coil; falls from maximum to zero in the second quarter turn; increases from zero to maximum in a new direction in the third quarter turn; and falls from maximum to zero in the last quarter turn. This is the same sequence of variation as the rate of vertical motion of the coil in its rotary path and explains why the electromotive force induced in the coil has this wave-like form.

From the foregoing account it is clear that the electromotive force varies in value from instant to instant according to the position of the coil on its rotary path. This position can be expressed in terms of the angular degrees through which it has rotated from its starting or zero position. So at zero position of the coil the electromotive force is zero; at 90 degrees the electromotive force is a positive maximum value; at 180 degrees it is at zero; at 270 degrees it is a negative maximum value, having changed direction; at 360 degrees it is zero again, the coil having then completed a full circle. This is depicted in Fig. 1.7, where the horizontal axis of the graph can be

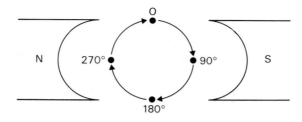

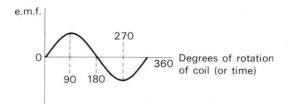

Fig. 1.7

considered to represent both time and degrees of rotation as the coil is rotating at a constant speed.

The electromotive force generated at any instant is related to the angle through which the coil has moved by being directly proportional to the sine of this angle; this is why this a.c. waveform is known as a *sine wave*. One complete wave (360 degrees rotation of the coil) is called one *cycle*; this is clearly made up of two half-waves or half-cycles, the current flowing in a different direction for each half-cycle. The next point to be considered is how frequently the cycles repeat themselves.

Frequency of alternating current

As the complete cycle of alternating current is produced by one complete rotation of the coil in its magnetic field, it is obvious that the rate of repetition of the wave-form depends on the rate at which the coil is revolving—that is the number of complete revolutions which it makes in a given period of time. For a single coil rotating in a magnetic field with two poles the number of cycles of alternating current and the number of complete revolutions is the same. The number of complete cycles per second is called the *frequency* of the alternating current. In the electrical system of the United Kingdom the frequency of most alternating current power supplies is 50 cycles per second (50 hertz). One complete cycle therefore occupies 1/50 second and one half-cycle occupies 1/100 second.

In the U.S.A. the frequency is usually 60 cycles per second, in which case a complete cycle occupies 1/60 second and one half-cycle occupies 1/120 second.

So far we have depicted only one coil rotating between two magnetic poles and giving rise to one sine wave; this is known as *single-phase alternating current*. Earlier in this chapter we considered just two sorts of electric current

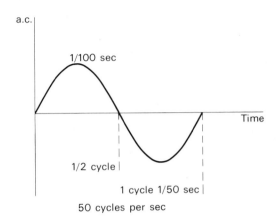

Fig. 1.8   50 cycles per sec

(i) direct current and (ii) alternating current. We can now extend our view a bit by considering that there is more than one sort of alternating current, the first sort being this single-phase alternating current produced by a single coil rotating at a uniform rate in a two-pole magnetic field.

Polyphase alternating currents

The persistent reader now knows about one sine wave and single-phase alternating current. Let us look at the production of a number of sine waves simultaneously—fortunately not a large number of them, but only three. This is called a *polyphase system* as the number of sine waves is more than one; it can be called specifically a *three-phase system* as the number of sine waves is only three.

If one coil of wire moving in relation to a magnetic field produces one sine wave of alternating current, it is not surprising that three sine waves may be produced by three coils moving in relation to a magnetic field. These three coils may be imagined grouped round each other and displaced equally from each other within 360 degrees as shown in Fig. 1.9.

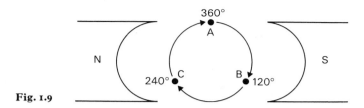

Fig. 1.9

As the coils are equally displaced from each other within a circle, they must be separated from each other by 120 degrees. From this it follows that when coil A is at the zero position in the magnetic field, as shown in Fig. 1.9, coil B must be at the 120 degrees position and coil C must be at the 240 degrees position. The coils rotate together and each has produced in it a separate a.c. sine wave of electromotive force. All the waves are of the same pattern, and all go up and down to peaks of the same height on the vertical axis, but they do not all reach their peaks at the same instant of time—i.e. they are not in step with each other. Waves which are *not in step* with each other are said to be *out of phase*; waves which *are in step* with each other are said to be *in phase*.

Why are these three sine waves out of phase? It is to be remembered that the magnitude and direction of the electromotive force produced in a coil depend on the angle at which the coil is situated in relation to the zero position in the magnetic field. When the coil is at zero position, the electromotive force is at zero value; when the coil is at 90 degrees, the electromotive force is at positive maximum; when the coil is at 180 degrees, the electromotive force is at zero again; when the coil is at 270 degrees, the electromotive force is at negative maximum; and when the coil is at 360 degrees, the electromotive force is again at zero.

It has been said that these three coils are disposed in the magnetic field thus: coil A at zero, coil B at 120 degrees, coil C at 240 degrees. It follows that at the instant in time when the electromotive force in coil A is zero in value, the one in coil B must be falling from a positive maximum (being 30 degrees past the 90 degrees position), and the one in coil C must be approaching a negative maximum (being 30 degrees away from the 270 degrees position). These three electromotive forces are shown in Fig. 1.10.

So it is possible to provide a generator with three coils which can produce three separate supplies of alternating current. The voltages provided by these three separate sources of electricity are out of phase with each other in the way that has been shown.

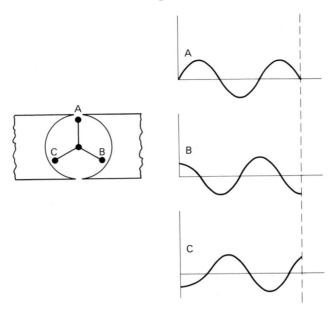

Fig. 1.10

Star-connected three-phase circuits

Three such separate sources of alternating current are not kept entirely apart when such a system is in use. If they *were* kept apart, it would be necessary to provide six output terminals to the generator and six conducting wires, two for each coil. Fig. 1.11 shows a sketch of such an arrangement. In practice a more economical system can be devised; this is explained below.

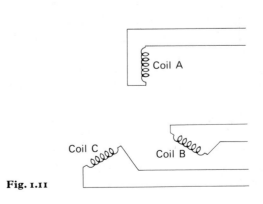

Fig. 1.11

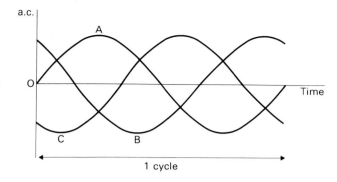

a.c.

A

O

Time

C   B

1 cycle

Fig. 1.12

Fig. 1.12 shows the three sine waves superimposed on one time-axis. Study of the graphs at the period of origin O shows that when one of the curves is at zero the other two have values which are equal and opposite; each is the same period of time (30 degrees of rotation) away from a maximum value, and each is at the same height on the vertical axis. This means that the sum of the currents represented by these three sine waves of electromotive force is zero, and this is true if all the sine waves are being equally used—i.e. in technical phraseology, all the phases are equally loaded. It is true not only for this instant of time at the origin of the graphs, but also for all the other instants of time along the horizontal axis.

Because of this it is not necessary to provide a generator in a three-phase system with six conducting wires. One end of each of the three windings is connected to a common centre point and four terminals are used as in Fig. 1.13.

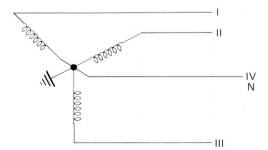

I

II

IV
N

Fig. 1.13

III

When this is done the generator windings are said to be *star-connected* or *wye connected*. Conductors I, II and III are connected to the free ends of the windings and conductor IV is connected to the common centre point as in Fig. 1.13. With this arrangement, if the electrical loads placed on each of the three phases are equal, the current flowing towards the centre in one of the windings is equal to the sum of the currents flowing away from the centre in the other two.

To look back at Fig. 1.12 will remind the reader that at any instant of time when one of the sine waves is below the horizontal axis, the other two are above it. The graphs are simply a form of illustration of a practical situation, and curves above and below the horizontal axis means currents flowing in different directions. So it seems fairly obvious from the graphs that this practical situation in regard to the windings can exist—that at any instant of time the current flowing towards the centre equals the current flowing away. This is so, provided that the electrical loads placed on the three phases are equal; in this ideal state of affairs each of the conductors I, II and III can act as a return path for the other two.

In practice, the electrical loads placed on the three phases may not be equal. In that case the fourth conductor IV (being common to all three windings at one end of each) acts as a common return path for current flowing from any of the windings to whatever external circuits are using the electrical power and back to the windings again.

The three conductors I, II and III are known as the three *lines* of the supply, and the fourth one IV from the common centre point (which is earthed) is known as the *neutral* cable. Such a system of distribution is known as a three-phase, four-wire system which is star-connected. It is a standard method of distribution of electricity.

Delta-connected three-phase circuits

The star-connected system of joining the three phases together is not the only one possible. Instead of forming a star, the phase can be connected so that in a diagram they look like a triangle as in Fig. 1.14. Since a triangle is similar to the Greek capital letter *delta*, this arrangement is known as *delta-connection* and it may also be described as *mesh connection*.

The wye-connected arrangement has certain advantages over delta-connection as a system of distribution. The machinery is cheaper to produce and there is less stress and liability to breakdown in regard to insulation.

Another important advantage of the wye-connected system is that distribution can be arranged to provide two different voltages simply by means of different connections. It can therefore easily meet the needs of different types of user and can supply power for the domestic consumer at

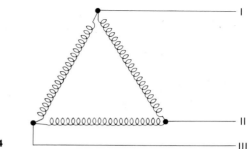

Fig. 1.14

one voltage, and for industry, hospitals and large institutions at a higher voltage. This is explained below.

DISTRIBUTION OF ELECTRICAL ENERGY

The uses of electrical energy constitute various electrical loads connected to the phases of the supply. The three conductors I, II and III in Fig. 1.13 are the three lines of the supply and IV is the neutral. Each load can be connected between any one of the lines and the neutral; this is shown at L_1, L_2 and L_3 in Fig. 1.15. These loads are obtaining their voltage from one of the windings and the voltage so obtained is called the *phase voltage*. In the United Kingdom it is 230–240 volts.

Another possibility is to connect electrical loads between any two of the three lines. This is shown for L_4, L_5 and L_6 in Fig. 1.15. These loads are obtaining their voltage from two of the windings and the voltage so obtained is called the *line voltage*. It will be remembered that these windings do not have their voltages in step with each other and the voltages do not come to a peak value at the same time. Because of this the line voltage obtained between any two of the lines is not twice the phase voltage obtained between any one of the lines and the neutral, but is a smaller value than this. It is in fact 1·7 times the phase voltage. If the phase voltage is 240 volts the line voltage will be 415 volts.

Thus it is possible to obtain two different voltages from a star-connected four-wire system. The lower phase voltage is suitable for operating electrical equipment which does not need very much electrical power. For example it is suitable for domestic use—for lighting and for operating various appliances such as electric fires, vacuum-cleaners and other things.

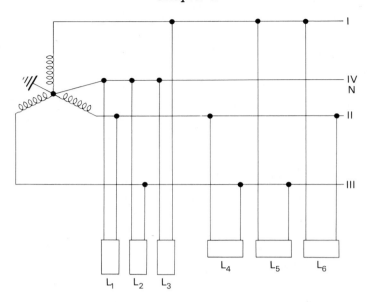

Fig. 1.15

The higher line voltage is supplied to users who need very much greater amounts of electric power to operate equipment in factories and hospitals. More will be said of this in the following sections on the use of electrical energy.

The electricity is generated at power stations using various forms of energy to drive the generators. The generators are not the simple equipment in terms of which the production of single-phase and three-phase alternating current has been described. Instead of moving coils of wire in a magnetic field, the generators (which are called alternators) move magnets in front of coils of wire wound on iron cores. So the basic principle is the same—that of relative motion between conductors and magnetic fields.

Each power station has a number of alternators and from these the electricity is transmitted along copper cables to where it is to be used, often over very big distances. From the point of view of expense and practicability, it is better if these cables can be as small in size and weight as is conveniently possible. The size and weight of a cable carrying electricity are determined by the current it must be designed to carry, bigger currents requiring thicker cables. Electrical power is proportional to voltage × current. It follows therefore that if a large amount of power is to be transmitted by means of a cable, the cable must carry a small current if the voltage is high and a big current if the voltage is low.

In supply systems the cables or lines receive the electricity from the alternators. The electrical pressure is raised to very high voltages, and the electricity is carried over the country at voltages of the order of 60–270 kilovolts. These high voltages allow the use of smaller cables. At electrical sub-stations the power is then converted to lower voltages by the use of transformers. It is supplied from sub-stations to users at the voltages which have been mentioned—in the United Kingdom, 230–240 volts for the phase voltage and 400–415 volts for the line voltage.

USE OF ELECTRICAL ENERGY

Relationship between power and current

When electricity is used to make a piece of equipment work, that equipment requires a certain amount of electric power if it is to work properly. This electric power is expressed in watts or in kilowatts.

An electric fire may be a 1 kilowatt fire if it has only one 'bar' or filament, and a 2 kilowatt fire if it is a bigger one with two 'bars'. A small electric bulb not giving a very intense light (such as would be fitted in a darkroom safelight in the X-ray department) is a 25 watt bulb. Bigger ones giving much more intense light are 100 watts and 150 watts.

Readers may care to imagine themselves in their homes using a lamp fitted with a 25 watt bulb. The lamp will be connected up to the mains supply in one of two ways. Either it will be a permanent installation in a room and the electricity will be brought to the bulb by means of wires emerging through a point in a ceiling or a wall; or it will be portable equipment connected to a wall-socket by means of its electric flex or thin cable.

In either case it may be assumed that the lamp is receiving its power at an electrical pressure or voltage which is 240 volts. When the lamp is switched on, electricity will flow along the wires—i.e. a certain quantity of electricity will flow at a certain rate. This rate of flow of a quantity of electricity is the electric current which flows along the wires when the lamp is operating.

Electric current is measured in amperes or amps, 1 amp being a rate of flow of 1 coulomb (a quantity of electricity) per second. For the 25 watt lamp (or any other piece of electrical equipment) it is possible to estimate the current that flows by dividing the number of watts by the number of volts of pressure at which the electricity is delivered.

Thus a 25 watt lamp on 240 volts mains draws a current of 25/240 amperes. This is just a bit more than 0·1 ampere—i.e. 0·1 coulomb per second.

If the 25 watt bulb is replaced by a 100 watt bulb, the lamp will give a brighter light. Connected still to the 240 volts mains, it will be using more electricity to provide this brighter light and will take more current from the mains at the same electrical pressure. This current will be 100/240 amperes—that is just a bit more than 0·4 ampere.

Suppose that the lamp is portable and is disconnected from the wallsocket, a 1 kilowatt electric fire being connected in its place. This new piece of equipment will obtain its electricity at 240 volts pressure just as the lamp did, but it will cause a different rate of flow along the wires and draw a different current from the mains supply. This current can be estimated in the same way as the current taken by the lamp (1 kilowatt being converted to watts) and is 1000/240 amperes. This is just over 4 amperes. Similarly, a larger electric fire with two 'bars' that needed 2 kilowatts of power to make it work would draw still more current. It would cause just over 8 amperes (2000/240) to flow along the wires from the mains.

Thus it is clear that more current is taken from the mains when equipment is operating at higher power—when lamps are giving brighter light and fires intense heat. In this, X-ray equipment is similar to other electrical devices and draws more current when it is using more power. The power used by the X-ray unit is related to its radiographic output. The values of milliamperes and kilovolts which the radiographer selects determine the current which the X-ray set takes from the mains when it is operating.

The milliamperes and the kilovolts are the electrical load which is placed on the X-ray tube. This can be turned into kilovolt-amperes (kVA) in a calculation which converts the peak kilovolts and the milliamperes into effective values and multiplies the two together. Thus a tube load of 50 mA at 80 kVp represents a consumption of power which is about 3·25 kVA. Suppose that the X-ray set were connected to the 240 volts mains supply. When the X-ray exposure is made with these tube factors the current that will be taken from the mains may be estimated by converting the kilovolt-amperes into volt-amperes and dividing by the value of the mains voltage. Thus the current is 3250/240 amperes, which is a little over 13 amperes.

Another combination of radiographic exposure factors will cause a different value of current to be taken from the mains supply. A tube current of 100 mA at 60 kVp means a consumption of power which is about 4·5 kVA. This in turn means a tube current of nearly 20 amperes taken from the mains.

So it can be seen that every time an X-ray set is used to make an exposure it draws current from the mains, and the value of this current will depend on the milliamperes and the kilovolts which are used. High values (high radiographic output) mean that large currents are taken from the mains;

low values of milliamperes and kilovolts (low radiographic output) mean that small currents are taken from the mains.

The current drawn from the mains for an X-ray tube-load clearly depends not only on the tube-load itself but also on the voltage of the supply to which it is connected. The calculations which have been done so far assumed that the X-ray set was connected to a 240 volts mains, i.e. to the phase voltage. If the X-ray set is instead connected to the 415 volts of the line voltage, then the same tube-loads result in smaller currents being drawn.

Thus taking the figures from the previous examples, a load of 3·25 kVA on the X-ray tube when the set is connected to 415 volts draws a current of 3250/415 amps—which is about 8 amps. A load of 4·5 kVA on the tube draws a current of the order of 11 amps when the set is connected to the 415 volts of the line supply.

Changes in the voltage clearly result in proportional changes in the current drawn by any given load in kilovolt-amperes or kilowatts.

Current loads and power losses

Mains voltage drop under load

When an X-ray set (or any other piece of electrical equipment) is in use and is drawing current from the mains supply, this current flows along conductors. There is, after all, no other way of bringing it to the piece of equipment concerned. As we seldom in life (and never in the physical world) get anything for nothing, some force must be expended in making the current flow through the resistance of the conductors which are carrying it. It is an inescapable fact that these conductors have resistance, and voltage is used up in making the current flow against it.

The question then arises as to the value of voltage required—how many volts will it take? This will depend on two things: (i) on how much current is to be made to flow, and (ii) on how much resistance is opposing it. The voltage (E) necessary to drive a particular current (I) through a particular resistance (R) is the product of the current and resistance:

$$E = RI.$$

Let us think again of an X-ray tube making an exposure with the conditions of 50 mA at 80 kVp: with the X-ray set connected up to the 415 volts of the line supply, this exposure (3·25 kVA) caused a current of about 8 amperes to flow from the mains. Suppose that the cables bringing the supply to the X-ray set have a resistance of 0·4 ohm for every 1000 yards of cable and that we have to deal with 500 yards of cable. The resistance of the cable is therefore 0·2 ohm, and to make 8 amperes flow along this cable

8 × 0·2 volts is required, i.e. 1·6 volts. This means that as soon as the X-ray exposure begins and a current of 8 amperes flows along the supply cables, the 415 volts of the mains fall (at once and for the duration of the exposure) to 415 − 1·6 = 413·4 volts. This fall in mains voltage by an amount necessary to overcome the resistance of the cables and send the current load along them is known as the *mains voltage drop under load*. It is an inevitable occurrence as soon as the X-ray exposure begins, and it is desirable that this voltage drop should be kept as small as possible; the voltage used up in this drop is really lost voltage so far as working the X-ray set is concerned.

If the X-ray set is to operate properly and obtain the power it needs, this voltage drop under load must not be too large a percentage of the mains voltage. In this particular case it is about 0·4 per cent and that is negligible. Let us consider factors which make it bigger and begin by recalling that the 3·25 kVA load on the X-ray tube drew a current of about 13 amperes when it was connected to the 240 volts phase voltage instead of to the 415 volts line voltage.

With the 13 amperes flowing, the mains cable of resistance 0·2 ohms will give rise to a voltage drop of 13 × 0·2 = 2·6 volts. This is something like 1 per cent of the 240 volts and certainly would not be considered significant. The little piece of arithmetic shows, however, that (for the same tube loads) the mains voltage drop gets bigger as the supply voltage is smaller because the smaller supply voltage means that larger currents must flow for the same amounts of power being used by the X-ray tube.

When mains voltage requirements are being considered in relation to the installation of X-ray sets, voltage drops in excess of 5 to 6 per cent of the mains voltage are to be avoided. They result in too low a voltage being left to work the X-ray set; this makes it impossible to obtain sufficient radiographic output even when the controls are set to give adequate exposure factors for a particular examination. Large voltage drops affect the kilovoltage, the milliamperage and the accuracy of timers, and can therefore lead to very poor radiographic results.

The arithmetical examples just considered were based on 50 mA at 80 kVp; these are not factors giving a very high radiographic output, as any radiographer will recognize. On many occasions the X-ray set will be used with factors much greater than these. Instead of currents of 8 amperes and 13 amperes such as we have considered, currents as high as 200–300 amperes may flow along the cables when the X-ray exposure is made. These high currents will flow for periods of time which are only momentary as the exposure intervals used with high milliamperes are very short. Nevertheless, the voltage drop under load will occur. With a mains resistance of 0·2 ohms, 150 amperes (for example) produce a 30 volts drop. This is about 7 per cent of the 415 volts line voltage.

From the foregoing paragraphs, the following important considerations may be extracted.

1 Resistance in supply cables gives rise to a fall in the mains voltage when the current being used by the X-ray set flows from the mains.

2 The value of this current depends on the conditions of operation of the X-ray tube (milliamperage and kilovoltage) and on the supply voltage. For the same tube factors, a higher supply voltage means a smaller current flowing. If the X-ray set is a major one giving high radiographic output, it should be connected to a higher supply voltage (to the line rather than to the phase voltage) in order to reduce the currents which it will draw from the mains.

3 The extent to which the mains voltage falls depends on the resistance of the mains and on the current flowing. For the same tube factors, a higher voltage entails smaller voltage drops than are associated with a lower supply voltage.

4 The resistance of the supply cables should be as small as possible. This is particularly important when very high currents are to flow, as a combination of high current and high resistance results in excessive voltage drop. When the currents are not large, cables may have higher resistance without giving rise to excessive voltage drops.

Perhaps it should be admitted now that while these considerations relating to mains resistance may be nothing but the truth, they are not the whole truth. They have made it seem that the only opposition to the flow of the current in mains cables is ordinary ohmic resistance. In fact, since these cables are carrying alternating current there are other elements (arising from the alternations of the current) which constitute opposition to the flow; these elements are grouped with resistance to constitute *impedance*—which may be simply defined as the total opposition to current in an a.c. circuit. (Impedance is measured in ohms.) However, in the case of the mains supply cables these other elements would be very small in comparison with the resistance; so we venture to leave them unexplored and to consider resistance only instead of the more complex term impedance.

In the installation of X-ray sets all these matters are taken into account very carefully. If they were not, it would be impossible to achieve efficient operation of the units.

Power lost in cables

A little earlier it was said that the mains volts which disappear as the voltage drop under load are lost volts so far as the operation of the X-ray set is concerned. This voltage used up in making the current flow represents lost power and its energy appears as heat in the cables. Power losses should be as small as possible so that the processes of transmitting power may involve as little waste as possible. It is also required that cables should not become excessively hot.

From these considerations it follows that major X-ray sets should be operated from the highest available supply voltage. As previously explained, for any given X-ray tube-factors a higher supply voltage results in a smaller current flowing along the cables. Since the heat produced in a cable is proportional to the square of the current flowing along it, doubling the supply voltage reduces the current by a factor of 2 and the heat by a factor of 4. So higher supply voltages result in a real saving in power losses and are essential where large amounts of power are to be used.

It is for the above reasons—reductions in voltage drops, in power losses and in the heat produced in cables—that the users of large amounts of power have their electrical loads connected across two of the lines of the supply, using the 415 volts line voltage. Equipment using only small amounts of power is satisfactorily connected across one of the lines and the neutral, using the 240 volts phase voltage, since even with this lower voltage the currents drawn will not be very great.

X-ray equipment and a three-phase four-wire system

In Fig. 1.16 the diagram representing a three-phase four-wire system of distribution has been shown again to indicate how it may be applied to X-ray equipment.

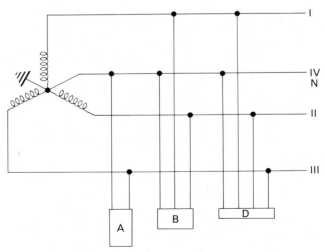

Fig. 1.16

At A is shown a single-phase supply—the 240 volts phase voltage provided by connection between one of the lines and the neutral. This will be used to provide power for X-ray equipment of low output—dental sets, small portable sets and mobile units of restricted radiographic output; this means a restriction to tube currents not greater than 50 mA and to tube voltages around 90 kVp as maximum. This equipment may draw currents up to about 15 amperes. Wall-sockets available in X-ray departments, in wards and in hospital theatres for using mobile equipment of this type usually provide currents up to 13 or 15 amperes at the 240 volts phase voltage.

Dental sets and small portable sets limited to 10–12 mA at 80 kVp maximum draw currents very much smaller than 13 amperes at the phase voltage—that is currents not in excess of 5 amperes. Some mobile equipment has much greater radiographic output than the factors mentioned in the preceding descriptions here, and mobile sets are available which can be used with a tube current of 300 mA at tube voltages up to 100 kVp. If these sets are to be operated at their full output on the phase voltage special wall-sockets and wiring suitable for carrying high currents must be available.

At B in Fig. 1.16 is shown connection between two of the line conductors I and II. This provides a supply at the line voltage (415 volts) suitable for operating major units which are permanent installations in the X-ray department. These are X-ray sets providing tube currents up to 500 mA and tube voltages up to 100–130 kVp. With these units there are many features (various control circuits, motors, lights, etc.) which do not require the higher line voltage and can be operated on the lower phase voltage. A connection between the neutral line and I to provide this voltage can also be seen in Fig. 1.16.

At D in Fig. 1.16 are seen connections from all three of the lines. These allow the supply to be fed to the primary windings of special three-phase transformers and to provide power for the three-phase X-ray equipment. This three-phase supply is at the 415 volts line voltage. In this case again the single-phase 240 volts phase voltage is needed for operating various auxiliary features. In Fig. 1.16 a connection between the neutral and I is shown to provide this.

Changes in the mains supply

Voltage changes

For the satisfactory operation of any X-ray equipment the mains supply must be stable both in voltage and in frequency. In practice complete stability is not achieved. As has been shown, the X-ray equipment itself produces a fall in the mains voltage as soon as the exposure begins because it is drawing a current which in the case of a major X-ray set may be very big. Other pieces of equipment which take currents for short intervals—for example, lifts—give rise to similar voltage drops which show themselves as sharp changes in the mains voltage supplied to the X-ray equipment.

In addition to these voltage changes which occur rapidly over short periods of time, there are changes which occur slowly over long periods of time. These changes are due to the differences in demand which exist at different times in the day and at different seasons. Examples are the big demand for industrial needs during a working day as compared with the demand during the night hours; the big demand early on a winter's morning when everyone is switching on electric fires and kettles as compared with the demand in the evening hours of a hot summer's day.

When there is a big demand for electricity the alternators at the power stations have more work to do. The extra work can mean that the alternators rotate at a slower speed. This reduced speed will decrease the voltage which is induced since it alters the rate of motion between the magnetic fields and the coils, and hence the mains voltage is lower than it should be.

The authorities supplying electricity make every effort to maintain the alternators at a constant speed so that the mains voltage is at its stated nominal value. Nevertheless, when the demand is great the alternators may rotate more slowly, and when the demand is small they may rotate more quickly giving rises to decrease and increase in the mains voltage.

In relation to a given X-ray set the voltage changes taking place may be summed up below:

1   Slow variations over long periods due to differences in demand. These variations occur outside the X-ray exposure.

2   Rapid variations in short intervals of time due to heavy loads being applied on the same supply cables. Such heavy loads include the operation of other pieces of X-ray equipment. These changes occur both outside the X-ray exposure and during it.

3   The voltage drop under load which occurs during (not outside) the X-ray exposure because it is *caused* by the X-ray exposure and by the current taken by the X-ray equipment itself.

All these voltage changes can affect the operation of X-ray equipment if no methods of compensating for them are used. Chapter 2 examines these matters further and explains both the effects of the changes and the compensating devices which are used.

Frequency changes

The differences in the speed of rotation of the alternators which occur slowly as the result of varying demands for electricity change not only the voltage of the mains supply but also its frequency. This must be so because the rate of repetition of the a.c. wave pattern (that is the number of cycles per second or the frequency) depends on the speed of rotation of the alternators. So when the alternators rotate more slowly the mains frequency falls, and when they rotate more quickly the mains frequency rises.

It is therefore not always possible for the mains frequency to be kept at its stated nominal value (50 cycles per second in the United Kingdom), and variations of plus or minus 5 per cent are allowed by law. Chapter 2 explains the important effects of frequency changes in relation to certain components in X-ray equipment.

It may be noted that in modern terminology the expression *cycles per second* is replaced by the internationally understood term *hertz*. The frequency in the United Kingdom is thus said to be 50 hertz.

Using electricity in hospitals

Since this book is about X-ray equipment and is written for the people using such apparatus, we are concerned mainly with electric power in hospitals. It is perhaps easy to take electrical safety for granted and to use the power with little understanding of how it is supplied to the hospital and without appreciating that the mains supply can be dangerous and in certain circumstances can be, and has been, lethal. So it was felt that some explanations and some safety rules should be included here.

In the United Kingdom, hospitals (unless they are small) take electricity from their local supply at 11 kV. Within the hospital grounds, three-phase transformers in a substation reduce this high voltage to 415 volts and 240 volts as mentioned on page 13. The primary side of a three-phase transformer is fed with three-phase current at 11 kv. On the secondary side, supplies are obtained through a star-connected three-phase four-wire system such as is illustrated in Fig. 1.15 and Fig 1.16. For loads up to 3 kW the single-phase supply at 240 volts is used. Loads over 3 kW should be fed by all three phase lines.

Earthing

From the hospital switchroom and its transformers, the supply is carried to other parts of the building by means of electrical wiring. This consists of insulated cables which are either run in steel conduits or steel trunking; or have a metal sheath integral with the insulation. The metal enclosures must be well earthed. This is done by joining to the mains earth connection all the steel conduits or trunking or metal sheaths which leave the switchroom.

The main earth connection consists of copper rods which are specified to have more than a certain resistance and to be of a required size. These copper rods are set into the earth. The neutral of the mains is also earthed at the transformer site by means of this earth connection.

Throughout the entire electrical installation in the hospital there must be continuity of connection to this earthing system. Earth-continuity ensures that there is a low-resistance path to earth and this provides electrical safety if faults occur. The intention of the earthing system is: (i) to make certain that in faulty conditions current will flow to earth and blow fuses or operate circuit-breakers; and (ii) to prevent excessive voltages developing on metal parts when there are faults and these metal parts are accessible to the user.

To use an X-ray set is to use mains electricity inside a metal container since it is not feasible to enclose the whole set completely in an insulating material. The metal case must be earthed and this is done through the three-core flexible cable which connects the set to the supply and through the earth-pin of the three-pin plugs which are used in wall-sockets.

Wall-sockets giving connection to the electrical supply can be checked by means of special equipment (earth-bonding testers) to make sure that there is earth-continuity throughout the system and that the resistance of the path to earth does not exceed 0·1 ohms. The checking should be done by a competent electrician and should be done regularly as part of proper maintenance.

Safety rules for radiographers

Radiographers commonly operate two main categories of X-ray equipment: (i) permanent installations fixed in departments; (ii) movable equipment which is used at various sites in the wards and theatres of the hospital. Electrical hazards are likely to be greater with the movable equipment because it undergoes more mechanical stress and hence it is more likely to have damaged cables, faulty plugs and loose connections. Furthermore, it is operated from many different outlet sockets and any of these may be in a faulty condition. However, there are certain rules to be observed by radiographers which are of positive help to increase safety.

1   All movable X-ray equipment should be checked regularly and often by an electrician.

2   The radiographer using the equipment should report at once any observed damage or defect so that an electrician may attend to it. Always *notice* your equipment and be on the watch for worn cables, damaged plugs, loose plug-tops and evidence of loose connections or of the cable pulling out of the plug. It is you who are at risk and not even to notice that you are using

faulty equipment or not to take positive action to correct defects is foolish indeed.

3 Radiographers should not put plugs into or pull plugs out of sockets which are live—that is, their switches are in the 'on' position. Turn the switch to 'off'.

4 Cables and plugs should be treated as kindly as if they were patients! The following points are to be noted for preserving plugs and cables and we must remember that their integrity is important to our safety. (a) Do not stretch a cable. (b) Do not run the X-ray equipment (or anything else) over a cable or plug. (c) Do not leave cables and plugs lying on the floor after you have used the equipment because someone else may run something over them. (d) Do not pull a cable into position by hauling on the plug or take a plug from a socket by heaving on the cable. (e) If you find that you must waggle a plug or a cable in order to make the equipment work, then stop and do not use the equipment until it has been checked and rectified by an electrician. The broken lead or loose connection indicated by the necessity to waggle may in fact be a situation which is very dangerous for you and any other person who uses the equipment.

Chapter 2
Components and Controls in X-ray Circuits

The first chapter of this book dealt with an essential to the use of X-ray equipment—the mains supply. The present chapter considers some circuit components which are needed for the controlled operation of an X-ray tube from this supply.

In order to make an X-ray tube produce X rays it is necessary (i) to heat its filament so that electrons are given off and (ii) to connect the X-ray tube to a source of high voltage so that the electrons move fast through the tube and thus have high kinetic energy; it is this kinetic energy which is converted to other energy when the electrons impinge on the target of the X-ray tube and X rays are produced. Important components of any X-ray set are therefore (i) the filament circuit through which the filament is heated and its electron emission controlled; and (ii) the high voltage source by means of which the electrons are given energy of motion across the X-ray tube.

Radiographers using X-ray sets need controls which alter features of the X-ray output. Many different types of subject and many different body parts present for radiographic examination. Sometimes a very penetrating beam is needed and sometimes one of much less penetrating ability; for examples, the first patient in a day's work may be a muscular young man who has injured his spine by a fall off scaffolding and the second a two-year child who has hit one finger with a hammer. Sometimes a more intense and sometimes a less intense beam is needed—for example compare the relative amounts of radiation required to radiograph the chest of an adult man and that of a new-born baby. Sometimes a very short time of exposure is essential because rapid motion is a characteristic of the subject; if for example a radiograph is one of a series showing blood and contrast agent passing through the heart.

These three—the penetrating power of the beam, the intensity of the beam and the length of time for which it is directed at the film through the patient—are important factors in the production of a radiographic image. Radiographers must be able to vary these factors in a wide range of radiographic techniques and they learn skill in selecting and combining them for any given case.

26

How are these three factors altered? The penetrating power of the X-ray beam is varied principally by change in the high voltage across the X-ray tube; this voltage is called the kilovoltage because it is thousands of volts. Raising the kilovoltage makes the electrons travel faster across the X-ray tube and the X rays produced are then more penetrating; and of course lowering the kilovoltage produces the opposite effects. So to alter the penetrating power of X rays a radiographer needs and uses a kilovoltage control. This kilovoltage control which varies the voltage across the X-ray tube and the penetrating power of the beam also incidentally alters the intensity of the beam. Higher kilovoltage increases intensity as well as penetrating power and lower kilovoltage results in a less intense as well as a less penetrating beam. A radiographer selecting the kilovoltage which seems appropriate to any particular X-ray examination, however, usually has in mind as a first consideration the effects on penetrating power: the changes in intensity seem almost incidental beside the fact that control of kilovoltage is so important to the image-contrast of the radiograph that is obtained.

A close control of intensity is given by alteration in the number of electrons which are emitted from the heated filament of the X-ray tube. To put it simply, making the filament hotter causes it to emit more electrons and conversely making it cooler causes it to emit fewer electrons. These electrons constitute an electric current flowing through the X-ray tube during the exposure; this current is called the milliamperage because it is measured in thousandths of amperes. The higher the milliamperage or current through the tube, the more intense is the beam of X rays emitted and the relationship is one of direct proportion; for example increasing the tube current by a factor × 2 doubles the intensity. So to alter the intensity of the radiation the radiographer needs and uses a milliamperage control, and this milliamperage control is part of the filament circuit.

The third important factor is the exposure time. By this radiographers mean the length of time during which the X-ray tube is energized from the high voltage source and the beam of X rays is directed towards the film. This period must be capable of being varied and so the radiographer needs and uses a timer in the X-ray equipment. This timer is connected to a switch which acts to start and stop the exposure—that is, it acts to start and stop the flow of current through the X-ray tube.

We can summarize these features by making a list as below.
1 Mains supply voltage
2 X-ray tube
3 High tension source
4 Kilovoltage control
5 Filament circuit and milliamperage control
6 Timer

Fig. 2.1 is a block diagram showing these features assembled together, all obtaining power from the mains supply. We must now consider in more detail what is within some of the blocks in the diagram.

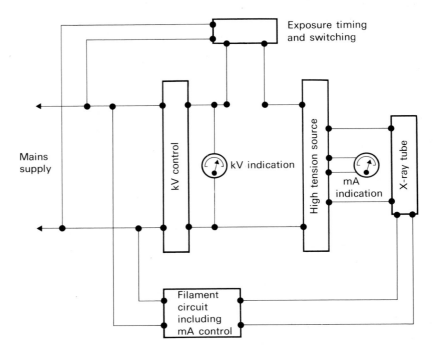

Fig. 2.1

X-ray tubes will be seen in Chapter 7 and timers and exposure switches are surveyed in Chapter 5. Here we will consider the high tension source, the control of kilovoltage and the filament circuit. Since it is important for the radiographer to be informed of the kilovoltage and the milliamperage which are used for the exposure after manipulation of the controls, the X-ray equipment must include devices which indicate these quantities. These indications appear as two further blocks in the diagram in Fig. 2.1 and will be explained within this chapter.

The diagram makes it clear that the several important components with which we are concerned obtain their power from the mains supply. From this it follows that variations which occur in the mains voltage (see Chapter 1, page 21) must have effects on the X-ray equipment. These effects and certain compensating devices used to minimize them are also described in this chapter.

THE HIGH TENSION TRANSFORMER

The turns ratio

The high voltage source which is used to drive electrons fast across an X-ray tube is a transformer always known as the high tension generator. Its task is to transform the voltage of the mains supply up to the thousands of volts required to operate the X-ray tube. This means that the transformer must provide a range of voltages from about 20,000 volts up to 150,000 volts (20–150 kV). It is a step-up transformer with two windings and it has many more turns in its secondary winding (to which the X-ray tube is connected) than in its primary winding (to which the supply is connected via the kilovoltage control at which we are going to look shortly).

How many more turns are there in the secondary winding as compared with the primary winding of this transformer? It is easy to calculate this from the ratio of transformation:

$$\frac{\text{Number of turns in primary winding}}{\text{Number of turns in secondary winding}} = \frac{\text{primary volts}}{\text{secondary volts}}$$

Assume that 400 volts are to be transformed to 100,000 volts. Then the ratios

$$\frac{\text{Secondary volts}}{\text{Primary volts}} \quad \text{and} \quad \frac{\text{secondary turns}}{\text{primary turns}}$$

(which are the same) must both be

$$\frac{100,000}{400}$$

This is 250/1. So for every one turn of the primary winding there must be 250 turns of the secondary winding. In practice this means a secondary winding with about 100,000 turns on it.

We must note that the little calculation which we have just done involved transforming 400 volts to 100,000 volts or 100 *kilovolts*. When X-ray equipment is used, the voltage across the X-ray tube has been traditionally expressed as *kilovolts peak*. As we have seen, the voltage waveform of the a.c. mains supply is a pulsating one, coming up to a peak value in each half-cycle in the pattern of change. In certain circuits, the voltage output from the high tension transformer which is applied to the X-ray tube is also pulsating. The term *kilovolts peak* refers to the highest kilovoltage reached in each cycle of pulsating voltage which the transformer delivers to the X-ray tube.

Kilovolts peak have been considered to be important values in having regard to the following points:

1   manufacturers testing X-ray tubes measure peak kilovolts across them.;

2   the features of electrical and radiation safety which are provided should
relate to the peak value of the highest voltage to be used;

3   there is a simple relationship between the peak value of the kilovoltage
applied across the X-ray tube and the maximum photon energy (or
minimum wavelength) in the heterogenous spectrum of radiation emitted
from it. So for a very long time the abbreviation kVp for kilovolts peak has
been in the language of radiology and on the controls and meters of our X-
ray sets.

The mains supply is expressed not as a peak voltage but as the useful or
effective value reached in the cycle of change; this is also known as the *root
mean square* (R.M.S.) value because it is the same as the square root of the
mean of the squares of all the instantaneous values in the cycle. The 400
volts of our calculations are 400 volts R.M.S. and the 100 kilovolts are 100
kilovolts R.M.S. The simple relationship between the effective and the peak
values is:

$$\text{R.M.S.} = \frac{\text{peak}}{\sqrt{2}}$$

To know the peak kilovolts which this transformer delivers, 100 kV R.M.S.
must be multiplied by the square root of 2 (1·41), which gives the answer
141 kilovolts peak (kVp).

In recent times those generators which provide a non-pulsating voltage
for the X-ray tube are being more widely used. These are the three-phase
high tension generators to which we referred on page 21. The voltage
waveforms across the X-ray tubes for which they provide power may be
slight ripples (in which the voltage falls to a value somewhat lower than the
peak and then rises to the peak again) or may be straight lines. If the tube
kilovoltage is always at a steady value or does not fall much during the cycle
of change on the a.c. mains, the term *kilovolts peak* loses some significance.
So the modern international practice is to use the term *kilovolts* (abbreviated
as kV) to express the voltage across the X-ray tube which is supplied from
the generator.

In this context the kilovolts which are stated are those values which are
reached at the top of the wave in a rippling voltage waveform and the extent
of the ripple is expressed in relation to these values. For example, a generator
with a 3 per cent ripple which is operating at a stated 100 kV has 97 kV as
the voltage in the trough of the ripple.

If an expression is wanted to relate to the photon-energies of the X-ray
beam, the one used is kilo-electron-volt (abbreviated to keV). The electron-
volt is a unit of energy: its definition is the work done on a single electron
which is transferred through a potential difference of 1 volt. Since the
energies of the photons in the X-ray beam are related to the energies of the

electrons which come from the filament and reach the target of the tube, it can be seen that kilo-electron-volts can be used to express the energies of the photons. Since an X-ray beam is composed of photons with many different energies, it is the average kilo-electron-volts which are used generally to express the quality of the beam of X-rays by a tube operating at a stated kilovoltage. The average kilo-electron-volts are always a lower value than the tube kilovolts.

The core

The core of the high tension transformer is rectangular in shape as shown in cross-section in Fig. 2.2. The plain rectangle is shown at (a) and if the core

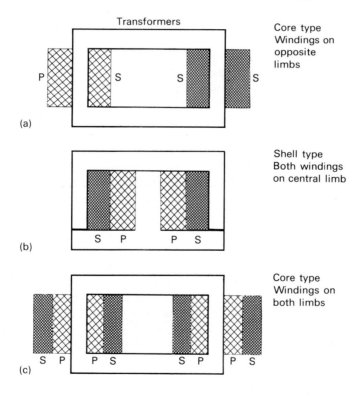

Fig. 2.2

(a) A step-up transformer of the core-type with windings on opposite limbs of the core.

(b) A step-up transformer of the shell-type with both windings on the central limb of the core, the secondary winding being over the primary windings.

(c) A step-up transformer of the core-type with both windings in two halves on opposite limbs of the core, the secondary winding being over the primary winding. The high tension transformer shown at the foot of the generator tank in Fig. 2.3 is of this type.

is like this the transformer is said to be of the core-type. In this type of transformer the iron core is nearly enclosed by the windings, for the windings are put on opposite sides of the rectangle as indicated in the diagram. This type of transformer is easily assembled and has a good cooling surface.

Another type of transformer core is shown at (b) in Fig. 2.2 and as can be seen this one has a central limb. A transformer with this sort of core is known as the shell-type. In this one the windings are put on the central limb and the windings are then nearly surrounded by the iron core. In this design there is a shorter magnetic circuit than the core-type has and little of the magnetic flux strays outside the core.

In our diagrams we have shown the windings by means of a lattice pattern which is the conventional way of drawing transformers. It saves drawing thousands of wire endings and, as the finer lattice indicates the winding with the greater number of turns, it enables the initiated to see at a glance whether a drawing depicts a step-up or step-down transformer.

In Fig. 2.2 at (c) is shown a core-type transformer with a step-up ratio. The primary winding and the secondary winding are both wound in two halves, each limb of the core carrying one-half of the windings. The secondary winding is wound over the primary winding on each limb. The high tension transformer in an X-ray set may be done like this and is rather more often of the core-type than of the shell-type.

The core is laminated. This means that it is made of thin separate sheets insulated from each other by a layer of insulating varnish. The core is built up by putting the sheets together; they must be clamped very closely or the transformer will hum when it is energized and this is not considered to be a helpful form of music while you work. The humming occurs because when the magnetic flux is maximum the laminations repel each other. Then as the magnetic flux falls to zero in the alternating current cycle the laminations come together, only to be remagnetized in the reverse direction which makes them repel each other again. Unless the laminations are held very tightly together, these vibrations result in a humming noise. The laminations can be clearly seen in Fig. 2.3.

Why have laminations instead of a solid block? The purpose of the laminations is to reduce eddy currents in the core; eddy currents are currents induced in the core by the changing magnetic fields of the transformer windings. Eddy currents appear as heat in the core of a transformer and they are wasteful of power. The laminations ensure that the core is discontinuous in the direction in which eddy currents are likely to be established and this makes it difficult for eddy currents to flow. The core is made of special iron alloys—silicon-iron and nickel-iron—and these materials help to reduce eddy currents. The core of the high tension transformer is earthed.

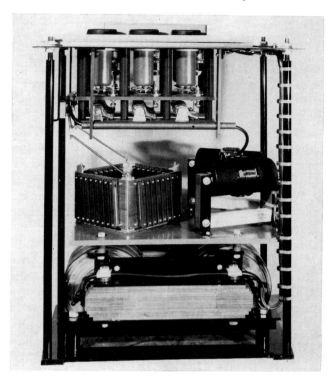

Fig. 2.3 The interior of a high tension generator tank with solid state rectifiers. At the top are seen the high tension switches and below these on the left are the banks of rectifiers. On the right beside the rectifiers are the filament transformers for the X-ray tube. At the bottom of the tank is the high tension transformer. *By courtesy of Picker International Ltd.*

The windings

The wire used to wind the transformer is obviously of different length in the two windings since the one has many more turns in it than the other. Length is not the only difference for the two windings are made of wire which is different in thickness. The primary winding consists of relatively fewer turns of thicker wire; the secondary winding consists of many more turns of very thin wire.

To explain the difference in thickness we must consider voltage and current relationships between the two windings. The secondary winding of the transformer provides kilovoltage and milliamperes for the X-ray tube; it supplies power in the form of a low current (even 1000 mA through the X-ray tube is only 1 amp) at a very high voltage. Its primary winding takes power in the form of a very high current (it may be 200 amperes or more) at mains voltage. Where very large currents are to flow the resistance of a wire along which the currents pass must be as low as possible—that is, the wire should be short and thick. If the resistance of the wire is high too much voltage will be needed to send a large current along the wire and too much power will be lost. Fortunately in the high tension transformer the winding which carries the large current has the shorter length, so it is not difficult to make the wire relatively short and thick.

If the secondary winding were made of the same wire it would be very thick as well as long and the result would be a great mass of copper wire. The equipment would be more costly and much heavier than it need be and the arrangement would be impractical. Because the secondary winding carries such a low current, the resistance of the wire can be much greater relative to the primary winding without too much voltage being needed to send the current along the wire and too much power being lost. So the secondary winding is made of thin wire wound in many turns.

The arm of the core which is to carry the windings has a sleeve of insulating material fitted over it. The copper wire of the primary winding is wound over this sleeve. When the first layer of turns has been made a special insulating varnished paper is put over it and then the next layer is wound. Another piece of the paper is put over the second layer of the windings and a third layer is wound. This process of layers of copper winding inter-leaved with insulating paper is continued until the primary winding is complete. The paper must be sufficiently stout to withstand the pressure of the secondary winding, which in due course is placed over the first on a separate insulating tube.

An earthed copper sleeve may be put over the primary winding when it is complete, the sleeve being insulated from the winding. In the event of insulation breakdown in the secondary winding, this copper sleeve serves to isolate the high tension from the primary circuit.

The secondary winding is wound on to an insulating sleeve placed over the primary winding. The secondary winding consists, as we have said, of very many turns of thin copper wire. This wire is coated with an insulating varnish and the turns are wound in many layers. The layers are separated from each other by thin paper prepared with wax so that it will insulate. This is to keep the layers separated from each other. The difference in voltage between any two of the layers remains relatively small (200–300 volts) and the potential difference between the beginning and the end of the long secondary winding is built up in stages through the layers. This method of construction lessens the risk of the insulation breaking down under high-voltage stress.

The secondary winding of the high tension transformer is wound in two parts and the centre point of the winding where the division occurs is earthed through the core; this point is known reasonably enough as the earthed centre point or the earthed mid-junction or the grounded centre of the high tension secondary winding. It is shown depicted in Fig. 2.4.

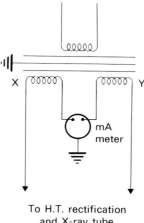

Fig. 2.4

To H.T. rectification
and X-ray tube

The purpose of winding the secondary in two halves and earthing the mid-point is to reduce the insulation which is necessary; hence to reduce the size and cost of the transformer and any high tension cables used to connect it to the X-ray tube. If the secondary winding were not split and were wound as a long continuous winding, the insulation required would be such as was necessary for the full peak kilovoltage which might exist across the two endings of the winding—for example 100 kVp available between points X and Y in Fig. 2.4. With the winding split and earthed at its mid-point, the voltage stress with respect to earth is halved. Although there remains 100 kVp between X and Y for the X-ray tube, one end of the winding (X or Y) is at +50 kVp in relation to the earthed core and the other end of the winding (Y or X) is at −50 kVp in relation to the earthed core. So it is necessary to provide only such insulation to earth as will be appropriate for 50 kVp.

Oil immersion

The high tension transformer is oil-immersed in an earthed metal tank. This is a readily identified part of an installation in an X-ray room because of the high tension cables which connect the transformer to the X-ray tube. The student has only to trace the cables back from the tube in its housing to see where the high tension transformer itself is housed. The oil is there to insulate the transformer and to cool it because when it operates it becomes warm because of the power it consumes; this state can easily be felt by a hand on the outside of the tank at the end of a busy morning. Special techniques are used so that the thin purified transformer oil is put into the tank and all the air is removed. The oil fills up all the spaces both in the tank and in the transformer itself and the tank is closed with a tight-fitting lid. The oil-filled tank which houses the transformer, the high tension cables and the shield enclosing the X-ray tube together form a continuous earthed metal shield over the high tension parts of the X-ray set.

Other insulating media

In most X-ray equipment oil is used for insulation of the high tension parts—the high tension transformer, rectifiers in the high tension system and the X-ray tube itself. Oil has a great advantage in that it acts to cool the parts immersed in it. However, in situations where the heat is likely to be less of a problem—for example in a small portable X-ray set or in a dental unit—other materials may be used. Such X-ray units operate with a low output and so do not develop as much heat as sets with higher output.

It is a common practice in small X-ray units to use a tank construction. This is a construction in which the high tension transformer and the X-ray tube are together in one housing surrounded by the insulating medium. The insulation may take the form of a plastic dip instead of the oil, the components being immersed in the selected plastic material when it is in a fluid state. Subsequently it solidifies and the high tension parts are surrounded by and embedded in a solid insulating medium. This may save some weight in comparison with oil but it is not suitable when the equipment is likely to develop much heat.

At least one high-powered mobile set on the market used an insulating resin-impregnated paper plus some oil. This allows the size of the tank construction to be smaller since the high tension transformer can safely be just over 2 cm away from the case at 125 kVp. If oil alone were used a 7·5 cm gap between the transformer and the sides of the tank would be necessary.

Transformer losses

In an ideal transformer the power obtained from the secondary winding and the power applied to the primary winding is the same. That is,

$$\text{watts input} = \text{watts output}.$$

In practice the ideal transformer (like many other ideals) cannot exist as a fact because the process of transformation would have to be 100 per cent efficient. This process is not 100 per cent efficient and the efficiency which is achieved is about 90 per cent, the actual figure varying from transformer to transformer. The lost 10 per cent is power lost as part of the price paid for the transformation process. In relation to other electrical equipment such as generators and motors, transformers are very efficient devices.

Because a transformer is made of windings on an iron core and works by electromagnetic induction, it has two sorts of circuit associated with it. There are (i) the electrical circuits which are the windings; and (ii) the magnetic circuit, which is the core. The power losses which occur in a transformer are divided into two separate groups: (i) losses in the electrical circuits, that is in the windings and (ii) losses in the magnetic circuit, that is in the core.

Losses in the windings

The power losses which arise in both the primary and secondary windings occur because the windings have resistance and power is lost as heat in the windings when current flows through this resistance. These power losses are usually called copper losses to denote that they are resistance losses in the copper wire of the transformer windings. They are kept as small as is practicable by choosing material for the windings with low specific resistance and by paying attention to the lengths of the windings and the thickness of the wire as indicated on page 34 of this chapter.

When the transformer is doing work (say when the high tension transformer which we are discussing is providing kilovoltage and milli-amperes for the X-ray tube), electric current flows through both its windings. This current is referred to as the load current and the transformer is said to be on load. If the transformer is providing the highest current that it can, it is said to be working at its highest current rating and to be on full load.

The copper losses in a transformer vary with the load because they are proportional to the square of the current flowing. In each winding the copper losses in watts equal I^2R, *where I is the current flowing and R is the* resistance of the winding; the total copper losses in watts are calculated as the sum of the losses in each winding. That is copper losses in watts = I^2R for primary winding $+ I^2R$ for secondary winding.

From this it follows that the copper losses will be greatest at full load. It shows that if the current flowing through the winding is big, the resistance should be small to keep the losses down to an acceptable figure.

Losses in the core

The power losses which arise in the iron core of a transformer are called iron losses. They arise through the magnetization of the core and they are classified as (i) hysteresis loss and (ii) eddy current loss.

Hysteresis loss

Hysteresis loss is the power used to maintain the alternations of the magnetic flux in the iron core. In their windings, transformers have alternating currents which are constantly changing in direction and this means that the core is magnetized first in one direction and then in the opposite way. Energy is used in establishing the magnetic field in each new direction and power is lost as heat in the core. Hysteresis loss may be kept small by the use of special alloys for the core. The materials used for the core are chosen so that the total iron losses (being the sum of the hysteresis losses and the eddy current losses) are a minimum.

Eddy current loss

Eddy current loss occurs because the changing magnetic fields associated with the windings induce currents in the core. These currents are called eddy currents and they too have been mentioned earlier in this chapter (page 32) because they are minimized by laminating the core. They are lost energy which is dissipated as heat in the core.

The total iron losses are made up of the hysteresis loss and the eddy current loss considered as a single entity. Like the copper losses, the iron losses are expressed in watts.

The iron losses derive from the magnetic flux in the core and this remains more or less constant whether the transformer is idle in the no-load state or is doing work and is on load. So, unlike the copper losses which vary with load, the iron losses in any given transformer remain more or less the same from no load to full load; they do of course vary between transformers with different characteristics of construction.

Transformer regulation

Earlier in this chapter (page 29) we used the turns/voltage ratios of transformation to estimate how many turns might be necessary in the secondary winding of a high tension transformer. It is important for the student to remember these ratios so we state them again here:

$$\frac{\text{Number of primary turns}}{\text{Number of secondary turns}} = \frac{\text{primary voltage}}{\text{secondary voltage}}.$$

It is equally important to remember two more facts about these ratios as follows.

1   If the ratios are true what do they mean? They mean that the voltage output of a transformer is independent of the current load, and for a given turns ratio, and a given voltage input, the voltage output will be the same whether the transformer is on no load or on full load or on any load between these two extremes.

2   The ratios are true only for the ideal transformer which is without transformer losses.

As we have indicated any practical transformer as opposed to the ideal one has power losses and the copper losses vary with the load, being greatest at full load and minimal at no load; a transformer with its primary winding connected up to a voltage source and its secondary winding not loaded (carrying no current) has only a negligibly small current flowing through its primary winding and of course no current in its secondary winding and hence negligibly small copper losses.

The copper losses arise because current must flow through the resistance of the windings. Voltage is required to make it do this. The greater the current that has to flow, the greater is the voltage used to send it through the transformer windings. The result of this is that with a constant voltage applied to the primary winding, the voltage available from the secondary winding (in theory independent of the current load, being determined by the ratio of transformation) in practice falls as the current load increases and rises as the current load decreases. Let us see what this means in relation to X-ray equipment.

We are considering here a high tension transformer of fixed ratio which is being used to operate an X-ray tube. Let us suppose that when 400 volts is applied to its primary winding, the ratio of the turns is such that 100 kVp is available from its secondary winding. As soon as the transformer is on load—that is providing milliamperes for the X-ray exposure—current flows through both its primary and its secondary windings, voltage is required to send the current through the windings and the theoretical 100 kVp is at once reduced by the amount of voltage necessary to do this. Thus the kilovoltage which is actually applied to the X-ray tube during the exposure is not 100 kVp but some value which is less than 100 kVp. Less by how much? The answer depends on (among other factors) the resistance of the windings and the milliamperage being used for the X-ray exposure. At the highest milliamperage which can be selected from the control, the greatest current will be flowing in the transformer windings and the fall in kilovoltage will be maximum; at the lowest milliamperage much less current will be flowing in the transformer windings and the fall in voltage will be least.

If this fall of the transformer voltage under load were not compensated by means of circuit arrangements in the X-ray equipment, when the radiographer varied milliamperes there would also be alteration in the kilovoltage applied to the X-ray tube during the exposure. The kilovoltage would fall as higher milliamperages and rise as lower milliamperages were selected. The arrangements made to compensate for this loss of voltage when the high tension transformer is on load are described in a later section of this chapter (page 57).

Those who manufacture X-ray transformers are expected to include among the specifications of a transformer a statement which indicates how much the voltage output falls when the transformer is on load. In practice they approach this the other way round and make tests to determine how much the voltage *rises* between the full-load and the no-load states of the transformer. An artificial load is set up in the testing department and a reading of the voltage at full load is taken and then a reading of the voltage at no load. The rise in the secondary voltage between full load and no load is then obtained by subtracting the first voltage from the second.

The ratio relating this rise in voltage to the full-load voltage is called technically the regulation of the transformer. Thus:

$$\text{Percentage regulation} = \frac{\text{no load voltage} - \text{full load voltage}}{\text{full load voltage}} \times 100.$$

For the high tension transformer in a diagnostic X-ray unit, the regulation is given for the transformer both when it is operating to give radiographic exposures (i.e. intermittent running) at its highest current and when it is being used for fluoroscopy (i.e. continuous running) at its highest current for continous loading. In radiographic use the regulation is much higher than the regulation in fluoroscopic use. Obviously in general terms a good transformer is one with low regulation, for basically the regulation is a statement of the voltage which is lost when the transformer is put on load.

Transformer efficiency

In the ideal transformer without any losses the power input and the power output are, as we have said, equal. In a practical transformer which is bound to have power losses the power input is somewhat greater than the power output.

$$\text{The power input} = \text{power output} + \text{total losses.}$$

The ratio of output to input gives the efficiency of the transformer and this can be expressed as a percentage.

$$\text{Efficiency} = \frac{\text{power output in watts}}{\text{power input in watts}} \times 100.$$

The level of efficiency achieved is 90 per cent or less depending on the transformer. The highest efficiency is obtained in very large transformers and the lowest in very small ones.

Transformer rating

Any transformer has limits to its useful output and manufacturers provide statements of what these limits are. Such statements concerning any particular transformer are called its rating. To try to operate a transformer beyond its rating—that is beyond the limits of power output and time which have been specified for it—is to risk making the transformer too hot and possibly thus damaging its insulation.

A high tension transformer in a diagnostic X-ray set providing power for the X-ray tube has different conditions of use. It may be required to provide a low current throughout sustained periods (that is periods of several seconds' duration repeated in a series if the X-ray tube is being used for fluoroscopy). In contrast to this the transformer may provide a high current for very short intervals (less than 1 second) in intermittent use for radiographic exposures; sometimes these short exposure periods may be repeated very rapidly indeed if the tube is being used for angiography.

So a statement in kilovolt-amperes of the power which a transformer can provide is not full enough to meet the needs for high tension transformers in X-ray sets. There are three ratings to be specified as follows.

1   The highest kilovoltage (no load) which the transformer can provide.
2   The maximum current which the transformer can give on continuous running.
3   The maximum current which the transformer can give for a period not exceeding 1 second.

The maximum current allowed on intermittent loading is always much higher than that allowed as a continuous load because over a very brief period the transformer can absorb more heat without a dangerous rise in temperature.

Other items specified in a transformer rating include the regulation on continuous and on intermittent loading and also conditions relating to rise in temperature, insulation and permissible overload.

THE RECTIFICATION OF HIGH TENSION

A high tension transformer provides for an X-ray tube a kilovoltage which is alternating. This means that the voltage changes in direction and each end of the secondary winding of the transformer is alternately positive and negative.

The simplest way to use a high tension transformer to work an X-ray tube is to connect the X-ray tube directly to the secondary winding, one pole of the transformer connected to the cathode of the X-ray tube and the other pole of the transformer connected to the anode of the tube. The arrangement is shown in a diagram in Fig. 2.5.

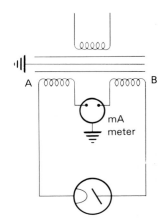

Fig. 2.5

In this arrangement the X-ray tube has alternating voltage applied to it. The transformer pole A in the diagram is first negative, then positive, then negative again and the transformer pole B is first positive, then negative, then positive again in a repeated cycle of change.

An X-ray tube in order to produce X rays requires that its filament should satisfy two conditions: (i) that it should be heated so that electrons are given off; and (ii) that it should be connected to a voltage source which makes it negative in respect of the anode so that electrons are attracted towards the anode. They then constitute a current through the tube and X rays are produced. It can be realized from what we have said that in Fig. 2.5 condition (ii) for the filament is met only when transformer pole A is negative; it is *not* met when the state of affairs is the other way round.

So the X-ray tube passes current only when A is negative and electrons flow through the tube from cathode to anode. When B is negative there is no electron flow in the reverse direction for two reasons: (i) the anode is not a heated electron emitter; and (ii) the heated filament is positive and its electrons will not be attracted away from it towards the anode.

The electric current thus flows through the X-ray tube in only one direction and, while the *voltage* from the transformer is alternating, the *current* is unidirectional—a word which is used to mean that a voltage or current does not change direction. This conversion from the alternating to the unidirectional is called rectification. Because the X-ray tube is achieving the change and is making the current flow in one direction only by means of a blocking action in the reverse direction, it is said to be functioning as a rectifier. This circuit in which the X-ray tube is connected directly to the secondary winding of the high tension transformer is called a self-rectified circuit (less usually a self-suppressed circuit because the reverse current is suppressed).

There are limitations (see Chapter 3) in using an X-ray tube in this way and these can be overcome by putting into the circuit (between the secondary winding of the high tension transformer and the X-ray tube) other devices which will act as rectifiers. The X-ray tube then finds itself with the filament always connected via the rectification system to a negative pole of the high tension transformer. The transformer, the rectifiers (if used) and the X-ray tube together constitute what is called the high tension generator. Chapter 3 considers various circuits in which these components are combined and compares the different arrangements. What we must do here is to describe the rectifying devices which are used.

The earlier rectifiers used were thermionic diode valves but in modern practice these are superseded by what are called solid-state devices (see page 45). Because the diode valves are disappearing we will not describe them in detail but we will use them to explain how a rectifying system for an X-ray tube works.

Diode valves pass current (as the X-ray tube does) through a vacuum; the solid-state devices pass electric current through a solid material which is why they have their somewhat odd-sounding name.

Thermionic diode valves

Construction and function

An evacuated tube with two electrodes in it is called a vacuum diode and an X-ray tube is one form of vacuum diode. Thermionic emission is the emission of electrons as a result of heat, and the X-ray tube works because of the thermionic emission of electrons from its filament. The X-ray tube passes current in one direction only and in blocking any reversal of flow it acts as a valve.

With these considerations in mind the reader who looks thoughtfully at the name *thermionic diode valve* may expect a thermionic diode valve to be very like an X-ray tube, having:

1   a glass envelope enclosing a vacuum;
2   two electrodes within the glass envelope, one of which is a heated filament;

3   a function to pass current in one direction only and to block any reversal of flow.

The reader would be correct for the thermionic valve is very like an X-ray tube and has in common with it the three listed characteristics. A thermionic valve operates to pass a current in one direction and to block a current in the reverse direction in essentially the same way as an X-ray tube does. The filament of a valve is heated by a step-down transformer and emits electrons. If the valve is connected to a voltage source in a complete circuit in such a way that its filament is negative in respect of its anode, the electrons from the filament are drawn across to the anode and the valve passes current. If the valve is connected to a voltage source in a complete circuit in such a way that its filament is positive in respect of its anode, no electrons will be drawn across and the valve acts as a block to current.

Fig. 2.6 shows two diode valves connected between the secondary winding of the high tension transformer and the X-ray tube. This is a simple circuit using rectifiers and it is chosen here as an uncomplicated illustration; other circuits are discussed in Chapter 3.

In Fig. 2.6 when X is negative both valves and the X-ray tube conduct and current flows in the circuit. Both the valves and the X-ray tube are obtaining voltage from the secondary winding of the high tension transformer and the division of the available voltage is this: the valves take all they need to enable them to pass the current and the X-ray tube takes all it can get after the valves have had their share. In practice this means that the valves take 1–2 kV each (forward voltage drop) and the X-ray tube has all the rest of the transformer voltage.

In the next half-cycle of the mains alternations, X in Fig. 2.6 becomes positive. The valves and X-ray tube all have their filaments connected thus

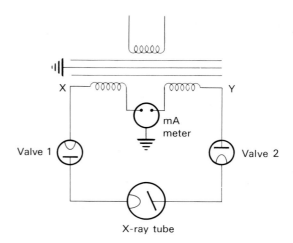

Fig. 2.6   X-ray tube

to a positive pole of the supply; none of them conducts. During this half-cycle therefore no current flows through the X-ray tube. The alternating mains supply has been rendered through the rectifying system as a unidirectional flow of current in the high tension circuit.

Solid-state rectifiers

In recent years there has been considerable development in the use of solid-state units to perform the functions previously undertaken by vacuum devices. As the name solid-state implies, conduction takes place by electron travel through solid materials as opposed to electron flow through a vacuum.

The solid materials used are semi-conductors. This means that their characteristics place them midway between metals, which are conductors of electricity, and non-metals, which mostly are non-conductors of electricity and are insulators. Semi-conductors can be made either to conduct or to insulate. Silicon and germanium are two elements which are semi-conductors. They can be used to construct semi-conductor or solid-state diodes to rectify the high tension for an X-ray tube in place of the vacuum diodes which we have discussed previously.

Fig. 2.7 has been drawn to show the circuit symbols of solid-state rectifiers replacing the vacuum diodes of Fig. 2.6. It can be seen that the solid arrowheads of these circuit symbols point in the opposite direction to the electron flow from the filament to the anode through the X-ray tube. The student may find it easier to remember which way round to draw these arrowheads if it is considered that the Arrowhead corresponds to the Anode of a vacuum diode and that electrons travel to the point of the arrows from the black layer touching the arrow tip.

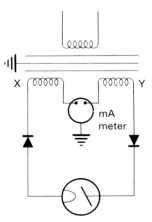

Fig. 2.7

N-Types and p-types

A semi-conductor or solid-state rectifier is made of two layers of material. One of these layers is a material which has in its atomic structure a great number of free electrons. A free electron is an orbiting electron in the outermost, incompletely-filled orbit of an atom; such an electron feels only a weak force from the atomic nucleus and can therefore easily be removed from the atom by a small amount of energy.

Materials with surplus free electrons can be produced by putting minute amounts of impurities into semi-conductors and these free electrons are able to move through the substance. Such material with many free electrons is called N-type material. We may think of the N as coming from the fact that the atoms are able to give negative charges; because the material gives electrons it may also be called donor-type material. Examples of N-type materials in semi-conductor devices are silicon and germanium with a minute amount of phosphorus as the added impurity to each element.

The second layer of a semi-conductor diode must be made of a material which has the opposite characteristic in regard to free electrons; it must have a deficiency of them. Such material has vacancies in its molecular construction into which free electrons can move. With pleasing simplicity, these vacancies are called holes. Material with holes is P-type material; the absence of electrons is equated with possession of positive charge and since the P-type material accepts electrons it may also be called acceptor-type material.

The semi-conductors silicon and germanium become P-type materials when small amounts of the elements boron or indium are added to them.

When a layer of N-type material is joined to a layer of P-type material electrons flow easily from the N-type layer (with its surplus of free electrons) to the P-type layer (with its deficiency of free electrons) but they cannot flow easily in the other direction. This is why the device is able to act as a rectifier—it has a low resistance to the passage of current in one direction and a very high resistance to the passage of current in the other.

In contrast to the vacuum diode which passes no reverse current, a solid-state rectifier does pass a very small current in the reverse direction. However, the reverse current is small enough to be considered negligible and the device rectifies an alternating current by acting as a sufficient block to reverse current flow.

Fig. 2.8 represents a layer of N-type material joined to a layer of P-type material and shows the direction of easy electron flow. The block to the reverse flow occurs at the *junction* between the two materials and this means that the region where the barrier exists is very thin indeed. The names junction diodes and barrier-layer rectifiers are given to these devices.

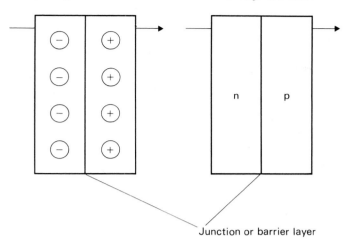

Junction or barrier layer

Fig. 2.8

We have mentioned the use of silicon and germanium in the production of solid-state rectifiers. Another semi-conductor element used is selenium but this is used somewhat differently; the N-type and P-type materials for the two-layer rectifier are not made by mixing the selenium with small amounts of other materials. Instead the P-type layer is made of pure selenium, which has a deficiency of free electrons. This layer is placed in contact with a layer of the metal cadmium, which has a surplus of free electrons and is therefore the N-type layer in the rectifier.

We have considered here the simple combination of one N-type and one P-type layer. This produces a barrier-layer rectifier which is the solid-state equivalent of a vacuum diode. By other combinations of N-type and P-type layers—in a sandwich of three layers or four layers—other devices can be produced which are the solid-state equivalents of triode valves, either vacuum triodes or gas-filled triodes. More is said of these in Chapter 5 for their use in exposure-switching and timing circuits.

Solid-state rectifiers in X-ray tube circuits

All solid-state high tension rectifiers in the X-ray tube circuit have certain advantages over diode valves. These advantages are as follows.

1   They have longer life, for they have no filaments to burn out. While they may be initially more expensive than vacuum diodes, it is considered that in the long run the expense will be justified by the lack of need for replacement.

2   They need no filament-heating transformers. This means that they are more economical of power because the power losses associated with heating

filaments are absent. It is also a cause of reduction in expense by the cost of filament transformers and equipment to control them.

3   They are more robust.

4   They are smaller in size—for example a silicon rectifier takes the form of a rod about the thickness of a finger while a vacuum diode has a thickness akin to that of a forearm.

5   Because of the smaller size of the rectifiers themselves and the absence of filament transformers, the high tension generator circuit can be enclosed in a smaller space and this provides equipment which is lighter and more compact. Thus it becomes possible to produce mobile X-ray sets which have full-wave rectification. The high tension transformer and the four rectifiers necessary may be enclosed in an oil-filled tank on the wheeled base of the unit and connected to the X-ray tube by high tension cables; or they may be enclosed with the X-ray tube in the oil-filled tank of the tube head so that high tension cables are not necessary.

6   The absence of filament heating for valves means that there is less heat in the tank enclosing the rectifiers and the high tension transformer. This is a further reason why the tank can be smaller for it is not necessary to give it such dimensions as would enable it to dissipate to the surrounding air the heat from the valve filaments (which are kept in the stand-by state all the time the X-ray set is switched on at the control panel).   In today's X-ray equipment solid-state rectifiers have replaced vacuum diodes in the high tension circuits. In older X-ray equipment vacuum diodes were the most commonly used high tension rectifiers.

Selenium rectifiers

Selenium rectifiers preceded silicon rectifiers in the high tension circuits of X-ray tubes. This use of selenium rectifiers was developed through the work of Messrs. Siemens–Reiniger–Werke AG Erlangen, Germany, who gave them the name barrier-layer rectifiers. They are very reliable if they are properly used and they need little maintenance.

A single barrier layer (that is, one P–N junction) of a selenium rectifier can withstand an inverse voltage which is only a few tens of volts but many junctions can be used to withstand the high inverse voltage in an X-ray tube circuit by stacking them so that there are several thousand selenium barrier layers. Thus 410 wafers (each wafer being one barrier layer) can be mounted in series, kept in close contact with each other by means of springs and held by insulating supports. Such an assembly forms a selenium cartridge about 20 cm in length with a wafer area of about 0·6 cm^2; this cartridge would be suitable for operation at 17–20 kVp. To cater for the full kilovoltage which must be rectified for an X-ray tube, a number of cartridges are connected in series. For example, a high tension generator circuit to operate at 300 mA and 125 kVp may require 32 cartridges making a total of something over 13,000 barrier layers. This seems a great number but the space they occupy is relatively small. The 32 cartridges could be mounted flat on a support in four groups of eight and the total dimensions of the banks of rectifiers would be about 40 cm × 30 cm × 4 cm.

Four vacuum diode valves would be required to achieve the same capacity. If a high tension generator with four vacuum diode valves were to provide the same output it could not be fitted into a transformer tank as small as would hold a unit with selenium rectifiers. This can be considered another way: a four-valve unit fitting into a tank of the same size as the selenium-rectified unit would have lower output—say, 200 mA and 100 kVp.

As seen on p. 44, thermionic diode valves have a low forward voltage drop of only 2–3 kV. In comparison with this, selenium rectifiers have a higher forward voltage drop, For example, the arrangements of 32 cartridges in four groups which we have mentioned might have a total forward voltage drop of about 20 kVp. This higher voltage drop forwards has an advantage if a fault develops in the high tension circuit which leads to the production of a very high voltage; this could be the result, for example, of breakdown in the insulation of a high tension cable. The cable then 'goes to earth' (the electric charge is dissipated to earth through the earthed metal sheath of the cable) and a high voltage develops in the circuit. The selenium rectifiers

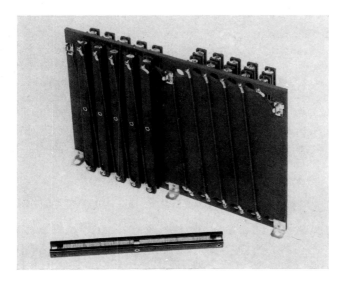

Fig. 2.9   Solid state rectifiers. *By courtesy of Picker International Ltd.*

reduce these high voltages by their forward voltage drop and hence they tend to be self-protective.

Selenium rectifiers must not be worked at too high a temperature, the maximum being 85°C. The oil in the tranformer tank in which they are immersed helps to cool them as it does the transformer and the selenium rectifiers are put towards the bottom of the tank, which is the coolest part. Selenium rectifiers are shown in Figs. 2.3 and 2.9.

Silicon rectifiers

Silicon junction rectifiers are a more recent development. The advantages of a silicon rectifier over a selenium rectifier are:
1   lower forward voltage drop;
2   very high resistance to reverse current;
3   the ability to withstand a higher inverse voltage, so a single barrier layer of a silicon rectifier can withstand some hundreds of volts instead of tens of volts as in the case of a selenium rectifier;
4   the ability to work at a higher temperature (200°C).

Because a single barrier layer of silicon can withstand some hundreds of volts, it is necessary to stack only several hundreds of silicon barrier layers (as opposed to the thousands of selenium ones) in order to rectify the kilovoltage used by the X-ray tube.

It is now possible to produce cylindrical cartridges of rectifiers capable of operating at up to 150 kVp and 1000 mA, the dimensions of such cartridges being 20–30 cm long × 20 mm diameter. The stacked rectifying units are contained within a ceramic tube which is hermetically sealed. The tube has metal terminal ends. The forward voltage drop and the reverse current of these silicon rectifiers are said to be negligible for practical purposes.

Silicon rectifiers are smaller in size than selenium rectifiers of the same rating. They are therefore popular with manufacturers in situations where there is little space—for example in mobile X-ray units.

In the circumstances of cable breakdown outlined previously (page 49) silicon rectifiers tend to be self-destructive as they cannot block the high voltage which can occur.

THE CONTROL OF KILOVOLTAGE

As we have said, radiographers must be able to control the kilovoltage across an X-ray tube because the applied kilovoltage determines the penetrating power of the emerging X-ray beam. This penetrating power must be varied by a radiographer through a range of kilovoltage from about 20 kV (for mammography) up to 100–130 kV (in high kilovoltage techniques). So that radiographers may command discriminating adjustment of exposure techniques, the changes in kilovoltage must be available in small steps of about 2 kV at each step.

The tube kilovoltage during the exposure is the output voltage of the secondary winding of the high tension transformer, to which the X-ray tube is connected either directly or through a system of high tension rectifiers. This output voltage may be controlled by changing the input voltage.

The variable input voltage for the high-tension transformer is obtained from another transformer which is connected across the primary winding of the high tension transformer. This is indicated in the diagram in Fig. 2.10 with the supplying transformer shown simply as a block T.

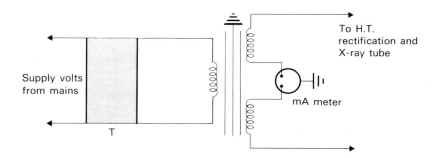

Fig. 2.10

Kilovoltage change is achieved by varying the output from the transformer at T and this output is applied to the high tension transformer as its primary (input) voltage. Since the high tension transformer is of a fixed turns ratio, when its primary voltage changes its secondary voltage (the tube kilovoltage) changes also. For example, if the transformer ratio were 250:1 as in the example we considered on page 29 in this chapter then a change of 8 volts on the primary side would result in a change of 2 kV (2000 volts or 250 volts × 8 volts) on the secondary side.

The transformer in the block T in Fig. 2.10 is such that changes of a few volts (for example the 8 volts we mention above) can be made in its output. It is a kind of transformer known as an autotransformer.

The autotransformer

An autotransformer is a type of transformer which has one winding only, and not two conductively quite separate windings as in the case of the high tension transformer. A transformer with two separate windings works on the principle of electromagnetic induction between the primary winding

and the secondary winding; the autotransformer with its single winding
works on the principle of self-induction. Because there is only one winding
the primary and secondary circuits are in metallic connection with each
other. This fact makes an autotransformer unsuitable for transforming high
voltages from one value to another or for stepping up voltages to high values.

Autotransformers can be used very successfully to step voltages both up
and down from the mains supply value so long as they are not used in high
voltage circuits. They can give a secondary output voltage which is variable
as we explain below and this feature makes them useful in the control of
kilovoltage in X-ray sets.

In comparison with two-winding transformers, autotransformers are
smaller in size, are economical of copper wire and cost less. These features
and the ability to provide an adjustable secondary voltage make an
autotransformer the most commonly used method of controlling kilovoltage
in diagnostic X-ray equipment.

Function of an autotransformer

The ratios of transformation which apply in an ideal transformer with two
windings also apply in an ideal autotransformer with its single winding. Fig.
2.11 depicts the single winding of an autotransformer.

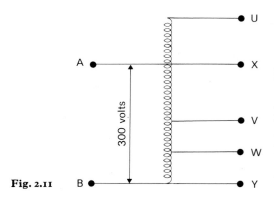

Fig. 2.11

Let us suppose that 300 volts are applied between the points A and B
(primary circuit). Ignoring transformation losses because this is the
theoretical ideal transformer, we know that the terminals X and Y will then
provide 300 volts for a circuit (secondary circuit) connected across them.
This follows because there are as many turns of the autotransformer
connected into the secondary circuit as into the primary circuit, and as the
turns in the primary and secondary circuits have a 1 : 1 ratio so also do the
voltages.

V is a terminal at the midway point between X and Y. If the secondary circuit is connected between V and Y instead of between X and Y, the turns ratio of the primary to the secondary circuit becomes 2 : 1 and the voltage ratio in the circuits is of course again the same as the turns ratio. So now with 300 volts across AB, 150 volts are available between the terminals V and Y.

W is a terminal at a point which includes only one quarter of the number of turns between A and B so the terminals W and Y provide a voltage for the secondary circuit which is only one-quarter of the applied voltage—in this case 75 volts are availalable between W and Y.

U is a terminal placed to include more turns between Y and U than there are between A and B. In the diagram, with the AB turns in the primary circuit and the YU turns in the secondary circuit, the turns ratio is 2 : 3. The voltage ratio is the same as the turns ratio, so that with 300 volts applied to the AB terminals 450 volts are available at the terminals Y and U.

Thus it is possible to construct an autotransformer to give a secondary output which is variable in fractions or multiples of the applied voltage; this is with the proviso mentioned in the previous section that an autotransformer cannot be used to transform voltages at very high values because the primary and secondary circuits are in conductive connection.

An autotransformer as control of kilovoltage

An autotransformer is constructed with its single winding wound on a laminated closed core. The winding has several tappings along it; these are conductors connected to the winding. The conductors lead out of the winding of the transformer and each conductor finishes in a terminal or 'stud'. These studs may be used to connect a variable number of turns of the autotransformer into its secondary circuit by means of a manual control which moves a rotary switch from stud to stud.

This stud-selector switch can be marked on the control panel of the X-ray set as the kilovoltage selector. Fig. 2.12 is a diagram showing the closed core with the winding on one limb, some tappings taken from the winding and the stud-selector control which can be moved from terminal to terminal so that a variable number of turns of the winding can be included in the secondary circuit.

This stud-selector switch gives a variable secondary voltage as the output of the autotransformer in the way described in the previous section of this chapter. This variable output voltage of the autotransformer is applied as the primary input voltage of the high tension transformer in the way described on page 51. Fig. 2.13 is a circuit diagram which is the same as Fig. 2.10 except that the block T in Fig. 2.10 has now had its secrets revealed and

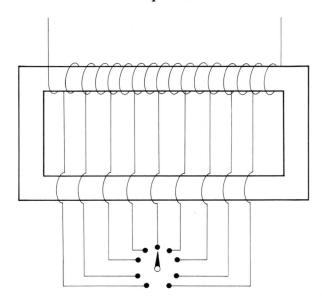

Fig. 2.12

is replaced in Fig. 2.13 by an autotransformer with tappings and a stud-
selector switch on its secondary side.

The diagrams show only a few tappings because we have sacrificed
realism for the sake of clarity. In practice there are many tappings for there
must be one tapping for every kilovoltage value used in the X-ray set. For
example, if the range provided by the kilovoltage selector is from 40 kV to
100 kV in steps of 2 kV, there must be 31 tappings.

In some X-ray units there may be a double selector: one is a coarse
control giving steps of 10 kV and the other is a fine control giving steps of

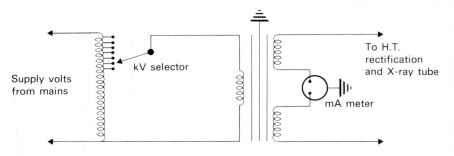

Fig. 2.13

1 kV. The coarse control has more turns of the autotransformer between its studs than the fine control has. On the coarse control there may be 10 or so turns of the winding between each stud and on the fine control the tappings for the studs are taken from adjacent windings of the autotransformer.

Continuous control of the kilovoltage

The system of kilovoltage control which has been described in the previous pages is one which results in kilovoltage being selected through a series of fixed steps. The radiographer uses the control to select kilovoltage prior to the exposure and it is not possible to change the tube voltage while the X-ray tube is being energized. This is not a significant limitation in a kilovoltage control used for diagnostic radiography. Periods of radiographic exposure are mostly too short for the use of a control to adjust kilovoltage in the intervals of time for which the exposures last. Radiographers do not alter kilovoltage during the radiographic exposure and it is therefore not necessary to provide a control which would allow them to do so.

When diagnostic X-ray equipment is being used for fluoroscopy the time intervals during which the X-ray tube is energized are longer than the instantaneous periods used in radiography. In some units fine kilovoltage control provided for fluoroscopic use of the X-ray tube is of a stepless type. This means that kilovoltage is not adjusted in a series of fixed steps but can be continuously controlled even when the X-ray tube is energized.

Such control can be achieved by using a Variac transformer.

Variac transformer in control of kilovoltage

The Variac transformer is an autotransformer of a particular type. It has a single winding which is wound on a cylindrical core. The insulation is removed along a track on the winding and a moving contact or brush passes over this track. This moving contact allows the ratio of turns in the primary and secondary circuits of the transformer to be varied.

Fig. 2.14 indicates how the transformer works. The cylindrical core is shown as a ring with the windings round it. The windings between P_1 and P_2 are the number of turns of the transformer which are in the primary circuit and the primary voltage is applied between P_1 and P_2. B is the moving contact or brush which rotates round the annular track where the insulation has been removed. Because there is no insulation between it and the windings, B makes electrical contact with the turn of the windings on which it presses when it is in any given position. The turns of the transformer

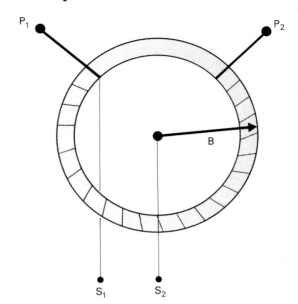

Fig. 2.14

which are in the secondary circuit vary for any given position of B, being most numerous when B is near to P_2 and least numerous when B is near P_1. Thus is it possible to obtain between S_1 and S_2 a continuously variable secondary voltage from this transformer.

For the control of kilovoltage across the X-ray tube, this variable output voltage is fed to the primary winding of the high tension transformer. This is in the same way as we have shown for the variable output of an autotransformer which gives change of kilovoltage in fixed steps.

On page 53 we described the operation of a kilovoltage control which was through a rotary switch moved by hand between different stud settings. To the radiographer such a manual control presents itself as a knob which must be turned in a clockwise direction to raise the kilovoltage and in an anticlockwise direction to lower the kilovoltage. The 'feel' of the control is of a positive clicking into position as the switch arrives at each setting.

Modern radiographers are accustomed to the ease of push-button settings through which adjustments may be quickly made and time and energy are saved. However, even if modern consoles present to the radiographer controls which seem very different from earlier versions, the basic control of kilovoltage remains essentially the same: variation to the input side of the high tension generator by controlling and altering the output from an autotransformer and applying that output to the generator which steps up the voltage required for the X-ray tube.

KILOVOLTAGE INDICATION

Given the need to vary kilovoltages used for radiographic exposures and the means to make variations, a radiographer's further requirement is to know the kilovoltage which is being selected by any given setting of the control. On the control panel of the X-ray set there must be indication of the kilovoltage values which are being used.

As we have described, the kilovoltage selector varies the voltage which is taken from the windings of an autotransformer. This voltage is applied to the primary winding of the high tension transformer and hence each setting of the selector results in a different kilovoltage existing across the X-ray tube, which is connected either directly or through a rectifying circuit across the secondary winding of the high tension transformer.

How does a radiographer know what kilovoltage is applied to the X-ray tube for any given position of the selector? The following are possibilities.

(i) Each setting of the selector is marked with a kilovoltage value—for example, the lowest might be marked 40 kV and the highest position might be labelled 100 kV, the settings between bearing intermediate values in steps of 1·5 kV. This method is known as a calibrated autotransformer. The word calibrated indicates that the settings have been marked in gradations or steps (i.e. kilovoltage values) with allowance for certain irregularities. We shall shortly consider what these irregularities are. On modern consoles the settings of the selector may be 'labelled' by kilovoltage values which are digitally displayed.

(ii) All the settings of the control are arbitrarily numbered in sequence from 1 upwards and the kilovoltage indication is given by means of a meter. This meter is called a pre-reading kilovolt meter because it indicates or reads the value of kilovoltage which will be applied to the X-ray tube when the exposure is made and it gives this information before the kilovoltage is actually applied to the X-ray tube with the start of the exposure.

The calibrated autotransformer

If all the transformers (and mains cables) worked with 100 per cent efficiency there would be no errors in marking truthfully each position of a kilovoltage selector switch with the number of kilovolts provided for the X-ray tube when each position was used; for with 100 per cent efficiency transformer ratios are true. Thus let us suppose that when the kilovoltage selector in Fig. 2.15 is at position A, 200 volts (R.M.S.) are taken from the autotransformer and are applied to the primary winding of the high tension transformer. If the turns ratio in the high tension transformer is 400:1 and there are no transformer losses, then the kilovoltage resulting from this position of the selector switch will be 200 × 400 volts (the product of the turns ratio and the primary voltage). This is 80 kilovolts. If we are to convert this to the peak value at the top of the a.c. waveform, we must multiply it by 1·41 and this gives 112·8 kV. This is the voltage for the X-ray tube when the kilovoltage selector in Fig. 2.15 is at position A.

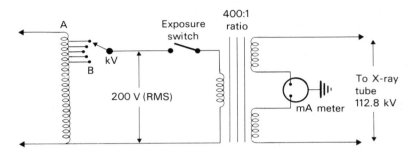

Fig. 2.15

We might therefore venture to mark position A with the value 112·8 kVp, but if we did our selector would not be truthful when the radiographer pressed the exposure switch, the transformer voltage was impressed across the X-ray tube, current flowed through the tube and X rays were produced. This is because when the X-ray tube is passing current, the current flowing through the tube is of course also flowing as a load current through the windings of the high tension transformer. These windings have resistance and voltage must be used to make the load current flow against this resistance. So the kilovoltage in fact available for the X-ray tube is *not* the calculated kilovoltage across the secondary winding of the high tension transformer. It is the calculated voltage *minus* the voltage used to make the load current flow through the windings. This voltage absorbed in overcoming the resistance of the windings is lost to the X-ray tube and is called the kilovoltage drop.

The kilovoltage drop in the transformer windings increases as the milliamperage is raised because the voltage (V) required to make a current (I) flow through a resistor (R) is the product of I and R:

$$V = RI.$$

If there are high tension rectifiers connected between the transformer and the X-ray tube, there will be some further kilovoltage drop associated with passing current through them. The total kilovoltage drop = kilovoltage drop in the transformer + kilovoltage drop in the rectifiers. The kilovoltage available for the X-ray tube in Fig. 2.15 from selector position A is the calculated kilovoltage *minus* the total kilovoltage drop.

Since the total kilovoltage drop varies with the X-ray tube current or milliamperes, the kilovoltage available from selector position A must also vary with the milliamperes; it will be lowest at the highest tube current and greatest at a tube current near zero. These are the irregularities which we mentioned on page 57 with reference to the calibrated autotransformer.

Anyone who has used modern X-ray apparatus knows that some X-ray sets give kilovoltage indication by means of selector positions marked with kilovoltage values. So how are these made to be truthful through the whole range of tube currents used?

A method employed is to add into the primary circuit of the high tension transformer a voltage which is matched to the voltage drop that occurs when the load current flows. This additional voltage offsets the kilovoltage loss and so maintains the kilovoltage available for the X-ray tube at the value stated for any given position of the selector.

The extra voltage required to offset the kilovoltage loss is obtained from the autotransformer when the tube current is selected. In this way the extra voltage can be matched to the kilovoltage drop. As we have seen, when milliamperage is increased the kilovoltage drop increases and a greater extra voltage is needed.

In Fig. 2.16 the control marked kVC is joined to the milliamperes selector; when this type of link is used, the one control may be said to be ganged to the other. When the milliamperes selector is changed to select higher tube current, the kVC control which is ganged to this selector changes in the direction towards H. This selects more voltage for the primary of the high tension transformer. When the milliamperes selector is moved in a direction to select lower tube current, the kVC control changes

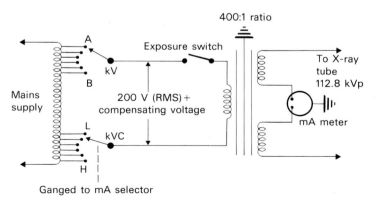

Fig. 2.16

with it and goes towards L in the diagram, thus selecting less additional voltage for the primary of the high tension transformer.

Thus with the kilovoltage selector at position A, which is to be marked as 112·8 kV (in practice 113 kV), the actual voltage applied to the primary of the high tension transformer is V volts—this being in our example 200 volts *plus* an extra voltage matched to the kilovoltage drop. The high tension transformer steps up V volts to a calculated kilovoltage of Y kilovolts in accordance with the ratio of transformation. During the exposure the actual kilovoltage available for the X-ray tube is 112·8 kV, which is Y kilovolts *minus* the kilovoltage drop.

The pre-reading kilovolt meter

The pre-reading kilovolt meter is a voltmeter which indicates to a radiographer the kilovoltage obtainable from the different positions of the kilovoltage selector. The meter is an a.c. (moving iron) instrument connected across the output of the autotransformer and so the voltage which energizes it is the voltage from the autotransformer which will be applied to the primary winding of the high tension transformer when the exposure begins.

As we saw in a previous section (page 58) the kilovolts peak which are available on the secondary side of the high tension transformer can be calculated as the product of the primary volts (R.M.S) and the turns ratio of the transformer, the result being multiplied by 1·41 to turn it into the kilovoltage available at the peak of the a.c. waveform. So the meter can have a scale which is calibrated to read thus:

(the various voltages from the numbered tappings of the autotransformer) × (step-up ratio of the high tension transformer) × 1·41 in kilovolts.

As we saw in the previous section, the actual kilovoltage which is applied to the X-ray tube when the exposure begins is lower than the calculated voltage because it is the calculated kilovoltage *less* the kilovoltage drop that occurs when the load current flows. So a pre-reading kilovolt meter indicating the kilovoltage before it is reduced by the kilovoltage drop gives a reading which misleads by being too high.

The degree of discrepancy between this reading and the actual kilovoltage impressed across the X-ray tube during the exposure varies with the selected tube current, as we have seen. The amount of kilovoltage lost changes with the load current in the secondary circuit of the high tension transformer. The discrepancy is greatest at the highest milliamperage used and least at the lowest milliamperage used from the milliamperes selector.

The manufacturer of the X-ray set is able to determine what the discrepancy is at each of the tube currents used. The actual tube kilovoltage when the X-ray tube is passing current is measured by special methods and is compared with the meter indication. It is then possible (for any given tube current) to know by how much the meter reading must be brought down to make its reading a truthful indication of the kilovoltage across the X-ray tube during the exposure. The meter reading is brought down by reducing the voltage across the meter through an arrangement known as the meter-reading compensator. Such an arrangement is shown in Fig. 2.17.

In the diagram the winding MC is a winding which is added to the autotransformer, but it is wound in a direction opposite to that of the main autotransformer winding. This winding has induced in it a voltage which is opposite in polarity to the output voltage from the main autotransformer; it is a counter voltage.

One lead from the pre-reading kilovolt meter is taken to the kilovolt meter compensator marked X in Fig. 2.17. This compensator is ganged to the milliamperes selector so that when the millamperes selector is moved the compensator selects a counter-voltage related to the milliamperage. The voltage across the pre-reading kilovolt meter is the output voltage of the autotransformer minus this counter-voltage. The counter-voltage is matched to the kilovoltage drop which occurs when the exposure is made and thus the voltage across the meter is reduced to bring its reading down so that it indicates the kilovoltage impressed across the X-ray tube during the exposure.

The radiographer must select the tube current and use the millamperes selector *before* setting the kilovoltage control and reading the kilovolt meter because it is only the act of moving the milliamperage control that enables the appropriate counter-voltage to be applied. If this point is forgotten and

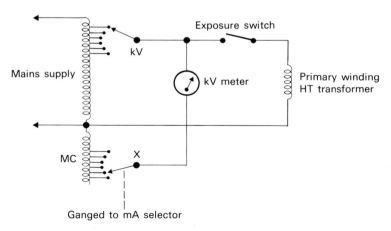

Fig. 2.17

the kilovoltage is selected first, the radiographer will find that as soon as the tube current is chosen by operating the selector switch, the kilovolt meter indication falls or rises because a different counter-voltage has been introduced. It will be necessary then to reselect the kilovoltage by moving the kilovoltage selector switch until the pre-reading kilovolt meter reads the kilovoltage which it is wished to use.

THE FILAMENT CIRCUIT AND CONTROL OF TUBE CURRENT

The filament transformer

In order to make an X-ray tube produce X rays its filament must be heated so that electrons are emitted. It is clearly very convenient to heat the filament by passing a current through it and not much power is needed to heat the extremely fine filaments of X-ray tubes to the necessary high temperatures.

The power is provided by a small step-down transformer called the filament transformer, to the secondary winding of which the filament of the X-ray tube is directly connected. Two filament transformers can be seen in Fig. 2.3, one for each filament of a dual focus X-ray tube.

The turns ratio

The filament transformer provides a secondary voltage of 8–12 volts and this sends a heating current of 4–8 amperes through the filament of the X-ray tube. This current raises the temperature of the filament to white heat. The primary winding of the filament transformer obtains its voltage from the mains supply via the autotransformer of the X-ray set. This voltage is about 240 volts across the primary winding. Since the secondary voltage is required to be about 12 volts, this step-down transformer must have a ratio which is around 20:1, the larger number of turns being in its primary winding.

The core

The core of the filament transformer is constructed similarly to that of the high tension transformer previously described (page 31); that is, it is laminated and made of a special alloy so that losses in the core may be minimized. Both the transformer windings of the filament transformer are put on one limb of the core, the secondary winding being wound on top of the primary one. The transformer is required to provide only a small amount of power (say 5 amps at 12 volts) and so the core and the windings are much smaller in size than the same features of the high tension transformer.

The windings

Since the filament transformer is a step-down transformer, the primary winding has more turns in it than the secondary winding, 20 times more turns if it is the 20:1 ratio which we mentioned. Ignoring any losses, the voltage applied to the primary winding is 20 times bigger than the voltage obtained from the secondary winding and the current flowing through the primary winding is 1/20 of the current in the secondary winding.

So this transformer has a primary winding consisting of many turns carrying a small current; its secondary winding consists of fewer turns carrying a larger (but not a very large) current. So we find that the filament transformer has thicker wire in its secondary winding than in its primary. This is the reverse condition to the one we saw in the high tension transformer.

The secondary winding of the filament transformer has only a very small voltage across it, but it is directly connected to the filament of the X-ray tube, and the X-ray tube of course has a very high voltage across it which is being provided by the high tension transformer. It is therefore necessary to provide high voltage insulation between the secondary and primary windings of the filament transformer. This is done by placing over the primary winding a tube or cylinder made of insulating material such as porcelain or ebonite which is of sufficient thickness to withstand high voltage stress. The secondary winding of the filament transformer is then wound over the insulating tube.

Oil immersion

We have seen that the high tension transformer is oil-immersed in an earthed metal tank, the oil functioning both to insulate and to cool the transformer. It is usual to put the filament transformer into the same tank (as in Fig. 2.3) so that the oil may perform the same functions for it too.

The control of tube current

The current which passes through the X-ray tube is altered by altering the number of electrons which are emitted from its heated filament; this number of electrons in its turn is altered by changing the temperature to which the filament is raised. So the current through the X-ray tube (the milliamperage used for the exposure) can be controlled by altering the heat of the filament. Small changes in the heat of the filament can result in large changes in the numbers of emitted electrons and hence in the X-ray tube current, especially at high milliamperes. Because of this, alterations in filament heat give a very sensitive control for the current passed by the X-ray tube.

The filament is heated as we have seen by electric power which a step-down transformer provides, the filament being directly connected to the secondary winding of this transformer. The heat of the filament is readily changed by altering the power in watts which is used in the secondary circuit of the transformer, the secondary power being altered by changing the voltage across the secondary winding of the filament transformer. The voltage across the secondary winding is controlled by changing the voltage applied to the primary winding.

The control set by the radiographer is in the primary circuit of the filament transformer and hence it is insulated from the high tension circuit into which the secondary winding is connected. It is therefore safe to handle. It functions to alter the voltage applied to the primary winding of the filament transformer and so to control the current passing through the X-ray tube (the milliamperes used for the exposure).

There is more than one method available for controlling the voltage applied to the filament transformer. In practice the one often used is control of voltage through resistors.

Fig. 2.18 shows a step-down transformer with its secondary winding connected to the filament of an X-ray tube and its primary winding supplied with a stable voltage source. This stable voltage comes from the mains supply via the autotransformer, and later sections of this chapter deal with the important matters of why it must be stable and how stabilization is achieved.

In Fig. 2.18 a resistor is connected in series with the primary winding of the filament transformer. The voltage across the primary winding is the supply voltage *less* the voltage drop in the resistor. The movable control at A allows more or less resistance to be included in the circuit. Thus more or less voltage is dropped across the resistor and the voltage across the primary winding of the transformer can be lowered or raised. Corresponding changes of voltage are produced across the secondary winding by the changes in the

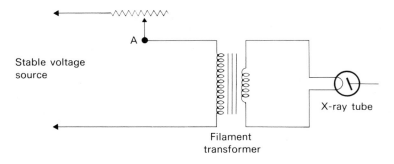

Stable voltage
source

A

X-ray tube

Filament
transformer

Fig. 2.18

primary voltage. Thus the filament heat is altered and the current through the X-ray tube is controlled.

This adjustable resistor gives stepless control of tube current and allows the milliamperage to be altered while the X-ray tube is being energized. It provides free control of the tube current within the limits set by the resistor. If the X-ray tube were not to be overloaded at high tube currents, it would need very careful setting because small changes in the position of the control then give relatively large changes in milliamperes. The ability to alter the tube current during the exposure which this stepless control gives is of no use when high milliamperes are used for diagnostic radiography, because the exposure intervals are then too short to allow any adjustments to be made to the controls. So this type of variable resistor may be used to control the tube current during fluoroscopy, when the milliamperages are low, the setting of the control is less critical and the periods are long during which the tube current flows.

For radiographic exposures, control of tube current may be achieved by the use of resistors in a way which is different. The system is shown in Fig. 2.19.

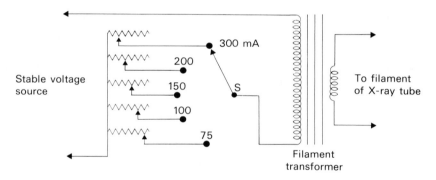

Fig. 2.19

In this circuit the single resistor which is variable is replaced by a number of separate resistors each of which has a fixed value. In practice there is a resistor for each value of tube current which is to be made available through the selector. Each resistor being of a different value, each has a different voltage drop across it. A movable selector switch shown at S in Fig. 2.19 allows any one of the resistors to be connected into the primary circuit of the filament transformer. Thus the voltage on the primary winding is altered to give different values of current through the X-ray tube. Each resistor has a value chosen to give a certain milliamperage as indicated in the diagram in Fig. 2.19.

This system is called pre-selection of tube current by resistance control and it gives variation of milliamperage in fixed steps. Selection may be through a rotary switch moved by the radiographer over a series of settings each marked with a different milliamperes value. Such a control may be found in older equipment. Today's selectors may present as settings of touch buttons or a series of push buttons each indicating a different tube current.

A manufacturer installing an X-ray set is able to give his customer the range of milliampere settings that the user wishes to use, but of course once the set has been installed a radiographer can use only the tube currents provided by the different settings: there is no free choice. In practice this is not very much of a limitation on the exposure techniques which are used.

Voltage stabilization for the filament circuit

In Chapter 1 (pages 21–22) the changes which occur in the mains voltage were explained as being of three types. These are:
(i) slow variations in voltage occurring outside the X-ray exposure;
(ii) rapid variations occurring both outside and during the X-ray exposure;
(iii) the fall in voltage which is *caused* by the X-ray exposure, occurs as soon as the exposure begins and lasts for the duration of the exposure.

From what has been said so far in the present chapter about the filament circuit and the control of X-ray tube current, it is clear that the voltage for the filament transformer must be a suitable one. The filament heat, which is such a sensitive control for the tube current, must be altered precisely by carefully changing the voltage on the filament transformer. The required precision is not there if the voltage supplied to the filament transformer is an irregular one.

A change in the filament voltage of about 5 per cent leads to a similar change in the filament-heating current and these changes result in a change in the X-ray tube current (the milliamperes) which is much bigger: 20–30 per cent. The graph sketched in Fig. 2.20 shows how steeply the X-ray tube current rises when plotted against filament-heating current.

Variations in milliamperes as big as 20–30 per cent cause noticeable variations in the densities of radiographs. So a radiographer using an X-ray set which permitted such uncontrolled changes to occur would not be satisfied with the results obtained from the equipment. It is only when the voltage on the filament transformer is stable that reproducible results follow every setting of the milliamperes selector.

The filament transformer obtains its supply from the mains via the autotransformer and in the absence of compensators and stabilizers all changes in the mains voltage cause changes in the filament voltage. Because it is so important that uncontrolled changes in filament voltage should not

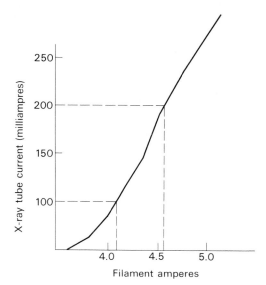

Fig. 2.20

occur, the X-ray equipment includes components functioning to prevent them.

Mains voltage compensators which are described from page 78 in this chapter are in the primary circuit of the autotransformer and can deal with mains voltage fluctuations occurring *outside* the X-ray exposure. They cannot deal with mains voltage changes which occur *during* the exposure.

Other devices are necessary to maintain a stable voltage on the filament transformer during the exposure and these devices are called, not surprisingly, stabilizers.

Various circuit arrangements are possible for the stabilization of voltage but it is not our purpose to review them here. The important points in regard to a constant voltage stabilizer for the filament supply in the operation of an X-ray tube are as follows:

1 the filament transformer must be supplied with a stabilized voltage that remains steady despite the variations in the mains voltage that can occur;
2 the stabilizer (as is shown in Fig. 2.21) is connected into the filament circuit on the primary side of the filament transformer;
3 the stabilizer is located to operate between the supply voltage taken from the autotransformer (on the input side of the stabilizer) and the milliamperes selector (which is on the output side of the stabilizer);
4 the stabilizer functions automatically and immediately to provide a steady voltage on its output side even when the input voltage varies;

5 the primary winding of the filament transformer is provided with a constantly maintained stable voltage despite the changes which occur in the voltage of the mains supply.

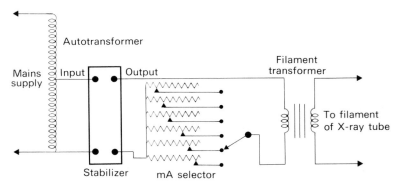

Fig. 2.21

Effects of changes in frequency

As well as being liable to changes in voltage which are inevitable, the mains supply as it is produced at the generating stations may be subject to changes of frequency (see Chapter 1, page 22). Some of the circuit components which are used to stabilize voltage for the filament transformer are sensitive to frequency: the result of a change in frequency is that the stabilizer ceases to perform the task to which it is dedicated and the output voltage of the stabilizer becomes unstable and varying. So the stabilizer might as well not be there. If the stabilizer is frequency-dependent, the circuitry of the filament supply includes what is called a frequency compensator. This device corrects for those changes in the output voltage of the stabilizer which may arise because the mains frequency has altered.

Space charge compensation in the filament circuit

A modern X-ray tube operating at high milliamperes has heavy electron emission from its filament. The electrons tend to form a cloud round the filament called a space charge and not all the electrons emitted from the filament are drawn across the X-ray tube by the anode voltage.

This situation means that when the anode voltage (the kilovoltage) is raised, more electrons from the space charge cloud are drawn across and the current through the tube (the milliamperes) increases, although the milliamperes selector switch has not been altered. When the kilovoltage is lowered, fewer electrons are drawn across to the anode and the tube current falls, again with unchanged position of the milliamperes selector. A given setting of the milliamperes selector results in fact in different currents through the X-ray tube according to the kilovoltage which is used. For example, one setting of the milliamperes selector switch could give 500 mA at 70 kV, 450 mA at 50 kV and 550 mA at 90 kV.

These figures mean that in order to obtain 500 mA at 50 kV the heat of the filament of the X-ray tube must be increased; and in order to obtain 500 mA at 90 kV the heat of the filament must be decreased. The manufacturer therefore includes circuit components which will do this, thus providing what is called space-charge compensation so that a given position of the milliamperes selector switch will give the same tube current over the whole range of kilovoltages used. Because what is needed is a means to alter the heat of the filament as the tube kilovoltage is changed, the space-charge compensator functions in the filament circuit.

Various systems have been devised to achieve this compensation and we propose to describe only one suitable circuit. Fig. 2.22 indicates the arrangement.

The secondary winding of a special compensating transformer (marked T in the diagram) is in series with the primary winding of the filament transformer (marked F in the diagram) and with the milliamperes selector (marked R in the diagram). As we shall see, the voltage induced in the

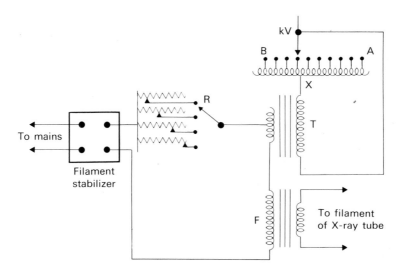

Fig. 2.22

secondary winding of the compensating transformer T can be either an additive voltage or a subtractive voltage.

The voltage applied to the primary winding of the filament transformer determines the filament temperature and is given by:

1 the voltage output from the filament stabilizer

minus

2 the voltage drop in the resistor R, which is the milliamperes selector;

plus or *minus* (as the case may be)

3 the voltage produced in the secondary winding of
the compensator transformer T.

One side of the primary winding of the transformer T is connected to a fixed point on the autotransformer marked X in the diagram. The other side is connected to the variable selector switch which is the kilovoltage control and moves over tappings on the autotransformer. With the kilovoltage control at X there is no voltage on the transformer T and this transformer does not then affect the voltage on the filament of the X-ray tube (the heating voltage). Let us suppose that this is the state of affairs when the kilovoltage selector is at 70 kV: and that with this voltage across the X-ray tube no space-charge compensation is necessary because the electrons being drawn across the X-ray tube are balanced by those being emitted from the filament—that is by the space-charge cloud—so as to constitute a current through the tube which is the selected milliamperes.

When the kilovoltage selector is moved towards B in the diagram corresponding to an increase in kilovoltage and it becomes necessary to decrease the filament heat, the voltage across the transformer T increases. The voltage from T and the voltage from the stabilizer in the filament circuit are in anti-phase to each other, so the voltage on T is a subtractive one in relation to the output from the stabilizer. This reduces the filament voltage and thus the filament heat with increase in kilovoltage across the X-ray tube. The reduction in filament heat is matched to the increase in kilovoltage and reduces the emission of electrons to balance the increased number from the space-charge cloud which the higher kilovoltage can collect to the anode. The X-ray tube current thus stays constant.

When the kilovoltage selector is moved towards A in the diagram corresponding to a decrease in kilovoltage and it becomes necessary to increase the heat of the filament, the voltage on the transformer T again increases. This time it is in phase with the voltage from the static stabilizer in the filament circuit and is therefore an additive voltage. The voltage on the filament transformer is thus raised as the kilovoltage is lowered, the increase in filament heat being matched to the decrease in kilovoltage. The X-ray tube current therefore stays constant.

SUMMARY OF THE FILAMENT CIRCUIT

In the foregoing sections we have considered various components in the filament circuit for the X-ray tube; through this circuit the milliamperes used for the X-ray exposure are controlled. It may be helpful here if we summarize them and give a diagram as in Fig. 2.23.

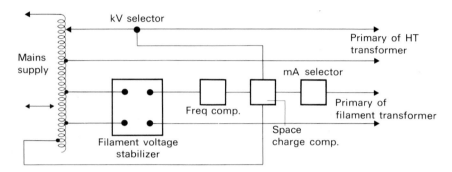

Fig. 2.23

Considered from the filament of the X-ray tube back towards the mains supply, the filament circuit comprises the following.

1   The filament transformer. This is a double-wound step-down transformer with a 20:1 ratio, its secondary winding supplying the filament with a heating current which is up to 4–8 amperes at 10–12 volts.

2   The milliamperes selector. This varies the X-ray tube current by controlling the temperature of the filament through alterations in the voltage applied to the primary winding of the filament transformer. The change in voltage is achieved by (a) a freely variable resistor (for fluoroscopy) or (b) pre-selected resistors of different value for each tube current used (for radiographic exposures). The resistors (whether freely variable or pre-selected) are in series with the primary winding of the filament transformer, the voltage on which is reduced by whatever voltage drop occurs across the resistor included in the circuit.

3   A space-charge compensator. This functions automatically to decrease the voltage on the filament transformer when the tube kilovoltage is raised; and to increase the voltage on the filament transformer when the tube

kilovoltage is lowered. This is necessary if a given setting of the milliamperes selector is to give the same tube current over the full range of kilovoltages used.

4   A frequency compensator if it is necessary. The compensator functions to provide a controlled voltage for the primary winding of the filament transformer if the output of the voltage stabilizer in the filament circuit varies with change in the main frequency. A frequency compensator is unnecessary if the filament stabilizer is not frequency dependent and does not change its voltage output with change in the frequency of the mains supply.

5   A voltage stabilizer. This is necessary to provide the filament transformer with a steady voltage despite variations in the mains voltage which occur. This is important because small changes in the filament voltage and thus in the filament heat can produce large changes in the X-ray tube current.

6   A source of alternating voltage. This is usually about 240 volts and is obtained from the mains supply via the autotransformer of the X-ray set.

MILLIAMPERES INDICATION

It is clear from the foregoing section that X-ray equipment is designed so that a radiographer can control the X-ray tube current which is used for the exposure. The radiographer should also have readable indication of the milliamperes flowing through the X-ray tube while the exposure lasts. Some designers of modern equipment may dispense with this indication and most radiographers regret it when they do. The usefulness to the radiographer of the milliamperes indication is reviewed in a later section of this chapter. Much X-ray equipment does provide indication of the tube current during the exposure and this is done by means of a meter called the milliampere meter.

The milliampere meter

The milliampere meter records the current passing through the X-ray tube. It is therefore measuring the current flowing in the secondary circuit of the high tension transformer.

Circuit connection

An earlier section of this chapter (page 34) described how the secondary winding of the high tension transformer is wound in two halves, the inner ends of the halves being connected to earth. This part of the high tension circuit is called the earthed mid-junction or grounded centre and the purpose of this earthing is to reduce the insulation which is required, as previously explained.

This earthed mid-junction is the only part of the high tension circuit which is virtually at zero volts in respect of earth. A meter placed here can record the current flowing through the secondary winding of the high tension transformer (which is the current flowing through the X-ray tube) and yet can safely be put on the control panel. Here it is easily read by the radiographer. So the earthed centre of the high tension secondary winding is a suitable place to connect the meter, giving the benefits of electrical safety and easy reading.

The two inner ends of the split secondary winding of the high tension transformer are joined through the meter by means of connecting wiring and the meter is placed on the control panel of the X-ray set.

The meter reading

The milliampere meter is a moving-coil meter. This instrument is chosen because it is accurate, it is easy to read because it has a linear scale (this is a scale with the calibrations on it spaced equal steps apart from each other) and it is relatively robust. A moving coil meter cannot read alternating current and it must be energized by current which passes through it in one direction only. Because of this, in certain high tension circuits (see Chapter 3) it is necessary to provide the meter with rectifiers.

The X-ray tube current is not a steady value. Because the alternating mains supply has a cycle of variation as we have seen in Chapter 1, the X-ray tube current rises and falls in waveforms (see Chapter 3) which may pulsate or may ripple. The milliamperes meter is energized by current which shows a pattern of variation in a repeated cycle of change.

In these circumstances a moving coil meter reads a value which is the *average* of the values in a cycle. This point is considered again in Chapter 3, for the relationship between the average and the peak values in the cycles of change is important and is different for different sorts of high tension generator providing power for the X-ray tube.

The meter scale

Since the radiographer must read the milliampere meter in order to check the performance of the X-ray set, this meter should be easy to read. It must record a wide range of values; for example from zero to 500 mA. But on a long scale such as this the tube current required for fluoroscopy is not easy to read because the calibration marks are close together and 4 mA or less will not move the meter needle far across the scale.

This difficulty can be overcome by giving the milliampere meter two scales—one for the low part of the range to be measured (for example 0–5 mA) and the other (scaled 0–500 mA) intended for use when the higher tube currents are employed. The two separate ranges are achieved by an arrangement such as is shown in Fig. 2.24.

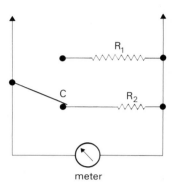

Fig. 2.24   meter

It can be seen that the meter has two resistors which can be connected in parallel across it by means of contacts at C. According to the position of C, either R_1 or R_2 is connected across the meter; R_1 is greater in value than R_2. These resistors are called shunts. The current flowing through the secondary winding of the high tension transformer flows *either* through the meter and R_1 *or* through the meter and R_2.

Let us suppose that the basic meter movement can measure up to 1 mA. This means that 1 mA passing through the meter produces full-scale deflection and moves the meter needle as far over the scale as it can go. It means also that if we try to pass more than 1 mA through the meter movement, we run the risk of damaging it, of burning it out by making it too hot and of bending the needle by making it go too hard against the stop at the end of the scale. When the meter is to be used to measure 5 mA, the contacts at C are in position to connect R_1 across the meter. The value of R_1 in relation to the resistance of the meter is such that 1 mA of the high tension secondary current goes through the meter and 4 mA go through R_1, which is lower in resistance than the meter movement. When 500 mA must be measured, the contacts at C are in position to include R_2 in the circuit. Then 1 mA of the high tension secondary current continues to go through the meter and 499 mA pass through R_2 which is much lower in resistance than the meter movement.

The contacts at C are operated by means of a switching system and the appropriate shunt is selected when the milliamperes are selected. Thus by means of shunts a basic meter movement of low range can be given two or even three scales. There is a different shunt for each scale or range of current, the shunts being lower in resistance as the range of the current to be measured becomes higher.

The milliampereseconds meter

The milliampereseconds meter is a meter which does as its name suggests and records milliampereseconds and not milliamperes. It indicates the product of the current flowing and the time for which it flows. It is a meter which measures a quantity of electricity or the electric charge.

In X-ray sets there is a need for milliampereseconds meters because when the exposure interval is very short an ordinary milliampere meter does not have enough time in which to register; this deprives the radiographer of opportunity to read it. It takes about 1 second for the moving-coil milliampere meter to give an accurate reading. If the exposure time is shorter than this, before the needle can reach the right place on the scale the tube current is cut off at the end of the exposure and the needle falls back to zero.

So that the radiographer may know the tube current on a very short exposure, the meters on the control panel include a milliampereseconds meter which records the charge which has passed through the X-ray tube. Knowledge of the tube current is then derived by dividing the milliampereseconds indicated on the meter by the exposure time. For example, if the exposure time is 0·04 seconds and the milliampereseconds meter reads 16 mAs, then the current through the X-ray tube is 400 mA. When the exposure stops and the tube current is cut off, the needle of the meter does not return to zero so that the radiographer has opportunity to read what it shows.

The meter movement

The movement of the milliampereseconds meter is essentially the same as that of a moving-coil milliampere meter with some differences of construction. In the moving-coil meter the current to be measured is passed into a coil of wire which is suspended in the magnetic field between the poles of a permanent magnet.

Current in the coil produces a magnetic field about the coil which makes it act like a magnet. The magnetic forces between the permanent magnet and the coil-magnet give a twisting force to the coil and (as it is constructed to be free to rotate) it rotates, putting tension on a spring as it does so and moving a pointer over a scale. The pointer movement is controlled by balancing the magnetic twisting force by the tension in the spring; the pointer comes to rest at a point on the scale which depends upon and indicates the value of the current flowing through the coil. Another spring provides a restoring force so that when the current which is being measured ceases to flow in the coil, the pointer is restored to zero.

In the milliampereseconds meter the two springs, one of which provides a controlling force and the other of which provides a restoring force, are left out. The coil rotates freely when current is passed through it and in this circumstance the extent of the rotation depends on the strength of the current and the time for which it flows. The final position of the pointer is proportional to the product of the current (milliamperes) and the time (seconds) and the meter reads milliampereseconds.

Since there is no spring to restore the pointer after the exciting current has died down, the pointer is moved back to zero by another method; a small unidirectional current at about 1·5 volts is put through the coil in a reverse direction. This may be done automatically when the exposure switch is put into 'prepare' for the next exposure, or it may be necessary for the radiographer to zero the meter by pressing a button situated near it on the control panel. It is best to do this *just before* the next exposure as the meter has a tendency to 'creep'; this means that the pointer tends to slide across the scale when the meter is not in use. Because the pointer is liable also to move slowly away from its position on the scale after use, the radiographer should read the indication as soon as the exposure has ended.

The meter scale

Milliampereseconds meters are often provided with double scales just as milliampere meters are. For example one scale may read 0–50 mAs and the other 0–250 mAs. The double scale is achieved by means of shunt resistors as we explained for the milliampere meter.

Circuit connection

The milliampereseconds meter is connected, like the milliampere meter, at the earthed centre point of the high tension transformer secondary winding. As shown in Fig. 2.25 there is a switch (marked S in the diagram) to connect either the milliampereseconds meter or the milliampere meter into the circuit.

When the exposure time selected is less than 1·0 second, the milliampereseconds meter is automatically connected into the circuit through S, which is moved to the appropriate position which is marked A in the diagram. When the exposure time is more than 1·0 second (or for fluoroscopy) the switch S is automatically in the place (B in the diagram) which connects the milliampere meter into the circuit.

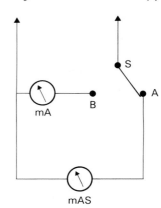

Fig. 2.25

Usefulness of milliamperes indication

The milliamperes indication tells the radiographer (a) that the X-ray tube has passed current; (b) that the exposure has taken place; (c) that the X-ray set is operating properly. So the radiographer should read the milliamperes indication for every exposure that is made. We have little sympathy for the one who, failing to notice that the milliampere meter or milliampereseconds meter has never recorded, woefully receives from the automatic processor several blank films in a radiographic examination. The strange behaviour which is lack of behaviour by the meter should have been noticed when the first exposure was attempted and the matter investigated then before further time and effort had been wasted.

A radiographer who reads the milliampere or milliampereseconds meter may save not only time and effort expended in the X-ray department by staff and patients but also wasted endeavour by an engineer who comes to put the equipment in order again after it has shown itself faulty. A radiographer who can give an informed answer about the milliamperes indication (Was it high? Low? Erratic? Steady? Anything at all?) can help the engineer towards a diagnosis of the fault. This is especially of value if the engineer must come some distance to the hospital and in any case engineers (like radiographers) are always busy and are grateful when radiographers can save their time.

The following indications on a milliampere (milliampereseconds) meter give clues to a knowledgeable radiographer about faults in the X-ray tube or its associated circuits.

1   No reading on the meter. This means that no current has passed through the X-ray tube. Provided that other causes of failure to obtain an exposure can be excluded (such as incorrect or incomplete manipulation of the

controls), the absence of tube current suggests a break in the filament of the X-ray tube; or failure at some point in the circuit supplying it; or a break in a conductor in the high tension cables connected to the X-ray tube. If the X-ray set 'makes all the right sounds' of contactors and microswitches operating and the anode rotating, so that a listening radiographer hears nothing to cause concern and believes that the exposure has taken place, absence of a reading on the meter indicates that the fault is in one of the possible situations mentioned above.

2 Intermittent failure in the tube current so that it comes and goes. This also suggests a broken filament in the X-ray tube, a break in the filament circuit or a broken conductor in a high tension cable. If the X-ray tube current can be made to come and go by varying the position of the X-ray tube and hence of the cables, then a broken conductor in the cable is strongly indicated.

3 If the tube current rises to a value somewhat above the expected one accompanied by a noise which is a high tension crack (it may not be very loud), then there is a fault in the insulation of a high tension cable (see Chapter 17 for further indications).

4 When the milliamperes increase erratically to a very high value so that the meter needle flies hard across the scale and may bend itself against the stop at the end, the radiographer sees the alarming indications of a gassy or incipiently gassy X-ray tube (see Chapter 7). The useful life of such an X-ray tube is at an end.

5 A low reading on the milliampere (milliampereseconds) meter suggests that there is a faulty filament boost (see Chapter 7) for the X-ray tube so that its temperature is less than it should be for the required X-ray tube current. This may persist throughout the exposure. Or it may exist at the beginning of the exposure and right itself as the exposure proceeds, thus showing that the filament boost is not timed correctly to be completely achieved before the exposure begins.

MAINS VOLTAGE COMPENSATION

In previous sections of this chapter (pages 62–72) we considered the filament circuit and the importance of a stabilized voltage for the step-down transformer which heats the filament of the X-ray tube. There are other parts of the X-ray unit where compensation is provided for changes in the mains voltage. We will now consider these.

As we have seen, the changes that occur in the mains voltage are:

1 slow changes over a period of time due to differences in demand on the supply at various periods in the day;

2 rapid instantaneous changes due to load currents being drawn on the same line by equipment which takes high current for short intervals;

3 the fall in mains voltage which occurs as soon as the X-ray exposure begins and is due to the load current drawn by the X-ray set itself for the exposure.

The changes under (2) and (3) above arise because the load currents flow against the resistance of the supply mains—that is, of the generators where the supply is produced and of cables and transformers between the generators and the hospital department where the X-ray set is in use. When current flows against resistance, voltage is used and this accounts for the fall in the mains voltage when load currents flow. The bigger the load currents are, the bigger the fall in voltage with a given resistance of the mains supply.

An X-ray set can be provided with a device to compensate for the mains drop under load which it causes as under (3) above. Such compensation protects various components from a fall in their supply voltages and the matter is considered further in a later part of this chapter (page 84). Slow changes over hours as under (1) above occur outside the X-ray exposure and are compensated by what is called the mains voltage compensator of the X-ray set.

The mains voltage compensator cannot prevent the mains voltage changes from taking place. What it can do (and is designed to do) is maintain a voltage output from the autotransformer of the X-ray unit which is unchanged despite the alteration in the applied primary voltage (which is the mains voltage) to the autotransformer. Reference to pages 53–55 in this chapter will remind the undaunted reader that the kilovoltage for the X-ray exposure is selected by means of a control which moves over tappings on the secondary side of the autotransformer (see Fig. 2.13). For any given setting of the autotransformer control to provide consistently the same kilovoltage, it is essential that the voltage output of the autotransformer is not changed by changes in the applied voltage; if it *is* changed, then a given kilovoltage setting will give a different and unexpected kilovoltage. With the kilovoltage selector in a given position, a rise in the mains voltage will result in a rise in the voltage output from the autotransformer and hence an increase in kilovoltage; a fall in the mains voltage results similarly in a lowered kilovoltage for the X-ray tube.

Mains voltage compensation can be achieved (a) by means of a manual control which the radiographer uses in conjunction with the reading of a voltmeter; (b) by an automatic method of compensation which removes the necessity for a radiographer to check the mains supply and use the control.

Both sorts of compensator compensate only for voltage changes which occur outside and not during the X-ray exposure.

.

Manually adjusted mains voltage compensator

As shown in Fig. 2.26 the manually adjusted mains voltage compensator consists of tappings on the autotransformer at one end of the winding. The tappings are on the primary side in the diagram but could be on the secondary side.

Each tapping ends in a terminal or stud and there is a movable selector switch which connects to any one of the studs. In the diagram the selector is

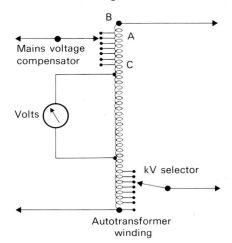

Fig. 2.26

in position to connect it to the stud marked A. Also shown in the diagram is a voltmeter marked *volts* which is connected across a fixed number of tappings of the autotransformer. This voltmeter is called the line voltage compensator meter. It is usually a moving-iron voltmeter and is without figures on its dial. Instead there is a mark on the dial—for example, a red line—and when the incoming voltage from the supply is at its correct value the pointer of the meter is against this reference mark on the scale.

Let us suppose that the selector switch is at A as it is in Fig. 2.26 and that in this circumstance the number of turns of the autotransformer included in the circuit is 240. The supply is at its correct value of 240 volts and the meter needle is at the reference mark on the dial. With 240 volts across 240 turns, the volts per turn ratio for the autotransformer is 1 volt per turn.

When the incoming voltage changes, so long as this volts per turn relationship can be retained at 1 volt per turn there will be no change in the voltage output from the autotransformer, which stable condition is the one we are trying to achieve. If the supply falls, for example to 235 volts, this will be shown by the pointer of the meter which will be below the reference mark. Seeing this, the radiographer moves the manually controlled selector switch towards C in the diagram. It will reach a stud setting which includes

235 turns of the autotransformer in the circuit. At that point 235 volts exist across 235 turns, the volts per turn ratio is again 1 volt per turn, the meter needle is back on the reference mark and the voltage change has been compensated.

Let us suppose now that the mains voltage rises to 245 volts. The meter will indicate this by having its pointer above the reference mark. The radiographer moves the selector switch towards B in the diagram and this brings more turns of the autotransformer into the circuit. With the selector switch at the stud which includes 245 turns of the autotransformer in the circuit, the volts per turn ratio is again back to 1 volt per turn, the pointer is at its reference mark and the rise in mains voltage has been compensated.

Maintaining the current to the autotransformer

The simple selector switch shown in Fig. 2.26 has the disadvantage that as it moves from the one stud to the next it breaks the current to the autotransformer for the period of time that it is between studs—that is, when the switch has been disconnected from one tapping and has not arrived at the next. In the X-ray set this discontinuity in the autotransformer current is prevented by a circuit arrangement of one sort or another.

To our own relief, we need not consider here more than one method and we give below a way of maintaining the current to the autotransformer when the switch is moved between studs.

Fig. 2.27 shows the arrangement. The selector switch has two poles which move together and are connected by a resistor. The poles are set so that when one is between studs the other is connected to a stud. The resistor which joins the two poles provides a pathway for the current to flow. Thus the autotransformer current does not have a discontinuous circuit whatever the position of the selector switch on the main voltage compensator.

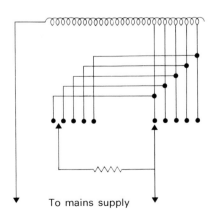

Fig. 2.27   To mains supply

Automatic mains voltage compensation

In some generators, compensation for changes in the mains voltage is made automatically by means of a special circuit. This is not to say that radiographers may with impunity disregard a mains voltmeter. Before a radiographic exposure is made, a glance at the meter is always needed for reassurance that the mains input to the autotransformer is as it should be.

The mechanism

As we have just seen in relation to a manually adjusted mains voltage compensator, the necessary operation is to obtain a correctly balanced voltage from the autotransformer by means of adjustment of the turns ratio. In the case of the manually operated device, this adjuster is a selector switch driven by the radiographer's hand as need arises.

In the mechanism now to be considered, the adjustor is a special contact, called a sledge, which can be made to move over a section of the transformer windings. Along this section, part of the insulation is removed from the windings so that the sledge contact travels on an electrically live track: its

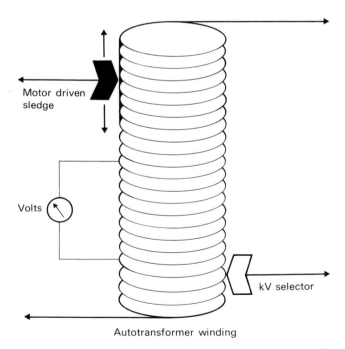

Motor driven sledge

Volts

kV selector

Autotransformer winding

Fig. 2.28 A diagram to illustrate the principle features of an automatic method of mains voltage compensation.

position along this track establishes the turns ratio of the autotransformer and so can be manipulated to obtain a consistently balanced output voltage from the transformer, independent of variation in the mains input.

The power which drives the sledge along its track on the windings comes from an electric motor. We have now briefly to consider the circuit which supplies a voltage to this motor and causes it to move the sledge in one or other of two directions, such as are indicated in Fig. 2.28. Fig. 2.28 is Fig. 2.26 re-drawn to show how the sledge and the stripped track may replace a moveable selector switch and tappings: it may help the reader if the two sketches are compared.

The circuit

The compensating circuit supplying power to the windings of the a.c. motor is—for the authors and readers of this book—a relatively complicated one. An idea of it is sketched in Fig. 2.29 which shows, firstly, an operational amplifier which has three pins.

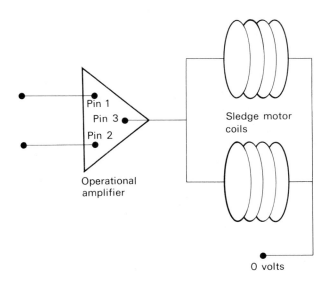

Fig. 2.29.

One side of the compensating circuit is fed to pin 1 of the amplifier; the voltage on pin 2 is a reference voltage. If the voltage on pin 1 does not correspond to the voltage on pin 2, then current flows from pin 3; if there is a correspondence of the circuit voltage and the reference voltage, then no current flows.

When current is present on pin 3, it is either positive or negative of the desired voltage, depending on the status of the circuit voltage relative to the reference voltage; that is, on whether there has been a rise or a fall of the mains voltage. In either circumstance, the current which flows from the operational amplifier is the agent which affects the production of a current through the coil of the motor driving the sledge; with the difference that a positive current from the amplifier will drive the sledge in one direction and a negative current will drive it in the opposite direction.

The sledge contact is driven along the autotransformer, one way or the other, until the correct balance of voltage is reached. In this event the voltages on pin 1 and pin 2 of the operational amplifier are restored to agreement and pin 3 ceases to provide any current. When this is so, there is no voltage on the motor and the sledge stays where it is, until a change in the mains supply triggers again the sequence of events just described.

Compensation for mains voltage drop on load

As we have seen, when an X-ray exposure begins the load current flows against the resistance of the mains supply and the mains voltage falls because of this; this is the mains voltage drop or line drop under load. It is *caused* by the X-ray exposure, occurs when the exposure begins and lasts for the duration of the exposure. The amount of this voltage drop, for a supply with a given resistance, depends on the load current, being greater for higher loads. The load current in its turn is proportional to the factors selected by the radiographer for the X-ray exposure. The greater the tube load in milliamperes and kilovolts, the higher is the current drawn from the mains supply.

It is possible to compensate for the mains voltage drop under load by providing a transformer which develops across it a voltage related to the load current and thus to the voltage drop which occurs. This transformer can be used to supply extra voltage which compensates for the change.

This special transformer providing line drop compensation compensates only for this fall in the mains voltage when the load is applied; it cannot compensate for any other mains voltage change.

Line drop compensation transformer

The special transformer which provides a voltage to compensate for the mains drop under load is a small current transformer with its primary in series with the load current. This is shown as T in Fig. 2.30.

The load current which flows from the mains supply flows also in the primary winding of this special transformer, just as it flows through the

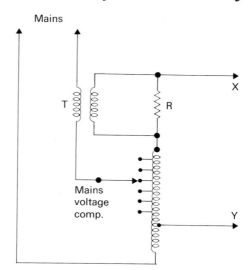

Mains

Mains
voltage
comp.

Fig. 2.30

primary winding of the autotransformer of the X-ray set. The secondary winding of the compensating transformer has a resistor in parallel with it; when current flows in the primary winding an induced current flows in the secondary winding which gives rise to a voltage developed across the resistor R. The voltage consequently available across the points X and Y is the on load 'booster voltage' to compensate for the line drop which occurs.

By selection of the transformer ratio in the compensating transformer and of the resistance in R, the extra voltage can be made to match the line voltage drop. For example, let us suppose that the X-ray tube load in milliamperes and kilovolts is such as to cause a load on the line of 50 amperes. This load of 50 amperes flows through the primary winding of the compensating transformer. If the ratio of the transformer is 20:1, the current flowing in the secondary winding of the compensating transformer is 50/20 = 2·5 amps. If the resistor has a value of 2 ohms, 2·5 amps passed through it gives 5 volts developed across the resistor. Let us suppose in contrast that the X-ray tube load is such as to cause a much smaller load on the line—for example 10 amperes. Then 10 amperes flowing in the primary winding of the compensating transformer results in 10/20 = 0·5 amperes flowing through the resistor of 2 ohms. The voltage developed across the resistor is only 1 volt.

Thus it can be seen that when the load on the line is light and the line drop is negligible, the booster voltage available at XY in the diagram is correspondingly very small. When the load on the line is heavier and the voltage drop consequently bigger, the booster voltage is greater too.

MAINS SUPPLY AND THE X-RAY SET

It may be helpful if we list the effects upon the X-ray set of changes in the mains supply, together with a summary of the compensators which are included in X-ray equipment to prevent these results from occurring unchecked, with mention of two other compensators for different purposes.

The changes in the mains supply may be (i) in voltage; (ii) in frequency. Voltage changes are:

1   slow changes over a period of hours because of the differences in demand at various times of the day;

2   rapid changes because some equipment on the same line draws a heavy current for a short interval;

3   the fall in the mains voltage caused by the X-ray set itself drawing current for the diagnostic exposure.

If there are no compensating devices at all in the X-ray equipment, voltage changes will cause the following effects.

(*i*) Change in the X-ray tube kilovoltage because there is alteration in the voltage supplied by the autotransformer to the primary winding of the high tension transformer.

(*ii*) Change in the X-ray tube current because there is alteration in the voltage supplied by the autotransformer to the tube filament transformer and hence in the heat of the filament. The change in milliamperes is the greater of the two effects because small changes in filament heat can produce large changes in the tube milliamperes. The change in kilovoltage occurring alone would probably not be noticeable in the radiographic result; the change in tube current can be great enough to be seen in the radiograph.

(*iii*) Change in the voltages operating many components in the X-ray set—timers, motors, relays of various sorts. These are less important to the radiographer than the other changes mentioned under (*i*) and (*ii*) above.

Changes in the mains frequency occur slowly and cause the following events.

(*i*) Any components driven by synchronous electric motors (for example the rotating anode of the X-ray tube) will run at an incorrect speed. In the case of the rotating anode, this will alter the rating of the tube and could lead to overload.

(*ii*) If a frequency sensitive type of stabilizer is fitted in the filament circuit of the X-ray tube, its voltage output alters. This changes the voltage applied to the primary winding of the filament transformer and alters the filament heat and hence the X-ray tube milliamperes. Small frequency changes can result in large changes of tube current. This is the most important effect on the X-ray set of a change in the frequency of the mains supply.

Various devices are included in X-ray equipment to minimize the effects of changes in the mains supply, both in voltage and in frequency. These devices are called compensators because they compensate or make up for the changes which have taken place. They prevent the effects which the changes would otherwise produce in the X-ray equipment. They do not prevent the changes from occurring in the first place. The devices are listed below and in the list we have put a page reference after each item to indicate where in this chapter the item is described.

Mains voltage compensator (page 78)

This may be manually or automatically adjusted. It acts to maintain a constant volts per turn ratio on the autotransformer of the X-ray set so that the voltage output of the autotransformer is not changed by alteration in the input voltage. It compensates for slow voltage changes occurring outside the X-ray exposure.

Line drop compensator (page 84)

This is a special transformer in series with the autotransformer. It functions to provide a voltage to be superimposed on the line voltage in such a way that this extra voltage is matched to the fall in the line voltage which occurs when the load current flows against mains resistance. This compensator compensates only for the mains drop caused by the X-ray set itself.

In the filament circuit for the X-ray tube are:

Voltage stabilizer (page 66)

The voltage stabilizer functions to provide a steady voltage at its output points despite variations at the input side. This stabilized output voltage is applied to the primary windings of the transformers which heat the filaments of the X-ray tube. The filaments of the X-ray tube are protected thus against all types of voltage change in the mains supply. This therefore makes the first two items in this list not *necessary* so far as the X-ray tube filaments are concerned. But a steady voltage for the filament is very important so the manufacturers, as Shakespeare's Macbeth in a more exciting context, plan to 'make assurance double sure' and put all these items to work for the filament circuit.

Compensator for frequency change (page 68)

This is necessary if the filament voltage stabilizer is frequency-dependent. In this state, if the mains frequency changes the voltage output from the stabilizer becomes variable and no longer maintained steady. The frequency compensator corrects for the variations and in effect restores a stabilized condition.

Also in the filament circuit is another compensator which acts in respect of the X-ray tube current and voltage and not in respect of the mains voltage. This is as follows.

Space charge compensator (page 68)

This is to prevent a change in the X-ray tube current when the radiographer selects a different kilovoltage. Basically it is a special transformer winding which puts into the filament circuit (a) an additive voltage to increase the filament-heating current when the kilovoltage is lowered; and (b) an opposing voltage so that the filament-heating current is reduced when the kilovoltage is raised.

In the primary control circuit of the X-ray equipment there is one more compensator to be mentioned. This is as follows.

Kilovoltage compensation (page 59)

This compensation maintains the kilovoltage for a given setting of the kilovoltage selector against the different voltage drops that occur in the high tension transformer when the radiographer selects different tube currents. Basically it is a sliding contact on the autotransformer of the X-ray set which is ganged to the milliamperes selector. When the tube current is raised, more voltage is selected from the autotransformer and when the tube current is lowered less voltage is selected from the autotransformer in such a way as to compensate for the different voltage drops at different current loads. Thus for a given setting of the kilovoltage control, the kilovoltage does not vary with the milliamperes selected.

Chapter 3
High Tension Generators

In previous chapters it has been seen that in order to make an X-ray tube produce X rays it is necessary to connect it to a source of high voltage. High voltage gives great kinetic energy to the electrons which leave the filament of the X-ray tube and bombard the anode; when the electrons are halted or slowed down this kinetic energy is converted to other energy, of which a small proportion is X rays and a large proportion is heat. What do we mean by high voltage? For diagnostic radiology the range of voltages used is from about 20 kilovolts to about 130 kilovolts.

These high voltages are obtained from a transformer which steps up the supply voltage from the mains voltage level to the kilovoltages which are necessary to make the X-ray tube work. This high tension transformer, together with other components such as rectifiers in the high tension secondary circuit, is known among those who use or make and service X-ray equipment as the high tension generator.

There are various circuits constituting different high tension generators for X-ray tubes. These range from the simple to the complex. It is the purpose of this chapter to describe the main ones and to indicate their usefulness in different sorts of X-ray equipment.

THE RATING OF X-RAY GENERATORS

The essential function of high tension generators in X-ray equipment is to provide such power as is needed by the X-ray tubes to which they are connected. So an important specification in the description of any generator is a statement on its power output. This statement is expressed in watts, the common unit of electric power, and since the power input of these generators is thousands of watts the practical unit used is the kilowatt (kW): 1000 watts is one kilowatt.

The kilowatt ratings of generators are established when the generators are operating to provide power: that is, the ratings are evaluated when generators are under load. The formulae which may be used for the calculations involve multiplying the kilovolts and the milliamps which constitute the load and this gives us a reasonable approximation for the power output.

In the case of a three-phase generator the formula which may be used is

$$kW = \frac{kV \times mA}{1000}$$

In the case of a single-phase generator the formula which may be used is

$$kW = \frac{0.7 \times kW \times mA}{1000}$$

This modification (the factor 0.7) is required for the single-phase generator because (as will be seen if you read this chapter through to the end) the voltage waveform for this type of generator is pulsating: it varies up and down between zero volts and a peak value. For a three-phase generator the voltage waveform is a ripple which falls from a peak to some value a little below it (for example, from 100 kV to 86 kV) and rises again to the peak. So for a three-phase generator at a given milliamperage and kilovoltage, the effective power output is greater than that obtained from the same loading applied to a single-phase generator, with its voltage falling all the way down to zero at three points in one complete cycle of mains alternations.

Generators may be compared by means of their kilowatt ratings. In doing this and in considering the ratings of all generators, the following important points must be noted.

1   The manufacturer states the highest milliamperage which the generator can produce. (Examples are 500 mA, 800 mA, 1000 mA.)

2   The manufacturer states the maximum kilovoltage which the generator can provide. (Examples are 125 kV, 150 kV.)

3   It must not be assumed that when the generator is loaded these maximum values of kilovoltage and milliamperage can be *simultaneously* obtained. In practice they will not be obtainable together. If the highest kilovoltage is to be used, then the maximum milliamperage available will be lower than the highest value stated for the generator. Similarly, if the highest milliamperage is to be used the available kilovoltage is lower than the maximum voltage output given for the generator. Thus a generator which is described as 1000 mA and 150 kV might in practice provide as follows:

1000 mA at 80 kV (80 kW)
800 mA at 100 kV (80 kW)
500 mA at 150 kV (75 kW)

4   The alert reader may notice that the kilowatt ratings given immediately above are not all the same: the first two are both 80 kW and the third is lower, being 75 kW or 94 per cent of the higher value. This is often found

and the kilowatt rating at 150 kV could be much lower than is given here: for example, it might be only 75 per cent of the higher value. This disparity results from the fact that the practice of reducing the milliamperage with rising kilovoltage is usually overdone so that there is excessive reduction, despite the theory that the 'isowatt principle' should apply to maintain equality for the kilowatt ratings.

5   Kilowatt ratings for generators are determined under load and it is convenient to test and state the rating at the voltage level of 100 kV. If this were done for the generator mentioned above as giving 800 mA at 100 kV, then its kilowatt rating can be calculated as below, assuming it to be a three-phase generator.

$$\frac{800 \times 100}{1000} = 80 \text{ kW}.$$

6   The kilowatt rating at 100 kV provides one point of comparison between generators. However, it is *just one level* and the relative placings of generators tested at 100 kV may change when they are tested at a higher kilovoltage. For example, at 100 kV generator A may have a higher rating than generator B but at 150 kV generator B may be able to provide a greater kilowattage. This could be important if you are selecting a generator which is to be installed, for example, in a room where chest radiography is to be done with high kilovoltages as a planned exposure technique. You need to know the output in kilowatts at a high kilovoltage level.

THE SELF-RECTIFIED HIGH TENSION CIRCUIT

The simplest form of high tension generator consists of a high tension transformer with an X-ray tube connected directly to its secondary winding. This is shown diagrammatically in Fig. 3.1 where it can be seen that the cathode of the X-ray tube is connected to one end of the transformer secondary winding and the anode of the X-ray tube is connected to the other.

As might be expected, this results in a piece of equipment which in relation to others is:

1   small,
2   light in weight,
3   inexpensive,
4   easily manœuvred,
5   simple.

These are the advantages of the arrangement and they have led to its use in portable and mobile equipment (see Chapter 9), for which these advantages

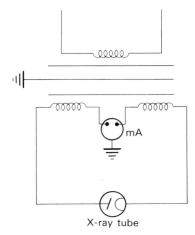

Fig. 3.1   X-ray tube

are naturally sought. In order to understand the disadvantages we must look at how the circuit works.

Limitations of the self-rectified circuit

The voltage supplied to the primary of the high tension transformer is alternating voltage and it varies in direction and magnitude in the way shown in Fig. 3.2(a). This means that during one-half of the a.c. cycle (period AB in the diagram) the filament of the X-ray tube is connected to the negative pole of the transformer and the anode of the X-ray tube is connected to the positive pole. In these circumstances the electrons liberated from the filament travel to the anode, current flows through the tube and X rays are produced.

Fig. 3.2(b) shows the waveform of the current through the X-ray tube during this half-cycle in the period of time AB. It is not the same shape as the sine wave of voltage; the tube current at first increases with the voltage from zero and then as the saturation point is reached it levels out to nearly a straight line, and finally as the voltage falls the current goes again to zero. During this half-cycle the X-ray tube is functioning to produce X rays.

In the next half-cycle the alternating voltage of the mains supply reverses as shown in Fig. 3.2(a) in the period of time BC. During this period the filament of the X-ray tube is connected to the pole of the transformer which is positive and the anode of the tube is connected to the pole of the transformer which is negative. In these circumstances there is no inducement to the electrons from the heated filament to go towards the anode. There is no flow of current through the X-ray tube and no X rays are produced.

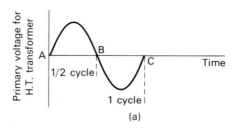

(a)

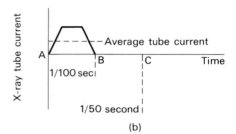

Fig. 3.2   (b)

During this half-cycle in which there is no current through the X-ray tube (period BC in Fig. 3.2(b)) the X-ray tube has acted to block a current that is trying to change direction, so that in fact the current flows through the X-ray tube in one direction only. Because the X-ray tube must always pass current in one direction only it converts the alternating current of the mains supply to a unidirectional current in the secondary circuit of the high tension transformer. Conversion of an alternating current to a unidirectional one is called rectification (a term sometimes used in the U.S.A. is commutation). When the X-ray tube does this it is functioning as a rectifier; this is why this circuit is called self-rectified and sometimes self-suppressed. The X-ray tube itself is doing the rectification and suppressing one half-cycle or half-wave of current.

It is to be noted that only one half-cycle in each complete cycle of the mains supply is used by the X-ray tube to produce X rays. Self-rectified high tension generators are therefore one type of half-wave generator.

The limitations of the self-rectified circuit for operating an X-ray tube derive from four important facts. These are:

1   that the peak voltage across the X-ray tube during the half-cycle when the tube passes current and produces X rays is not the same as during the half-cycle when the tube does not pass current and does not produce X rays;

2   that the peak value which the tube current reaches during the cycle is three times the average value;

3   that the rating of a given X-ray tube (that is the power which may be

applied to it during operation) is more limited when the tube is placed in a self-rectified circuit than when it is used in any other type of high tension generator;

4 that there is greater strain on cables used to connect the X-ray tube to the high tension transformer if the circuit is a self-rectified one than there is in circuits which use other rectification systems.

The explanations of these facts are given below.

Difference in peak voltage

The two half-cycles of voltage from the high tension transformer are distinguished according to whether the X-ray tube is or is not passing current and producing X rays. The half-cycle during which the X-ray tube passes current and produces X rays (period AB in Fig. 3.2(b)) is called the useful half-cycle for obvious reasons (sometimes the forward half-cycle). The half-cycle during which the X-ray tube is not passing current and not producing X rays (period BC in Fig. 3.2(b)) is called the inverse half-cycle; one of the meanings of *inverse* is *opposite in nature or effect*.

During the inverse half-cycle the secondary voltage of the high tension transformer is applied to the X-ray tube *but no secondary current is passing*. This means that during this half-cycle the transformer is doing no work, there is no load current passing through its windings, and the voltage applied to the X-ray tube is a 'no load' voltage.

During the useful half-cycle, current flows in the secondary circuit and the high tension transformer is doing work since it is passing current through the X-ray tube. The voltage applied to the X-ray tube from the transformer is therefore an 'on load' voltage; it is smaller than the 'no load' voltage by the voltage drop that occurs when current is made to flow through the windings of the transformer. This voltage drop is the voltage used in passing the load current against the resistance of the primary and secondary windings; it is equal to the product of the resistance and the load current.

$$E = RI \quad \text{or} \quad \text{volts} = \text{ohms} \times \text{amps}$$

The magnitude of the voltage drop is therefore influenced by the magnitude of the load current flowing through the transformer windings. This load current in the high tension transformer of an X-ray set is the X-ray tube current or milliamperage.

Fig. 3.3 shows the waveform of the X-ray tube voltage in a self-rectified generator and it can be seen that during the inverse half-cycle (period BC) it comes to a higher peak than during the useful half-cycle (period AB). The inverse voltage of the non-conducting half-cycle is thus always greater than the useful voltage of the conducting half-cycle, and the difference between

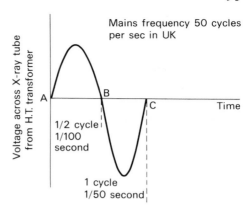

Fig. 3.3

the two becomes greater with the X-ray tube current supplied by the transformer. It may be about 20–30 kVp.

The radiographic output of the X-ray tube (quantity and penetrating power of the X rays) is related to the highest voltage in the useful half-cycle. The insulation required and therefore the size, weight and cost of the equipment are related to the highest voltage in the inverse half-cycle because this is the greater of the two. It is uneconomic to have a very big difference in voltage during the two half-cycles, for the result of that is that the user must pay more and accept greater size and weight in the equipment, without enjoying a commensurate improvement in the radiographic output of the X-ray unit. Typical for a self-rectified generator is a 1·5 to 2·0 kW rating, with 20 mA the upper limit for tube current and 80 kV the maximum voltage.

Average and peak tube currents

The current through the X-ray tube is recorded by means of a milliammeter which is a moving coil meter. When energized by a current which is subject to a cycle of change (as the X-ray tube current is except in very special cases) such a meter must record some steady value; it cannot follow each instantaneous variation. A moving-coil meter records a steady value which is the *average* of instantaneous values during the cycle.

Because the milliammeter is a moving-coil meter and records an average value, the X-ray tube current as an exposure factor is always expressed as an average value. That is what the meter reads and this is what radiographers have become used to considering and discussing in their work. It is a practical procedure to accept and to use the meter reading, so we need hardly be surprised if the fact that it is an average value is often forgotten and the question of what the peak value is during the cycle is never asked. It is after all seldom necessary to ask this question ; but in seeking an explanation of some of the limitations of a self-rectified circuit we must consider it.

Fig. 3.2(b) illustrates the waveform of the tube current during one complete cycle of the mains supply. It shows (i) that the current varies from zero up to a maximum value which is nearly constant for a time and then down again to zero; and (ii) that only half of the period of time of one cycle is occupied by the variations in the current.

Because the current occupies only half of one complete cycle, the maximum value reached during the cycle can be considered to be about three times the average value which the milliammeter records. This factor relating the average value and the peak value of the X-ray tube current during the cycle exists for all half-wave generators.

The average value of the milliamperage determines the radiographic output (quantity of X rays) and the total heat produced during the exposure. The rise in temperature of the focal spot and target of the X-ray tube is, however, a function of the peak milliamperage. So in a self-rectified circuit any given value of milliamperes read on the meter must result in a rise of target temperature which is produced by a peak milliamperage which is three times greater; for example 20 mA on the meter means a peak milliamperage of 60 mA. Any given tube load as an exposure factor thus produces at the tube focus a much greater temperature rise than would be the case if the peak current were much closer to the average. This limits the milliamperage which can be used in a self-rectified circuit.

Limitation of X-ray tube rating

An X-ray tube operated in a self-rectified circuit has a very low rating (see page 255 in Chapter 7) compared with its rating when it is supplied from other types of high tension generator. This is because when it is self-rectified the tube must never be so loaded that its anode becomes hot enough to be an electron emitter. The reason why the X-ray tube must operate with its anode relatively cool is this : during the inverse half-cycle when the filament is connected to the positive pole of the transformer and the anode is connected to the negative pole, if the anode is emitting electrons then those electrons will be drawn towards the filament and a reverse current will flow through the X-ray tube. So long as the anode is cool enough not to emit electrons there is no chance of a reverse current during the half-cycle of inverse voltage.

The target of the X-ray tube must therefore not be allowed to become hot enough for thermionic emission of electrons, and the only way to keep it cool enough is to operate the X-ray tube at a low rating in terms of kilovoltage and milliampereseconds. A reverse current is damaging to the

X-ray tube because the unfocused electron stream may destroy the cathode and the glass envelope of the tube. Furthermore current through the tube may escalate to a high value. The bombarding electrons make the filament hotter, and as a result on the next useful half-cycle the filament emits more electrons than previously and the milliamperage rises. This makes the hot anode hotter so that in its turn it emits more electrons, and on the inverse half-cycle the reverse current has increased to make the filament hotter still. So the milliamperage on the forward half-cycle and the reverse current on the inverse half-cycle continue to increase, each making the other larger.

Strain on high tension cables

It is usual in self-rectified circuits to employ what is called a tank construction (see page 333 in Chapter 9). This means that the high tension transformer, the filament transformer and the X-ray tube are all housed together within an oil-filled earthed metal shield; it is unnecessary to use high tension cables to connect the X-ray tube to the secondary winding of the high tension transformer. Eliminating the cables is a solution to the problem of the extra strain on high tension cables if they are put into a self-rectified circuit.

This strain arises because, when the X-ray set is in use, in a self-rectified circuit an alternating voltage is applied to the cables from the transformer such that the voltage between the inner conductors of each cable and its earthed outer metal sheath alternates between the positive peak value and the negative peak value. Between these metal parts of the cable—the inner conductors and the outer sheath—is the insulating medium and when the voltage is applied across this it undergoes stress. The alternation in the voltage results in alternation in the way the stress is applied to the atoms of the insulator. The energy involved in this makes the insulator warm, with a consequent reduction in its insulating property.

This means (i) that the maximum kilovoltage which may be applied to a high tension cable must be lower when the cable is used in a self-rectified circuit than when it is used in other forms of generator; or (ii) that for a given maximum kilovoltage the high tension cable must be thicker in a self-rectified circuit than in other generators.

Applications of the self-rectified circuit

The advantages and the disadvantages of the self-rectified high tension generator are listed below.

Advantages

Its use results in an X-ray set which is:
1 small in size,

2   light in weight,
3   relatively inexpensive,
4   simple to operate,
5   easy to transport and manœuvre.

Disadvantages

It can be used only for X-ray sets which are low-powered and give a limited radiographic output. The limits on the radiographic output arise because:
1   the kilovoltage across the tube is bigger on the inverse half-cycle than on the useful one and the difference between the two becomes greater as the milliamperage is raised;
2   the peak value of the tube current in the cycle is about three times greater than the reading on the milliammeter, and the temperature rise at the focal spot of the X-ray tube is a function of this peak milliamperage;
3   the anode must never become hot enough to emit electrons because if it does there can be reverse current through the X-ray tube;
4   there is a greater strain on high tension cables if they are used and this results in a lower kilovoltage rating for any cable of a given size and weight.

These features make the circuit suitable only for low-powered X-ray sets. So it is used for dental sets, in which a high radiographic output will not be required and advantages 1, 2, 3 and 4 will be sought; and for portable equipment, in which all the listed advantages will be attractive and the disadvantageously small X-ray output is accepted as the price of the advantages.

THE SINGLE PHASE FULL-WAVE RECTIFIED CIRCUIT

A high tension generator circuit which enables the X-ray tube to use *both* half-cycles in the alternating current cycle of the mains supply is described as a full-wave rectified circuit. In such a circuit the alternating voltage and current from the secondary winding of the high tension transformer are so rectified in relation to the X-ray tube that throughout the cycle the filament of the tube always finds itself connected by a continuous pathway to the *negative* pole of the high tension supply.

It needs a bridge of rectifiers for the X-ray tube which may be arranged as shown in the diagram in Fig. 3.4. The bridge consists of four banks of solid state rectifiers: in Fig. 3.4 each bank is depicted with a circuit symbol indicating a rectifier and the banks are labelled B1, B2, B3 and B4. The banks form a square with one bank of rectifiers to each of its sides and with two opposite points (at A and D in the diagram) connected to the X-ray tube and the other two opposite points (at X and Y in the diagram) connected to the secondary winding of the high tension transformer.

For one cycle of the mains supply, Fig. 3.5 shows at (a) the voltage across the secondary winding of the high-tension transformer; at (b) the voltage across the X-ray tube from the rectifiers; at (c) the current through the X-ray tube.

Let us assume that during the first half-cycle (period AB in Fig. 3.5(a)) the upper pole of the secondary winding of the transformer is negative in respect of the lower; in Fig. 3.4, X is negative in respect of Y. The rectifiers B1 and B2 can pass current for the X-ray tube, and electrons flow from X through B1, the X-ray tube and B2 to the lower pole of the transformer winding at Y. During this half-cycle X rays are produced; the voltage and current waveforms for the tube during this period AB are shown in Fig. 3.5 at (b) and (c).

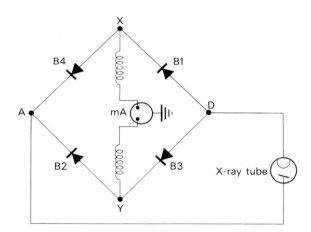

Fig. 3.4

In the following half-cycle (period BC in Fig. 3.5(a)), the voltage on the transformer winding changes direction and the lower pole of the secondary winding of the high tension transformer becomes negative in respect of the upper; in Fig. 3.4, Y is negative in respect of X. The rectifiers B3 and B4 can pass current for the X-ray tube. Electrons flow from Y through B3 the X-ray tube, and B4 to the upper pole of the transformer winding at X. During this second half-cycle X-rays are produced; the voltage and current waveforms for the tube in this period BC are shown in Fig. 3.5 at (b) and (c).

During both halves of the a.c. cycle the X-ray tube passes current and produces X rays. On the high tension transformer the voltage is alternating; for the X-ray tube the rectifiers make it unidirectional and the filament of

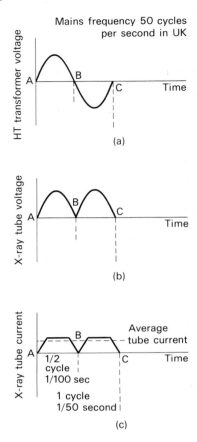

Fig. 3.5

the tube finds itself always connected by a conducting pathway to the pole of the transformer which is negative.

The operation of this circuit as two separate half-wave circuits is shown in Fig. 3.6.

Features of the full-wave circuit

Voltage waveform

In a full-wave circuit the X-ray tube passes current during both halves of the a.c. cycle, for the alternating voltage existing on the transformer secondary becomes a pulsating unidirectional voltage for the X-ray tube. This is illustrated in Fig. 3.5(a) in which it can be seen that the transformer voltage varies 'on both sides of the line' which is the axis of time; this means

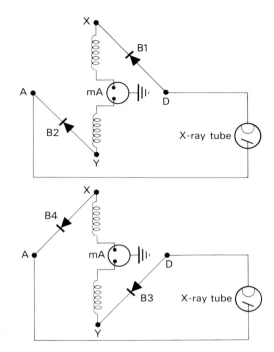

Fig. 3.6

that the voltage changes direction as time goes by. The X-ray tube voltage, however, has both half-waves above the line in Fig. 3.5(b) and is therefore seen to be not changing direction.

During both half-cycles the transformer is doing work and is providing current for the X-ray tube, so the voltage during both halves of the cycle is an 'on load' voltage. The transformer voltage therefore reaches the same peak during both halves of the cycle; it can be seen in Fig. 3.5 that one is not bigger than the other.

So in this circuit the problem of an inverse voltage which is bigger than the useful voltage does not exist. Both half-waves of voltage are useful for the X-ray tube and both come to the same peak value. The distribution of the transformer voltage between the rectifiers and the X-ray tube is this:

1   during the half-cycle that rectifiers B1 and B2 pass current, each of these banks takes one or two of the kilovolts available from the transformer and the X-ray tube takes all the remaining voltage; rectifiers B3 and B4 cannot pass current and in this half-cycle they find the transformer voltage an inverse voltage which is shared between the two banks.

2   during the half-cycle that rectifiers B3 and B4 pass current, each of the two banks takes only one or two of the kilovolts available from the transformer and the X-ray tube takes all the voltage that remains; in this

half-cycle rectifiers B1 and B2 cannot pass current and they find the transformer voltage an inverse voltage which is shared between the two banks.

Average and peak tube currents

In a full-wave rectified circuit both half-waves of the alternating cycle are used by the X-ray tube to produce X rays and current passes through the tube throughout the period of time occupied by one cycle. This can be seen in Fig. 3.5(c) and Fig. 3.6. Because the current has a waveform which is almost a sine wave with both halves on one side of the time axis, and because the current passes throughout the cycle, the maximum value reached during the cycle is about one and a half times the average value which the milliammeter records.

So in a full-wave bridge circuit the average and the peak values of the milliamperage are much closer together than they are in a half-wave circuit. This means that for the same reading on the milliammeter the milliamperage comes to a peak value which is lower in a full-wave circuit than it is in a half-wave circuit; for example 100 mA on the meter means a peak of 150 mA in a full-wave circuit and of 300 mA in a half-wave circuit.

It will be remembered that the rise in temperature at the focal spot of the X-ray tube is a function of the peak milliamperage, while the average value of the milliamperage determines the radiographic output (quantity of X rays) and the total heat input. Any given tube load as an exposure factor produces a temperature rise at the focal spot which is less for a full-wave than for a half-wave circuit. This means that higher milliamperages can be used in full-wave circuits on short exposures without overloading the X-ray tube.

Rectification for the milliammeter

It will be recalled from Chapter 2 that the milliammeter in an X-ray set is a moving-coil meter connected at the earthed centre-point of the secondary winding of the high tension transformer. It is placed there because that is a very convenient place to put it as we explained in Chapter 2 and it is a moving-coil meter because this instrument has the required characteristics in being accurate, relatively robust and easy to read.

Having a moving-coil movement, this meter can register unidirectional current only; it cannot deal with alternating current. In this regard there is a difference for the meter between a half-wave high tension generator and a full-wave one. In a half-wave self-rectified circuit with the X-ray tube doing its own rectification the meter at the centre-point of the secondary winding finds itself energized by current which flows through the winding in one direction only. When the X-ray tube conducts during one half-cycle, current flows through the transformer winding, through the meter and through the tube. In the next half-cycle the voltage on the transformer winding reverses and if a load current were to flow through the winding it would do so in a reversed direction; but in fact during this half-cycle no load current flows because the X-ray tube cannot conduct. Thus no current flows through the meter. So although the transformer voltage is alternating, the transformer is 'on load' only every other half-cycle and the current through its windings and through the meter is unidirectional.

In the case of the full-wave circuit the transformer is 'on load' during both halves of the cycle, for the X-ray tube passes current throughout that period of time. The voltage which for the X-ray tube is made unidirectional, with unidirectional current passing through the tube, exists on the high tension transformer as an alternating voltage, and the current through the transformer winding reverses in direction with each half-cycle. Thus the milliammeter at the centre-point of the transformer winding finds itself dealing with alternating current.

In order that a moving-coil meter may continue to be used it is necessary to arrange for the current to be rectified so that it always passes through the meter in one direction. This is done by surrounding the meter by a bridge of rectifiers as shown in Fig. 3.7.

The rectifiers form a square which has two of its opposite points connected to the meter and two of its opposite points connected to the two halves of the high tension secondary winding. In the diagram the arrowheads (both for the dotted-line arrows of the current and the bold ones for the

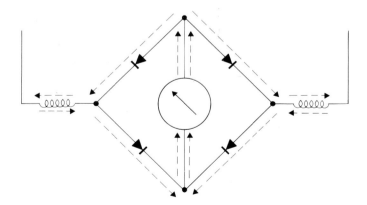

Fig. 3.7

rectifiers in their circuit symbols) point in the direction of conventional current flow. It can be seen that the current reverses in direction through the transformer winding but always goes the same way through the meter.

X-ray tube rating

When it is used in a full-wave rectified circuit a given X-ray tube has a higher rating than when it is used in a half-wave circuit which is self-rectified. The reason for this higher rating is that the average and peak milliamperages during the cycle have come closer together as explained in the preceding paragraphs. The same meter readings (average milliamperage) result in a smaller temperature rise at the focal spot on short exposures when the high tension circuit is a full-wave one because the peak milliamperage is smaller.

Because the total heat input is a function of the average milliamperage, one would expect the improved rating to be much less marked on longer exposures (when the total heat input is important) than it is on short exposures (when the temperature rise at the focal spot is the limiting factor). The ratings discussed in Chapter 7 show this to be so in accordance with expectation. On continuous running (fluoroscopy) the difference in rating disappears.

Rating of high tension cables

Earlier in this chapter we referred to the strain on high tension cables which have an alternating voltage applied to them. In any half-wave generator circuit an alternating voltage is applied to the cables; in a self-rectified circuit this voltage alternates between the two maxima of negative and positive voltage.

In a circuit with full-wave rectification the cables are better off for there is no alternating voltage applied to them. Since the rectifiers are interposed between the secondary winding of the high tension transformer and the cables, the voltage is rectified before it reaches the cables; they thus have applied to them the unidirectional voltage supplied for the X-ray tube. A given pair of cables therefore has better insulating properties because of the reduced strain and a higher rating when used in a circuit with full-wave rectification.

Shortest available exposure times

Because a fully rectified generator circuit allows high milliamperages to be employed, an X-ray set in which it is incorporated will be used with short exposure times. Let us consider the shortest available time of exposure with such a piece of equipment.

Exposure switching and timing devices are discussed in detail in Chapter 5. It suffices here to say that timing and switching systems are devised which permit periods of exposure in integral half-cycles. This means that the shortest possible exposure lasts for one complete half-cycle of the mains supply. What period of time is this?

In the United Kingdom the frequency of the mains supply is 50 cycles per second. The full-wave circuit enables the X-ray tube to use both halves of each cycle and thus the X-ray tube uses 100 half-waves (or 100 impulses of current) in 1 second. If the exposure lasts just while one complete half-wave of current passes through the tube, the duration of the exposure is 0·01 second. So this is the shortest exposure time which can be used with a single-phase fully rectified high tension generator which has conventional exposure switching related to the mains frequency.

At this point it is worth considering what we mean by 'the exposure time'. Do we mean the period of time during which the X-ray tube is energized from the high tension transformer? Or do we mean the period of time during which the X-ray tube is producing useful X rays? Useful X rays in diagnostic radiography are those which reach the film and produce photographic density on it when it is developed, thus forming an image. Tube voltages less than about 40 kilovolts result in radiation which (except in special circumstances) is not able to produce density in the radiograph, for it is too lacking in penetration to reach the film and is absorbed by the X-ray tube wall, the interposed filtration, the patient's body and other structures.

In one complete half-wave of tube voltage, the kilovoltage is at zero twice and at peak value once; most of the time it is somewhere between these two extremes (see Fig. 3.5b). For part of the time the X rays are thus being produced by voltages across the X-ray tube which are considerably below the peak and are lower than 40 kilovolts.

The period of time occupied by one half-wave (0·01 second in this single phase circuit on a 50 cycles per second supply) is the period of time during which the X-ray tube is energized from the high tension transformer. The period of time during which the tube produces useful X rays is clearly shorter than this and is about 0·003 second for a sinusoidal waveform.

This is the effective exposure time and it is much shorter than is appreciated by radiographers, who are accustomed to meaning by 'exposure time' the period during which the tube is energized. It is usually not important for them to realize the difference, but appreciation of this point does lead to a better understanding of the relative merits of certain high tension generator circuits.

Applications of the fully rectified circuit

Advantages

The advantages of a full-wave rectified circuit are that:
1   it confers on the X-ray tube a higher rating than can be obtained from any half-wave circuit;
2   it enables the X-ray set to be used with much higher milliamperages and kilovoltages. Thus an X-ray set which incorporates a full-wave high tension circuit has greater maximum permissible X-ray output (quantity and penetrating power) in comparison with any half-wave circuit.

Disadvantages

The disadvantages of this generator when it is compared with a self-rectified arrangement are that:
1   it is relatively more expensive;
2   it is more complex;
3   it is heavier and larger.
Some mobile X-ray sets with full-wave rectification given by solid-state rectifiers use a tank construction and this eliminates the size, weight and cost of high tension cables; but such equipment would obviously not be as small, light and inexpensive as a simple self-rectified circuit embodied in a tank construction.

The single-phase full-wave rectified generator which we have been discussing is used for X-ray sets which are permanent installations in departments and also in mobile sets to be used from wall sockets in wards and theatres. Those generators installed in departments are categorized as follows:
1   medium power generators with outputs between 25 kW to 50 kW, 300 to 500 mA and maximum kilovoltage 125 kV;
2   high power generators with outputs between 60 kW to 80 kW, 600 to 1000 mA and again 125 kV as a typical maximum kilovoltage.

They are satisfactory for all general radiography, the high power group obviously being the more versatile of the two. Both groups are limited in use by two considerations. First of all, they cannot be used for examinations which require a rapidly repeated series of exposures since the maximum rates of repetition to be expected from them are in the region of 1 to 2 exposures per second. The other limiting factor is that the shortest time of exposure that can be used with the equipment on a 50 hertz supply main, with conventional exposure switching related to the mains frequency, is 0·01 second. Time-intervals down to a few milliseconds are not available.

SOME CIRCUIT COMPARISONS

In the previous sections full-wave (two pulse) and half-wave (one pulse) high tension circuits have been compared in relation to the rating of X-ray tubes and cables, the permissible radiographic outputs to be expected of them, and the types of X-ray equipment in which they are used. The circuits will now be briefly considered in relation to power dissipation and to the comparability of their radiographic outputs, given the same settings on the controls.

It can be said that:

1   with any given milliamperage setting for the X-ray tube, the half-wave circuit will take from the mains more current than the full-wave circuit (this is because the peak milliamperage is higher in the half-wave circuit);

2   because of the higher current drawn from the mains, the half-wave circuit gives rise to bigger voltage drop on the supply and bigger power losses as heat in the cables and in transformer windings;

3   because the peak milliamperage is higher in a half-wave circuit for a given average milliamperage (meter reading), the filament of the X-ray tube must be hotter and this may shorten the life of a tube;

4   given the same settings on the controls, the radiographic outputs of the two circuits are equivalent. For example, exposure factors which are 0·5 second with 50 mA (25 mAs) at 60 kVp may be used on a half-wave X-ray set or a full-wave set with comparable radiographic results.

Many people when they are given this last point to consider theoretically come to the erroneous conclusion that with a half-wave circuit it would be necessary to set the timer of the X-ray set for 1 second in order to achieve 25 mAs with 50 mA; they argue that the half-wave set uses one half-wave in every cycle and is therefore passing current for only half the period of exposure, whereas the full-wave set is using both half-waves and is passing current throughout the period of exposure.

Yet if it were in fact true that half-wave generators need twice the time to produce a given radiographic result, radiographers going about their practical duties in the X-ray department would be required, during their consideration and discussion of exposure factors, to include mention of the high tension circuit which had been used, whether half-wave or full-wave. The truth is that, given the same exposure settings, half-wave and full-wave circuits supplied from a single-phase mains with sinusoidal variation are radiographically equivalent; the milliammeter is reading an average value which is the same in both cases, and the half-wave circuit conducting for only half the time has a peak milliamperage which is twice that of the full-wave circuit.

THREE-PHASE FULL-WAVE RECTIFIED CIRCUIT

It will be recalled from Chapter 1 that the electrical supply obtainable from the mains is delivered to users by means of a polyphase system of distribution which involves four lines or conductors; there is one line for each of the three phases of the supply and one neutral line which can act as a common return path for each of the other three.

Electrical equipment may be connected up so that it is using one of the lines and the common neutral return path (the phase voltage); or so that it is using two of the lines (the line voltage). In both cases the equipment is operating on single-phase supply; it does not have to be designed so that it can use more than one sine wave of a.c. voltage at a time. So far, the X-ray equipment which we have considered is single-phase equipment, as is shown in the diagrams of current and voltage waveform which illustrate this chapter; there is not more than one wave of current passing through the X-ray tube at a given time.

Now available is equipment with special transformers and other features so that it can be connected up to all three phases. Such equipment is known as three-phase equipment. X-ray generators of this type have come into more general use in the last ten years.

An X-ray set which uses all three phases of the supply is necessarily more complicated than one which operates on single phase voltage. It is therefore more costly. Features of the primary circuit—such as exposure switches and kilovoltage control—must be provided for three circuits instead of for only one; the autotransformer has triple windings and there are three primary windings and three secondary windings for the high tension transformer.

Fortunately we need not concern ourselves in this book with detailed consideration of the intricacies of the primary circuit, and for the secondary circuit we need look only at a simple version and a simple diagram. The general principles of operation are little different from those of the generator circuits previously described, and it is not difficult to understand how the circuit works.

Fig. 3.8 shows a simple version of a three-phase high tension generator (for the present ignore in the diagram the section of the circuit drawn with a broken line and the two capacitors).

The triple primary windings of the high tension transformer are in delta connection and the triple secondary windings are star or wye connected. A minimum of six rectifier banks is used in the secondary circuit and these (as will be seen) provide for the X-ray tube full-wave rectification of the three-phase a.c. supply. In modern equipment these three-phase high-tension generators almost all have 12 banks of rectifiers but for the moment we will stick with the six banks in order to explain how it works. If you can stay with us until page 113 you will hear further about the circuits with arrangements for 12 banks.

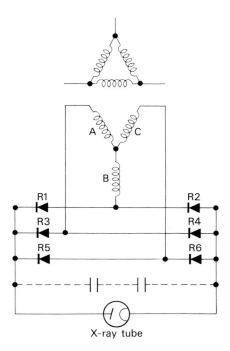

Fig. 3.8   X-ray tube

When the three-phase supply was described in Chapter 1 it was mentioned that the voltages in the three phases were not in step with each other. For all three phases, the waveforms are of the same pattern which repeats itself at the same frequency, and the peak values of each cycle are the same; but the voltages do not go through their maximum and minimum points together at the same instants in time. They are out of step with each other in such a way that when the voltage in one phase is at zero, the voltage in one of the others is just past the positive maximum and the voltage in the third is approaching the negative maximum.

Each of the three primary windings of the high tension transformer draws its voltage from a different phase. This means that at any given instant of time the voltages in the primary windings of the high tension transformer are different from each other. Similarly the voltages in the secondary windings are different from each other.

The simple way to describe how the circuit operates is to consider that at any given instant of time the X-ray tube is being provided with voltage from whichever two of the transformer secondary windings have the higher voltages, the winding with the least voltage in it being regarded as inactive in supplying the X-ray tube with current; the rectified voltage supplied to the X-ray tube is approximately equal to the sum of the two higher voltages.

Since the voltages in the three windings rise and fall one after the other as time goes by, it is not always from the same pair of windings but from successive combinations of pairs among the three windings that the X-ray tube obtains its voltage. Each winding in turn falls into a period of inactivity as the voltage in it drops down towards the zero point in the cycle. Thus in Fig. 3.8 the combinations could be first of all windings A and B, with C inactive; then B and C, with A inactive; then A and C with B inactive; then back to A and B, with C inactive, and so on.

Two transformer windings are thus providing the current for the X-ray tube at any particular instant of time, and with the appropriate bridge of rectifiers they form what is essentially a single phase full-wave system of rectification. Let us begin our consideration of this by imagining an instant of time when the transformer windings A and B are supplying the X-ray tube, and winding C is the one with the least voltage and is idle.

In that part of the a.c. cycle when the outer pole of A is negative, electrons flow from A through R4 (they always go in a direction opposite to the way the arrowheads point in the circuit symbols of solid-state rectifiers), then through the X-ray tube from cathode to anode and through R1 to the lower pole of B, which is positive at this point in the cycle. Why do the electrons not go from A to R3? Because R3 is connected the wrong way round to pass the current easily; electrons cannot go in the direction the arrowhead points. Coming from the X-ray tube, why do the electrons go through R1 and not R3 or R5? Because R1 is the only way to the lower pole of B to which they are *positively* bound to go.

In the next half-cycle of alternating voltage, the polarity reverses and the lower pole of B becomes negative. Electrons then flow from B through R2 (why not R1?), then through the X-ray tube from cathode to anode, and through R3 (why not R1 or R5?) to the upper pole of A which is positive.

The voltage on winding A falls as time goes by, and the voltage in winding C grows until it reaches a point such that A is the winding with the smallest voltage across it. It then for a time becomes the inactive one, and the X-ray tube is supplied by windings B and C. In that part of the cycle when the outer pole of B is negative and of C is positive, electrons flow from B through R2, through the X-ray tube and through R5, to the upper pole of C. In the next half-cycle of alternating voltage when the polarity reverses, the outer pole of C becomes negative and of B becomes positive. Electrons then flow from C through R6, through the X-ray tube and through R1 to B.

The voltage on winding B falls in its turn as time goes by, while the voltage on winding A grows until a point is reached at which winding B has the least voltage. Windings A and C then supply the X-ray tube, while winding B is inactive. In that part of the alternating voltage cycle when the outer pole of A is negative and of C is positive, electrons from A flow through R4, through the X-ray tube from cathode to anode and through R5 to C. In the next half-cycle the polarity reverses and the outer pole of C becomes negative. Electrons flow from C through R6, through the X-ray tube from cathode to anode and through R3 to A.

The voltage on C falls as time goes by and the voltage on B grows until the C winding has the least voltage across it. The X-ray tube is supplied by windings A and B with winding C inactive; which is where we came in as we began this explanation and the cycle of events repeats itself as before.

To summarize this explanation:

Windings A and B work as a system with R4, R1, R2, R3.
Windings B and C work as a system with R2, R5, R6, R1.
Windings A and C work as a system with R4, R5, R6, R3.

Features of a three-phase high-tension generator

Voltage waveforms

In a three-phase circuit such as this the alternating voltages from the three phases of the mains supply are fed into a triple high tension transformer. Here the voltages exist on the secondary windings as three phases of alternating voltage stepped up to the peak values required by the X-ray tube in operation. The waveforms of the supply from the secondary windings of the high tension transformer are shown in Fig. 3.9 at (a). For the X-ray tube the alternating voltages are rectified through the rectification system so that, as can be seen in Fig. 3.9(b), all the half-waves of voltages are on the positive side of the time axis, the voltage for the X-ray tube being unidirectional; through the rectifiers the filament of the X-ray tube always finds itself connected to a negative pole of the supply.

It will be noted that during the period of time occupied by one full cycle of voltage changes, the X-ray tube has six half-waves of useful voltage applied to it. This can be contrasted with a single-phase system having full-wave rectification, which gives two half-waves of useful voltage in one complete cycle.

The student should note that these six half-waves of useful voltage per cycle in comparison with two half-waves are an important and fundamental difference in a three-phase generator as compared with a single-phase generator.

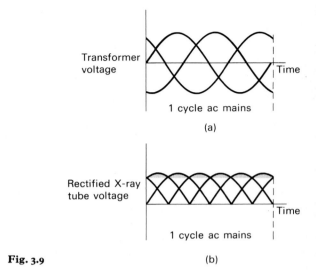

Transformer voltage

Time

1 cycle ac mains

(a)

Rectified X-ray tube voltage

Time

1 cycle ac mains

Fig. 3.9   (b)

Another important and fundamental difference is that the tube voltage never falls to the zero point in the cycle as it does in a full-wave single-phase generator, in which each half-wave of voltage varies in the cycle from zero up to maximum (the kilovolts peak used for the exposure) and then down to zero again. As we have shown, in a three-phase generator the X-ray tube takes its voltage from whichever two transformer windings have higher voltages than the third; each winding as the voltage in it falls below a certain value becomes the inactive one.

So the voltage across the X-ray tube takes the rippling form shown by the shaded section in Fig. 3.9(b). It varies from the maximum in the cycle (the kilovolts used for the exposure) to some value less than the maximum but it does not fall all the way down to zero.

How far does the voltage fall in fact? What is the difference between the maximum tube voltage at the crests of the ripple and the minimum tube voltage at the troughs of the ripple? It is not possible to give an exact answer to these questions for the voltage changes are a complex matter. They are influenced by various characteristics in the high tension transformer; by current surges in the circuit; by the length of the transition periods during which the current in each transformer winding dies out as the winding becomes inactive, and shifts to the next winding which is due to supply useful voltage for the X-ray tube. The waveforms we have shown in Fig. 3.9 are the ideal theoretical ones. In practice the pure half-wave shape is distorted to greater or less extent depending on various circuit characteristics.

This book is not intended to be an opportunity for going deeply into complex electrical phenomena in these circuits; that is a path along which we might find it difficult to walk, our readers might not care to accompany us and it is in any case unnecessary to go. So here the answer to a question on the magnitude of the voltage changes in the cycle is a general one: in practice the voltage does not fall below 80 per cent of the peak value, and this can be expressed another way by saying that there is a 20 per cent ripple. In theory the ripple may be stated as less than this, being given as 13·5 per cent for a theoretical value.

By certain methods the ripple can be made much smaller than 20 per cent. Capacitors in the broken line part of the circuit in Fig. 3.8 are connected across the output from the high tension transformer and rectifiers. These capacitors serve to reduce the ripple; the high tension generator charges the capacitors and the X-ray tube takes its energy from them as from a reservoir and not directly from the transformer. Because they function to reduce ripple, the capacitors are described as smoothing capacitors.

In order to improve in practice the ripple factor for 6-pulse generators circuits have been devised in which two separate sets of transformer windings are used on the secondary side, each with its own six banks of rectifiers. As before, the primary winding is delta-connected and both the secondaries are star (wye) connected. The arrangement is seen in Fig. 3.10(a): it is described as a six-pulse delta wye wye generator with 12 banks of rectifiers.

The *theoretical ripple* is still 13·5 per cent but the ripple in the *practical* conditions of load has been brought nearer to 13·5 per cent than could be achieved with only one set of secondary windings and six rectifier banks as shown in Fig. 3.8. This is a worthy practical result for the extra cost and complexity.

Most commonly encountered today for generators with 12 banks of rectifiers is a different arrangement for the two sets of transformer windings on the high tension side of the generator. One set is star (wye) connected and one set is delta connected (instead of two wyes). This delta wye delta configuration for the transformers is shown in Fig. 3.10(b). The two separate generators are out of step with each other, and the peaks of voltage from the star-connected generator are inserted as time elapses between the peaks of voltage from the delta-connected generator.

It is not surprising that this circuit arrangement results in twelve half-waves of voltage for the X-ray tube during the period of time occupied by one complete cycle of mains alternation. The ripple of the tube voltage is very small and is said to be theoretically about 3·5 per cent. This is a considerable improvement on 13·5 per cent.

We can here explain some terminology. The half-wave generator supplies one half-wave or pulse per cycle; the full-wave single-phase generator

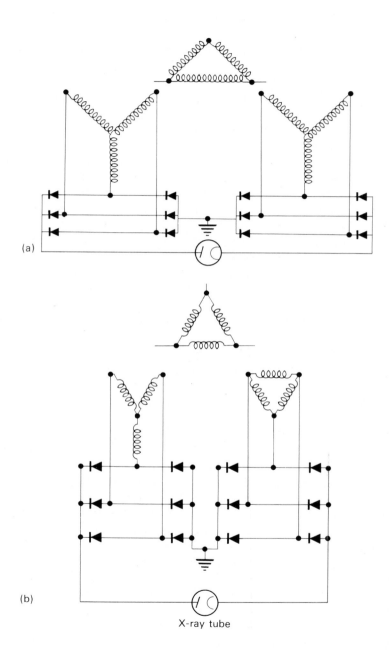

(a)

(b)

X-ray tube

Fig. 3.10

supplies two half-waves or pulses per cycle; the full-wave three-phase generator with 6 banks of rectifiers supplies six half-waves or pulses per cycle; the three-phase generator with 12 banks of rectifiers can supply six or twelve half-waves or pulses per cycle. All these generators are now described by convenient shorthand expressions as one-pulse, two-pulse, six-pulse and twelve-pulse generators respectively.

Average and peak tube currents

In a three-phase high tension generator circuit (as in a single-phase generator) there is a difference between the average milliamperage during the cycle (which the milliammeter reads) and the peak value which is reached. But the magnitude of the factor relating the two is not so great as in single-phase circuits. We saw that in a single-phase half-wave rectified circuit the peak tube current is about three times the average; and that in a single-phase full-wave rectified circuit the peak tube current is about one and a half times the average—that is, the separation between the two has become smaller. In three-phase circuits the separation becomes smaller still and it will be smaller in a twelve-pulse generator than in a six-pulse generator because the twelve pulses give a tube voltage with a smaller ripple.

We do not quote here a figure which relates the average and the peak milliamperages in three-phase equipment because it is not possible for us to do so. The exact value of the figure will depend on the waveforms of current and voltage in the circuit as well as on the frequency of the pulses, so it is a complex matter. Let us suffice to say that the average tube current in the cycle comes closer to the peak, and the smaller is the ripple in the voltage the closer together will be the average and the peak values of the milliamperage.

X-ray tube rating

To consider the rating of an X-ray tube when it operates in a three-phase generator, the comparisons which must be made for a given X-ray tube are between (i) its rating in a single-phase full-wave generator circuit and (ii) its rating in a three-phase full-wave generator circuit. In Chapter 7 some ratings for X-ray tubes are noted in detail and the facts which emerge for the comparisons to be made here are:

1   that on *shorter* exposures the X-ray tube has a *higher* rating on the three-phase generator;

2   that on exposures *longer* than 0·5 second the X-ray tube has a *lower* rating on a three-phase generator;

3   that at 0·5 seconds the rating for the two circuits is the same.
What is the explanation of this difference in rating?

Taking the short exposures first, we must refer to the fact that the rating of an X-ray tube which is given an instantaneous loading is limited by the temperature rise at the focal spot. This temperature rise is a function of the peak power, and hence of the peak milliamperage as a factor in peak power. The single-phase circuit results in a peak milliamperage which is one and a half times greater than the average; and the three-phase circuit results in a peak milliamperage which is closer to the average than that. Because of this, the same meter reading (average milliamperage) for the X-ray tube results in a smaller temperature rise at the focal spot in the three-phase circuit (lower peak) than it does in a single-phase circuit (higher peak).

On longer exposures the total heat input becomes important, and this is a function of the average power rather than of the peak power. So we must consider now as a factor in average power the average (or more properly the root mean square) value of the tube voltage. In single-phase circuits the relationship between the peak and the root mean square values of the kilovoltage is (as every radiographer ought to know)

$$\text{R.M.S.} = \text{peak}/\sqrt{2} \quad \text{or} \quad \text{R.M.S.} = 0\cdot71 \text{ peak};$$

in three-phase circuits the relationship is R.M.S. = 0·95 peak. From this it follows that for the same voltage rating in kilovolts peak, a given X-ray tube is subjected in a three-phase circuit to a higher root mean square voltage and in the single-phase circuit to a lower root mean square voltage; for example 100 kVp means 95 $\text{kV}_{\text{R.M.S.}}$ in a three-phase circuit and 71 $\text{kV}_{\text{R.M.S.}}$ in a single-phase circuit.

So a higher average power is dissipated in the three-phase circuit, the total heat input to the X-ray tube is greater, and the tube rating is lower on long exposures.

At exposures intermediate between the short and the long there is a gradual transition in importance between the peak power and the average power as factors in rating. So there are some periods when the ratings for single-phase and three-phase operations are the same; we find this at 0·5 second in the example we consider in Chapter 7.

Shortest available exposure times

It can be seen in Fig. 3.9 that during the period of time occupied by one complete cycle of the alternating mains, the X-ray tube receives six pulses of voltage and current if it is operating in a three-phase six-rectifier generator circuit. On a 50 cycles per second supply there will therefore be 300 pulses in 1 second and one pulse in 0·003 second. The period of time represented by one half-wave is therefore 0·003 second or 3 milliseconds, and this can be contrasted with 0·01 second of a single-phase generator.

This minimum period of 3 milliseconds represented by one half-wave is the shortest available exposure time when conventional exposure switching related to the mains frequency is used. The exposure time in this context is the time during which the X-ray tube is energized, for that is the interpretation which radiographers give to the term. The time during which the tube produces useful X rays, which is much shorter than 'the exposure time' in the case of single-phase equipment, ceases in the case of three-phase equipment to be markedly different from the time during which the tube is energized. This is because the tube voltage does not drop to zero in the cycle, but ripples down from the maximum to some value which is below that to an extent determined by the magnitude of the ripple. For example, a 13·5 per cent ripple results in a value for the lowest voltage which is 86·5 per cent of the maximum; a 3·5 per cent ripple gives 96·5 per cent of the peak voltage as the lowest figure.

The tube voltages thus do not fall to a point below which they can produce useful X rays. The tube current similarly has a rippling waveform and does not fall to zero at two points in each half-cycle as it does with single-phase equipment. This means that for the same exposure time on the timer, and with the same milliamperage and kilovoltage settings, three-phase generators give quantitatively greater output of X rays than single-phase generators do.

A three-phase twelve-pulse generator does better still and improves on the six-pulse generator, for the ripple of the voltage waveform is smaller and the tube voltage falls only a little way below the peak value in the cycle; theoretically to not lower than 96·5 per cent of the peak voltage. With this sort of equipment very short exposures are available. If the exposure switching is conventional and related to the mains frequency, the shortest exposure time is about 1·0 millisecond. In cases where special electronic switching is used (see page 171 in Chapter 5), exposure times can be reduced to less than 0·5 millisecond as a minimum value.

Applications of three-phase generator circuits

Disadvantages

Three-phase generators are:
1   more expensive;
2   more complex in circuitry;

3   larger and occupy more space.

It is easy to see that the triplication of transformer windings, control circuits and switching systems, etc., must cause these disadvantages to exist. Probably the disadvantage which has been greatest in practice is the one to which we have given first place—namely the cost.

Advantages

1   Because the load is distributed equally over all three phases of the supply when the X-ray exposure is made (instead of a heavy load being imposed on just one of the phases) conditions are more favourable for drawing large amounts of power. So three-phase high tension generators can supply higher milliamperages (for example 1000 mA and above) for the X-ray tube than single-phase generators can. It follows from this that three-phase generators must be used with X-ray tubes capable of taking the high energies they can provide, if the financial outlay involved in this equipment is not to be wasted.

2   A greater quantity of X radiation is produced per kilovolt and milliampere of the control settings for three-phase generators in comparison with single-phase generators. This advantage of more radiation output can be used to decrease exposure times when movement in the part examined must be encountered; for example in gastrointestinal and in cardiac radiology. Or to increase the tube-film distance when it is wished to make dimensions in the radiographic image nearly the same as the true dimensions of a structure being examined; for example, in pelvimetry. Or when it is wished to use the benefit of reduced geometric unsharpness by putting the X-ray source a long way from the subject: for example in radiography of the internal structures of the skull.

3   With conventional switching related to the mains frequency, shorter minimum exposure times are available on the timers of three-phase X-ray sets as compared with single-phase units.

The alert reader may note that we have said nothing about the *quality* of the radiation output from a three-phase high tension generator in comparison with that from a single-phase generator. There should in theory be a difference. The rippling form of tube voltage (as opposed to the pulsating form) should result in a beam of X rays from which are absent those components of low energy which owe their production to the tube voltages in the cycle which are a long way below the maximum kilovolts peak. With these low energies absent, the X-ray beam should be of higher *average* energy than another beam produced at the same kilovolts peak, but from a single-phase generator with its voltage waveform that varies between peak and zero values as we have seen. This beam of higher average energy will be effectively more penetrating and in theory it should result in a radiographic image which is flatter in contrast. It should also give a smaller dose to the patient, since certain low energies that do not contribute to the image and are absorbed in the patient's superficial tissues are not present in the beam.

However, there seems to be some disagreement as to whether in practice qualitative differences in the beams from the two types of generator are of any significance at all. It is probably true to say that for the radiographer in the X-ray room such qualitative differences as do exist make very little difference to radiographic techniques. Relative doses to the patient could be investigated by a physicist and we hesitate to make pronouncements on them here.

Choice of three-phase generator

By way of review of available equipment based on three-phase generators, we can distinguish three categories in a rank of ascending power output as follows.

1. 50 kW to 70 kW

These are six-pulse generators usually, with 700 mA as a typical upper limit and a maximum kilovoltage which is not above 150 kV. The minimum exposure time is most usually 0·01 second and the fastest repetition rate for exposures will not be above 8 per second. In practice the rate can be expected to be often much slower than this: for example no faster rate than 2 per second. These generators are suitable for all general work and for some angiography (peripheral, abdominal).

2. 70 kW to 100 kW or 125 kW

These are 12-pulse generators which can give 1000–1250 mA and have an upper voltage limit of 150 kV. The shortest exposure time is 0·003 second and the rate of repetition at its fastest is not less than 8 per second. Such generators are obviously a suitable choice for angiography undertaken with fast serial film-changers but the repetition rate of 8 per second makes them unsuitable for pulsed cine-filming. Their high power output of 100 kW commends them for installation in very busy accident and emergency departments and in orthopaedic departments.

3. 130 kW to 200 kW

Among three-phase generators, those in this group are 12-pulse and can give 1200 mA or beyond as a maximum tube current and 150 kV as the voltage limit. Their shortest exposures are down to 0·001 second and even to 0·0001 second and the repetition rates available are not less than 80 per second. Such fast rates clearly make these the generators of choice for pulsed cine filming and their purchase is justified if much of this is to be done.

VOLTAGE WAVEFORMS IN HIGH TENSION GENERATORS

So far we have considered for the X-ray tube two waveforms of voltage from a high tension transformer. These are:

1   a pulsating voltage which is a theoretical sine-wave of voltage varying from zero up to a peak value (the kilovoltage selected for the exposure) and down again to zero;

2   a rippling voltage which has theoretical sine waves of voltage with the peaks inserted between each other so that the voltage across the X-ray tube varies from the peak value (the kilovoltage selected for the exposure) to some value which is not lower than about 80 per cent of the peak.

If the up-and-down variation of the rippling voltage is not greater than 5 per cent (that is, the voltage does not fall to lower than 95 per cent of its peak) the X-ray tube is said to be provided with 'constant potential'—by which is meant a voltage that does not change its value in a pattern repeating in cycles. The expression 'constant potential' is clearly a courtesy title for a rippling voltage which (as we have seen) does change its value cyclically; but it is nevertheless a term which is often used for such a voltage despite its inexactitude.

However, circuits have been devised which can provide the X-ray tube with a voltage which is truly of constant form. If a graph is made to show what happens to such a voltage as time goes by (see Fig. 3.11) the result is neither a wave nor a ripple but a straight line, which indicates that the voltage does not change in value through repeated cycles.

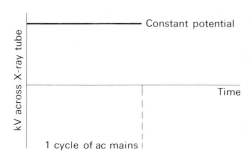

Fig. 3.11

A CONSTANT POTENTIAL CIRCUIT

A generator which provides constant potential for the X-ray tube makes use of high-tension vacuum triode valves in the X-ray tube circuit. Two such triodes are connected between the output from the secondary windings of the generator and the X-ray tube itself: one triode is on the cathode side of the X-ray tube and the other is on the anode side as is indicated in Fig. 3.12.

The actions of these triode valves are modified by control circuits so that the triode valves can perform in two essential functions:

1 to act as switches so that the tube circuit is closed (switched ON) for the start of the exposure and opened (switched OFF) to terminate it;

2 to stabilize and balance the kilovoltage output from the high tension generator so that the voltage existing across the X-ray tube is without variation, as its graphical depiction as a straight line in Fig. 3.11 shows.

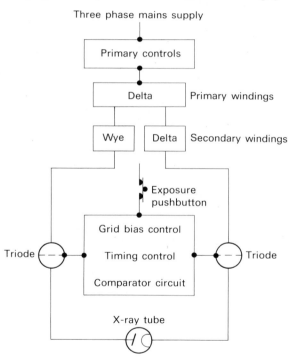

Fig. 3.12

The vacuum triode valve

As its name shows, the vacuum triode valve has three electrodes held within a vacuum. These electrodes are: (i) a cathode which is a heated filament and emits electrons; (ii) an anode which is a cylindrical metal plate surrounding the filament so that it can receive the electrons; (iii) a third electrode interposed between cathode and anode.

This third electrode is called a grid and it consists of a spiral or rings of wire surrounding the cathode. The relative placings of the three electrodes are such that the spiral of wire is nearer to the cathode than to the anode. The three electrodes are in a vacuum within a glass envelope.

The third electrode is called a grid because it can be made to act as a barrier to electrons as they pass from the filament to the anode. If the grid has a voltage applied to it which is negative in respect of the cathode, the electric field between the grid and the cathode makes it difficult for electrons to get through to the anode. If the grid is made more and more negative, fewer and fewer electrons pass to the anode. The grid can be made so negative as eventually to stop the electrons sufficiently for the valve to be non-conductive; it then will not pass current and acts in a circuit like an open switch.

If the triode is non-conductive because of a very negative voltage on the grid, it can be made conductive extremely quickly by reducing the negative grid voltage. It then becomes as a closed switch in a circuit. The important point here is that this is a switch which can be operated very quickly indeed. There is no mechanically moving part to the switch, with associated inertia, for the switch is closed or opened simply by decreasing or increasing (for ON or OFF) a negative voltage on the grid of the triode valve.

Once the switch has been closed by making the triode conductive, if the grid voltage is made increasingly less negative more and more electrons pass through to the anode and the triode passes current more and more easily. Thus alteration in grid voltage enables the triode to function not only as a switch, but also as a device which will pass current more or less easily following the changes in voltage on its grid.

This in effect is to change the resistance of the valve: with increased negative voltage on its grid, the valve passes current with difficulty and acts as a high resistance—that is, there will be a big voltage drop across the valve; with lower negative voltage on the grid, the valve passes current more easily and acts as a lower resistance—that is, there will be less voltage drop across the valve. Thus the valve can be made to absorb more or less voltage simply by alterations in voltage on its grid, and changes in the valve's effective resistance can be made instantaneously and in fine degrees of intermediate resistance through the controlling influence exercised by this grid voltage. This controlling voltage applied to the grid is called the grid bias voltage.

To sum up the capabilities of the triode valve we have described, we enumerate them below:

1   the triode valve can be made to act as an ON/OFF switch (passing current or not passing current);

2   it can be made to absorb different amounts of voltage;

3   the changes of function as given in (i) and (ii) above can be achieved by altering the grid voltage, and because this is simply a change in electrical characteristics the required effects in the valve can be brought about instantaneously.

Now let us consider how these triode valves perform in the high tension generator which we are describing.

Triode valves as switches

In Fig. 3.12 two triode valves are inserted between the X-ray tube and the output from the three phase generators. While they are non-conductive they block the way, and although the high tension transformer is energized as soon as the exposure switch is put to 'Prepare', no current passes to the X-ray tube. The exposure cannot begin until the triode valves are made conductive.

When the exposure switch is moved through 'Prepare' and achieves the closed position, the grid bias voltage on the valves is reduced through the electronic control circuits. The valves become at once conductive, kilovoltage is applied to the tube and the exposure begins. At the end of the exposure, the grid bias voltage required to make the valves non-conductive is reimposed through the control circuits; the valves become open switches in the secondary circuits of the high tension transformers and the exposure stops.

Thus the valves function as switches. They have, however, in this circuit other functions. These relate to the stabilization of the kilovoltage across the X-ray tube and are explained below.

Triode valves in kilovoltage stabilization

Fig. 3.12 shows some circuit arrangements for a three-phase generator with the system of controls which we are describing. The diagram indicates secondary windings of which one is wye connected and the other is delta connected. These separate secondary windings each have their own group of rectifiers in a six bank arrangement. The X-ray tube is connected across the output from the wye-delta windings with one triode valve connected on the side with the wye windings and the other triode valve connected on the side with the delta windings. Also shown in the diagram is the grid bias and timing control joined to the grids of the triode valves. As already explained, these controls function to make the triode valves act as ON/OFF switches for the start and termination of the exposure.

To help the triode valves in stabilizing kilovoltage so that all ripple is removed, the circuit for the control of grid bias also includes an arrangement of components which can make a comparison. The comparison is between the voltage outputs from the two triodes and the circuit functions to maintain a constant potential between the two by alterations in the grid bias voltages. When the voltage output from the triodes is balanced on the anode and cathode sides of the X-ray tube, the voltage waveform for the X-ray tube becomes a straight line.

Some considerations

A constant potential generator of the type which we have just described has a high power output which is in the range 130 kW to 150 kW. Over 1200 mA can be expected as the upper limit for the X-ray tube current and 140 kV as the highest voltage. Very short minimum times of exposure are available (down to less than 0·001 second) and fast repetition rates at up to 80 per second. These are of obvious application in cine filming and in angiography.

There are some disadvantages with this generator. One is that the triode valves may need replacement at frequent intervals (as does any hot-filament tube) and they are almost as costly to renew as are X-ray tubes. Disadvantageously limiting may be the fact that the high tension cables which connect the X-ray tube to the generator should not exceed 9 metres in length. This problem arises because long cables have associated with them a significant capacitance effect. This means that they store energy and this stored energy extends the exposure beyond the termination time, even although the high tension connection to the X-ray tube has been switched OFF. This is clearly not tolerable in its effect on the accuracy and consistency of very short exposures.

THE FALLING LOAD GENERATOR

Principles of the generator

In utilizing the output from a high tension generator for medical radiography the ultimate significant limitation comes from the characteristics of the X-ray tube. The reasons for this are fully explained in Chapter 7 and the tube's rating chart defines these limitations graphically.

Such a chart is illustrated again in Fig. 3.13. It depicts the maximum load applicable to one focus of a particular X-ray tube, having—in respect of this focus—an effective focal area of 1·0 mm and operating from a supply of 50 hertz. The lower chart refers to a single-phase high tension generator and the upper to a three-phase generator. For the present purpose we need refer to only one of these: the reader is asked to consider the lower chart.

Let us imagine that we wish to obtain an exposure of 400 mAs at 80 kVp.

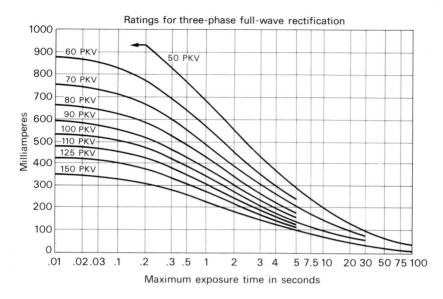

Ratings for three-phase full-wave rectification

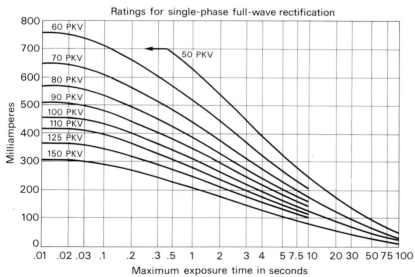

Ratings for single-phase full-wave rectification

Fig. 3.13

Reference to the chart shows that the highest tube current at which we may operate is 300 mA. If we try to raise the current to 400 mA we find that the exposure limit is limited to approximately 0·75 seconds and that we are short of 100 mAs for our projected technique. Thus we must accept that in these circumstances an exposure time of 1·5 seconds is the minimum we can obtain.

It is to be noticed, however, that in employing this combination of millampere-seconds we are operating along the lower part of the 80 kVp curve on the chart. If we can utilize the whole curve we shall find that we obtain 400 mAs in a shorter period of time. The aim of the falling load generator is to employ the whole curve.

Fig. 3.14 illustrates the principle of a falling load generator. In Fig. 3.14 part of a similar kilovoltage curve from the lower chart in Fig. 3.13 is again depicted. The diagram shows that the exposure begins at a tube current of 600 mA, which is close to the maximum on the curve, and that this current is dropped to 500 mA when the 600 mA 'line' reaches the curve. The current is dropped to 400 mA when the 500 mA line in its turn reaches its maximum point on the exposure axis. Thus, the tube current is progressively reduced at intervals—each of which comes just within the tolerance of the X-ray tube for the current concerned—until the desired total of 400 mAs has been compiled. A glance at the exposure axis shows that the total exposure interval has been 1 second, which is a very acceptable reduction from the original 1·5 seconds.

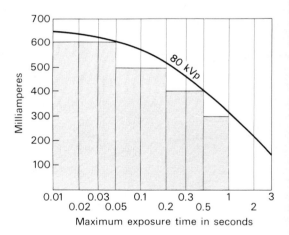

Fig. 3.14   Maximum exposure time in seconds

Practical features of the falling load generator

Although in theory a falling load generator may operate on the maximum tube load (as depicted in Fig. 3.14), in the interests of the X-ray tube some margin for error must be allowed in practice. This means that the aim is to work this generator on 80 per cent of the maximum load. On short exposures (say 0·1 second or less) the effect of this is to downrate the falling load generator in comparison with the rating of an identical generator which is without the falling load feature. An identical generator with conventional loading would allow use of a higher tube current on a short exposure time.

The tube current is stepped down at pre-determined intervals following initiation of the exposure: for example, current-reductions might be made at 0·1, 0·25, 0·5, 1 and 2 seconds. The amount by which the current is decreased at each step is a pre-determined percentage of the current at the starting point of the exposure. This initial value of the current is decided in accordance with the characteristics of the X-ray tube concerned: it might be as much as 1000 mA or as low as 200 mA.

The tube current

The 'straight-line' drop of the tube current between one level and the next which is depicted in Fig. 3.16 is not a realistic representation of what actually happens. The reader may remember that the current through an X-ray tube is controlled by altering the temperature of the cathode filament (see Chapter 2, page 63) and that this change is effected through the agency of the voltage across the filament transformer. Of course, as the voltage drops, the filament does not instantaneously lose the full amount of heat as Fig. 3.14 would have us believe. In fact the filament needs 20 milliseconds to decline in temperature to the required degree. This means that the filament emission and therefore the average current through the X-ray tube actually change with time in the manner of the curve indicated in Fig. 3.15.

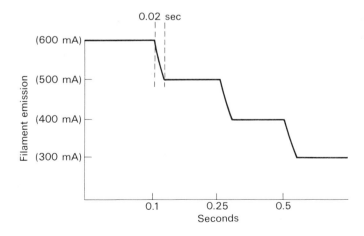

Fig. 3.15

The tube kilovoltage

Changes in the value of the current through the X-ray tube must not be made without taking account of the associated effect on the kilovoltage across the tube. Elsewhere in this book (see Chapter 2, page 57) we have shown that—in the absence of any compensation—as the load current in a circuit rises, the voltage will fall; and conversely. In the case of a falling load generator it is therefore necessary to provide a means of holding the kilovoltage at the preselected value, despite successive reductions in the current through the X-ray tube.

This may be done easily enough by introducing a number of resistors in the primary of the high tension transformer. Since the voltage drop associated with the load current is proportional not only to the current but to the simple resistance of the circuit, we can prevent any rise of kilovoltage across the X-ray tube by means of appropriate increases in resistance, at intervals corresponding to the points at which filament emission is lowered and the tube current reduced.

In practice an insignificant variation from the set kilovoltage necessarily occurs with this form of control. This is because the period which the filament requires to die down in temperature continues severally after the introduction of each resistor appropriate to maintain voltage. The effect is a very brief drop across the X-ray tube of about 10 per cent of the selected kilovoltage. As filament emission falls during the succeeding 0·02 seconds, the kilovoltage mounts on a steep curve to return to the set value. Fig. 3.16 graphically sketches the changes in kilovoltage with time and may be compared with the corresponding curve for tube current in Fig. 3.15.

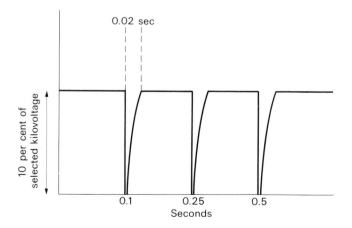

Fig. 3.16

The introduction of appropriate primary resistors is not the only available method of levelling kilovoltage in the case of a falling load generator. On pages 121–124 of this chapter, a high tension circuit is described which employs secondary electronic switching by means of triode valves; these valves further function as absorbers of different amounts of voltage in the selection and stabilization of kilovoltage. Such a circuit is appropriate to a falling load generator, as the kilovoltage is maintained against a variation from any origin, whether a random fluctuation or the upswing associated with a diminished load. However, this is a costly system and such equipment is necessarily expensive.

Evaluating the falling load generator

A falling load generator requires, in conjunction with it, an automatic timer for without automatic timing there is no benefit in the falling load feature. The programming of an automatic timer is facilitated with a falling load generator and this fact has been said to be the one big advantage for such a generator.

Another important point on the choice of such a generator and the nature of the work to be done is that on short exposures (say, shorter than 0·4 second) there may be little or indeed no advantage offered by the system. It is therefore not justifiable to consider installing such a generator in an X-ray room which is being set up for radiography mainly of the chest.

In order to explain the lack of advantage on short exposure-times, we ask the reader to consider the period of time for which the tube current is maintained at its initial high value. Let us call this time, which is the duration of the first and highest step of the milliamperage, t seconds. The graph in Fig. 3.14 shows t seconds as 0·05 second but in fact it may be much greater than this and about 0·1 second or more. Since the tube load is constant until the period t seconds has passed, it is obvious that for exposures shorter than t seconds there is no falling load advantage since the load is not in fact falling.

Obviously the greater the number of falling steps that can be accomplished in the exposure time, the greater is the advantage to be gained from using a falling load generator. So the reader may be wondering at what time after t seconds does the second step drop down to the third? The graph in Fig. 3.14 shows the second step falling to the third at 0·2 second. Again this is an optimistic figure and in fact it may be 0·4 second after the start of the exposure before the tube current has reached its third value in the descent as time goes by.

We may also consider the question of wear on the X-ray tube as being of some significance, since replacements are expensive in terms both of money and of frustration when an X-ray unit is out of action. All falling load exposures begin at a high milliamperage and obviously will do so even for examinations which can quite satisfactorily be undertaken with relatively low milliamperage and do not require short times of exposure. If the work undertaken is mostly in such a category, then the X-ray tube will be unnecessarily loaded with a high current on many occasions. Its useful working life may be thus curtailed.

So the conclusion to all this discussion must be that a falling load generator is a good choice only when most of the work to be undertaken implies the use of heavy milliampereseconds loadings and long exposure times. A busy orthopaedic clinic examining spines, for example, would be in this category.

From another point of view, one advantage for this generator and the automatic timing used with it is that the settings of the controls by the operator become simpler. The reader should continue with the next section for further consideration of that matter.

ANATOMICALLY PROGRAMMED GENERATORS

Radiographers have been traditionally accustomed to selecting and setting three separate factors in operating a generator to produce a radiograph. These factors are the settings of kilovoltage, milliamperage and time. Modern equipment provides a considerable range of settings in each of these three variables and today's radiographers for any given examination may be choosing one out of about 19,000 possible combinations. It is perhaps as well that we are not constantly aware of this or we might find the decision most perplexing, even with the aids of sound training and experience.

Modern circuitry has moved to a simplification of these selections. A falling load generator with automatic timing in conjunction with it is an example of such simplification in the required settings of the controls. Using this generator, a radiographer does not choose kilovoltage, milliamperage and time separately and sets only one instead of three controls. The one is kilovoltage and the individual selections of tube current and time have disappeared.

Turning somewhat aside from falling load generators, we find today other generators which have automatically programmed modules. These bring simplification to the point of providing a number of pushbutton settings. Each pushbutton is designated as appropriate to a particular anatomical part or region or to a particular radiographic projection: there may be as few as 8 settings or as many as 49. When the chosen pushbutton is pressed, the circuitry associated with it automatically sets the appropriate factors of kilovoltage and milliamperes if there is automatic timing or milliampereseconds if there is not and automatically selects the appropriate focal spot on the X-ray tube which is to be used.

The particular control-settings to which each pushbutton is committed (or dedicated, in the terminology of the manufacturers) are pre-set when the equipment is installed. The pre-settings are the choices of the purchasers, who are thus able to express preferences as to the exposure technique which will be applied from each labelled pushbutton. A facility is provided to give limited adjustment upwards (plus) or downwards (minus) for kilovoltages and milliamperage when the patient is not of 'average' build.

The anatomically programmed generator has certain advantages which may be enumerated as follows.

1   Consistent exposure techniques are used and this should, with automatic processing, help to ensure that consistent radiographic results are obtained even in large departments employing many radiographers with various extents of experience.

2   Radiographers should be able to complete examinations more speedily as they do not have to spend time consulting whatever technique charts might otherwise be used, whether displayed in the X-ray room, recorded in their pocketbooks or retrieved from the stores of their minds.

3   Radiographers operating unfamiliar equipment may work with greater certainty and speed and obtain more satisfactory results.

4   In a fluoroscopic room, if anatomical programming is used for spot-filming, there is an obvious benefit when examinations are changed (for example, a patient being fluoroscoped to investigate a possible gastric ulcer is succeeded by one undergoing an oral cholecystogram). To achieve the necessary changes in the exposure settings by pushing just a single button is clearly useful.

On the disadvantageous aspects there are certain points to be considered.

1   Radiographers may find the range of the selections not wide enough to embrace all the examinations which must be made in a busy X-ray room.

2   The radiographer must obviously use judgement on the selection of the plus-minus facility to adjust for the patients' physical build and perhaps also to adjust for certain known pathologies (such as osteoporosis, fluid-filled pleural cavities, disuse atrophy of muscle tissue). Such a limit on the exercise of their expertise may be objectionable to highly-trained radiographers who may dismiss with derision any notion of this automated equipment. 'Well, it's for any fool to use, isn't it?' 'It just makes it easy for the untrained and that's no good thing.' 'I am not going to have my exposure techniques dictated to me by a microprocessor.' These are predictable comments.

3   Well trained and experienced radiographers must be expected to have a full understanding of the radiographic image since the production of

radiographs is their professional concern. To this end, they must understand the selections of kilovoltage, milliamperage and time as these combine to influence the optimum results in radiographic quality. It is more difficult to teach such understanding if students are using equipment which deprives them of knowledge of the selections made and does not require them to have this knowledge in order to produce a good radiograph.

Perhaps some of these objections are overcome in the most versatile examples of this modern equipment. Some generators allow choice between an anatomically programmed (organ programmed) mode or one which permits free selection of radiographic exposure factors. There are also multi-programming systems which allow operators to key in their own choice of data.

Purchasers who are concerned about finances need to know that anatomically programmed generators can be expected to cost more than equivalent generators which are without these features of control. This difference in price may be an increase of about 50 per cent.

MODULAR GENERATORS—SHARED GENERATORS

Generators described as modular generators have been devised in order to extend the usefulness of an installation. One generator is linked to several control consoles. Each console controls the generator for the particular work to be done where the console is sited and the functions of the consoles need not be related to each other. Each console has its own separate settings, displays and controls so that each functions to direct one or more X-ray tubes associated with it and to effect radiographic exposures. The consoles do not need to be close to each other and a console may control a whole assembly of equipment in a diagnostic room housing one X-ray tube or several X-ray tubes.

Such a modular generator, as an example, may provide five separate unit consoles as satellites to a master console and through them four X-ray tubes may be controlled. This type of arrangement is sketched in Fig. 3.17. Each console stores the selected data of the settings made on it and this information is passed to the generator immediately before the exposure. The action of lifting the exposure handswitch engages the generator to that console and until the handswitch is replaced no other console can take the generator. After the exposure the generator becomes free again for use by any of the other units in the system. In these arrangements, the unit consoles may be anatomically programmed, while the master console may allow free selection of exposure factors. The satellite consoles can call up the factors on the master control.

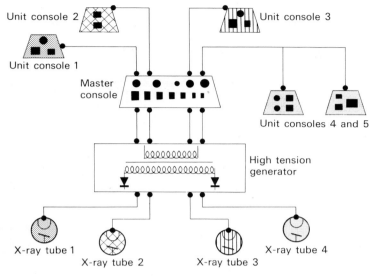

Fig. 3.17

Another arrangement for sharing a generator is sketched in Fig. 3.18. This has been described as a duplex system in which one generator has two separate sets of controls. Each set of controls can (i) switch the system ON/OFF; (ii) select the ability to set exposure factors; (iii) pass this ability to the other set of controls; (iv) reserve the generator to its own use when the handswitch is taken up and keep that condition until the handswitch has been replaced. The two sets of controls are thus effectively equivalent and there is no master control. A good siting for a duplex arrangement such as

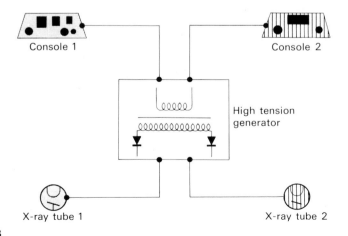

Fig. 3.18

this would be two adjacent X-ray rooms which share a control room in which both sets of controls are located. Such a plan clearly permits maximum co-ordination in the uses of the generator.

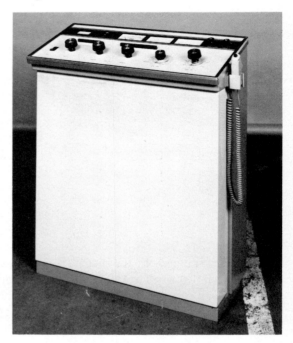

Fig. 3.19   A modern generator which is microprocessor controlled. *Illustration by courtesy of Medical X-ray Supplies Ltd and Shimadzu Medical X-ray.*

Considerations for shared generators

The installation of equipment-systems which involve the use of satellites and the sharing of generators between two or more examination units or X-ray rooms requires careful consideration by those responsible for the choices made. Unless wisely planned, the arrangements can result in such frustration among the users as to bring the reverse of what the manufacturers may claim for the systems: that they improve and rationalize radiological diagnosis. The points in favour of such systems are given below.

1   A shared generator may be of help where there is great limitation of space. A room which it would be infeasible to use if it must contain the generator as well as the controls and the equipment to be operated may become acceptable if the generator is housed elsewhere and the controls are embodied in a small satellite console.

2   Use of one generator to provide power for several X-ray rooms may, if finances are stringent, allow the purchase of a more expensive generator than might be otherwise considered. Thus may improved work-capacity be gained.

3 There may be a wish to simplify control-settings in several X-ray rooms. This simplification might be wanted so that a uniform operating technique could be applied over limited combinations of factors. A modular generator with anatomically programmed unit-consoles achieves uniformity of practice very easily.

4 It may be wished to exploit a generator to its full capacity. If that is the end in view, then sharing the generator between several units is a logical step to take.

To avoid difficulties which may arise, the following points must be considered.

1 A radiographer who is trying to produce radiographs of a patient who cannot or will not easily co-operate needs immediate access to the generator. If access is delayed because another unit has engaged the power, frustration results. There can be waste of time and energy for the radiographer and the patient who may have little enough of these commodities to spare. To waste the energy of seriously ill patients may bring results which are grave in more senses than one; and to waste the energy of radiographers is unfavourable to good economics in the employment of skilled staff.

2 Long-term procedures such as fluoroscopy should be excluded from sharing a generator.

3 Rooms for paediatric examinations should be excluded from sharing a generator.

4 It may be judged that the master control should be accessible at all times, especially if factors on a satellite console must be re-set through the master control. It then becomes important for the master console and the satellite to be close to each other.

5 Workloads must be carefully planned if a system of sharing is to work easily and effectively. Small departments may be less able than are busy ones to achieve a selective distribution of their work.

6 The close interdependence which the system implies can lead to disastrous ineffectiveness if there are changes in the departmental lay-out, in the use of the rooms or in the workloads. Shared generators can limit flexible adaptation to new circumstances.

7 Increasing the number of units or X-ray rooms that share the generator tends to increase the complexities of the situation and certainly increases the extent of the planning and the careful distribution of the workloads that must be undertaken. It has been said in general that sharing a generator between more than two X-ray rooms is not to be recommended.

8 If the saving of money is a prime consideration, the finances must be carefully examined in detail. A shared generator is more expensive than its standard equivalent and its cost must be considered in relation to that of generators which might be selected if a shared one is not chosen for the units

which are to be equipped. The comparable servicing costs must be taken into account. When all the detailed accounting has been done, the results are likely to show little or no significant financial advantage. They can in fact often show that the shared generator is a more costly system than separate conventional generators.

9   When a shared generator is out of action because it is being serviced or has broken down, the working units which share it are all out of action too. If the department is a small one, this situation can bring a big reduction in its capacity: for example two busy X-ray rooms unable to function might be complete inactivity for two thirds or one half of the X-ray department.

Chapter 4
Fuses, Switches and Interlocks

FUSES

The purpose of a fuse is to safeguard electrical equipment from the effects of abnormally high current. Excessive current is damaging to any equipment which is not designed or intended to carry it. It is also, of course, damaging to a fuse but electrical equipment is generally expensive to replace and fuses are cheap.

When current passes through a resistor, heat is produced which may be great enough to melt the resistor and thus break the continuity of the circuit. It is on this principle that a fuse operates. A fuse is simply a metal resistor or wire connected in series with the equipment which it is intended to protect. When the current in the circuit exceeds the rated value of the fuse the temperature of the wire becomes high enough to melt it and the fuse burns out and opens the circuit. We commonly say that the fuse 'blows' as the result of the excessive current.

Rating of fuses

Fuses are rated according to the value of the current which they will conduct without burning out. Thus, most of us have seen, and perhaps used in our own homes, fuse wire of differing thicknesses. The domestic user often buys a variety of three kinds on a card: first is a very thin wire for lighting, rated at 5 amperes; next is a thicker one for heating, rated at 15 amperes; finally at the bottom of the card comes an even stouter wire which is rated at 30 amperes and suitable for the circuit of an immersion heater, for example.

It is very important that anyone who repairs a blown fuse should use wire of the appropriate rating which, as a rule, is designated on the fuse. On the domestic scene, for instance, to put the 5 ampere wire into the circuit of the immersion heater would at once necessitate a repeat of the exercise; the fuse would blow unnecessarily. However, the reverse error of putting the 15 or 30 ampere wire into the lighting system would be worse, since equipment of low current-carrying capacity would not then be protected from excessive loads. The correct rating is one which is slightly higher than the maximum current which the circuit is expected to carry. In no circumstance should other conductors, which may be handy—such as paper clips and safety pins—be employed in place of the proper fuse. It is a simple job to change a fuse but it should not be attempted in any circumstance without first switching off the supply voltage.

A fuse occasionally operates because of fatigue—the gradual thinning of the wire which occurs with use—and in these circumstances when the fuse is replaced the equipment concerned functions satisfactorily. However, a repaired fuse which blows again almost at once indicates the presence of some fault in the circuit which is responsible for the abnormally high current. The equipment in question—whether a domestic item or an X-ray unit—should not be used again until it has been investigated by a qualified electrical engineer.

Fuse units

Fuses are made in many varieties of shape and size as well as of current rating. Even if we consider only the X-ray equipment in our own departments we find probably at least ten dissimilar kinds of fuse used by different manufacturers and even for various circuits in the one generator. Knowing where the fuses are situated in a generator or other item of X-ray equipment is perhaps one of the most useful pieces of knowledge which a radiographer may possess. For instance if a tilting table were to be driven accidentally against an obstruction (the footswitch is sometimes such a victim), it is probable that a fuse in the table's circuitry will blow, because of the overload on the motor; if there were no fuse in the circuit the motor could burn out in these circumstances. It is good housekeeping to have in the X-ray department some spare fuses of appropriate types.

The word *fuse* is usually applied to the complete fuse unit and includes in fact several separate structures. These are described below. In circuit diagrams a fuse is depicted by the symbol shown in Fig. 4.1.

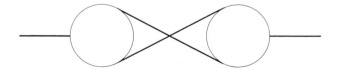

Fig. 4.1

Fuse element

The fuse element is the actual resistor, that is, the wire which melts when it is subjected to a current overload. The current-carrying capacity of the fuse is determined by the character of this wire: its diameter and the metal of which it is made which may be tin, tin-lead alloy, aluminium, lead or copper.

Fuse link

The fuse link is the part of the fuse which comprises the element and its container or carrier. Fuse links come in many varieties. A small glass cartridge with metal end caps sealed to the internal wire (see Fig. 4.2) is typical. In some examples of this kind the glass tube contains a piece of paper on which is printed the rating of the fuse; this prevents the element from

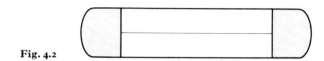

Fig. 4.2

being visible but the paper will singe when the fuse blows and its condition then becomes obvious. Ceramic cartridges include a colour or other indicator for the same purpose. In some cases the element is not enclosed or is readily accessible and the carrier can be rewired. Enclosed fuse links are safer since there is no open spark when the fuse blows.

Fuse contacts

Fuse contacts are contacts which either are attached to or are integral parts of a fuse link. In Fig. 4.2 the metal caps at the ends of the glass tube are the fuse contacts. Fuse contacts engage with fixed contacts, such as metal clips, in the equipment concerned. On the domestic fuseboard and others the fixed contacts are situated deeply within porcelain fuse bases.

SWITCHES AND CIRCUIT BREAKERS

A switch is a convenient and safe practical method either of allowing electric current to flow in a circuit or of preventing current from flowing. A circuit breaker is a device for breaking an electric circuit when the current in the circuit is too high. A circuit breaker does the same job as a fuse and is used instead of a fuse but its manner of operation and often its appearance are more like those of a switch. It is for this reason that switches and circuit breakers are together in the same section of this chapter, although each has an essentially different purpose.

There are many categories of switch. Even if we consider only those found in X-ray equipment the student radiographer can easily name several which are needed for an X-ray unit: the mains supply switch on the wall of the room; the on/off switch for the generator; the selector switches on the control table; and not least the exposure switch. These are but a few of them.

Exposure switching is a specialized subject which is fully discussed in the next chapter. At present we shall consider:

1   large, manually operated switches suitable for the mains supply;
2   magnetic relays which can be used to operate one or more sets of contacts automatically and thus to make or break electrical circuits;
3   circuit breakers which utilize relays in protecting electrical circuits from overload
4   the high tension switch.

Terminology

Student radiographers may be confused by the technicalities implicit in some of the words which appear in this chapter. For this reason the following short explanations of a few terms are given.

Electric circuits are completed by continuity between two or more metal *contacts*. In the United Kingdom the word *switch* usually implies the manual operation of contacts; in a relay the contacts are operated electromagnetically. A *relay* is an electromagnetic device which often operates many sets of contacts for different circuits carrying small currents. A *contactor* is a larger type of relay carrying fewer and heavier contacts for a higher current.

It is common in the case of heavy-duty switches for industry and those which handle the more moderate voltages of the mains supply for domestic and other purposes, to construct an enclosed composite unit which consists of a switch in series with a fuse or fuses. The term *fuseswitch* is applied to such a composite unit if the fuse is contained in or is mounted on the moving member of the switch (British Standard 3185 : 1959). A *switchfuse* is a similar composite unit in which the fuse is not part of the moving member of the switch. A fuseswitch is more compact than a switchfuse. Size for size, it carries heavier cables and allows more space for manipulating these to their respective terminals.

The moving limb of a switch carries—predictably enough—a *moving contact* which engages a *fixed contact* in the fixed part of the switch.

Mains supply switches

The mains switch is—or should be—situated on the wall of the X-ray room close to the generator (the control table). As its purpose is to provide a means of isolating *all* the X-ray equipment in the room from the supply voltage, the mains switch should be easily accessible to the radiographer. To reach the switch it should not be necessary to cross the room or to negotiate an assault course among free standing accessory equipment. If the switch cannot be sited near to the radiographer's normal position at the control table then it should at least be near the door of the room.

As we have said, the purpose of the mains switch is to enable all the X-ray equipment in the room to be switched off from one point during maintenance work or in an emergency. On one occasion when it was in normal use for conventional radiography a fluoroscopic table began to tilt spontaneously. The radiographer immediately threw the mains supply switch to 'off'. Unfortunately a switch in the auxiliary circuit which supplied the table drive and the tubestand brakes was incorrectly positioned on the wrong side of the mains switch and the table continued to tilt, to the radiographer's surprise and alarm. The interval before the supplementary switch was found and operated was happily brief; the table was halted when it and the inclining rather than reclining patient were still together. However, the delay might have been critical and would not have occurred at all if the mains switch had been correctly sited so as to isolate all the X-ray circuitry.

Operation and structure of the switch

Mains supply switches are similar in operation to a *knife switch* which is depicted in Fig. 4.3. Movement of the conductive, connecting arm or blade completes—or breaks—the circuit at the switch (fixed) contact; the last is usually described as a *pole* in a switch of this kind. The switch in the sketch is a *single pole* switch; its circuit symbol is shown beside it.

Many switches in everyday use, including mains switches, are of the *double pole* variety. The connecting arm is duplicate in structure, being a pair of parallel blades which are moved by means of a single lever and engage

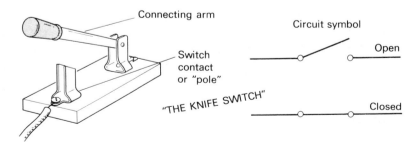

Fig. 4.3 *Reproduced from Basic Electricity by kind permission of The Technical Press Ltd.*

with similarly duplicated contacts. This type of switch is safer because it breaks both mains conductors (see Chapter 1) simultaneously. Triple pole switches breaking three lines (3 phase) at once are also in use. Small, inexpensive switches which are sometimes fitted to domestic table lamps may break only one line: a switch of this kind should be connected so that it breaks the 'live' and not the neutral conductor.

Fig. 4.4 is a sketch diagram to indicate the practical arrangement in a common type of double pole, heavy duty switch. The parallel U-shaped copper blades are mounted on a bar of insulating material which is rotated

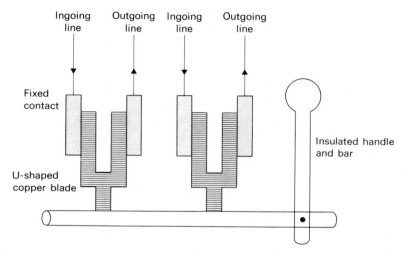

Fig. 4.4   Construction of a double pole switch. Fig. 4.5 shows the actual appearance of such a switch.

by means of the switch handle and this carries the blades into—or away from—the fixed contacts of the switch. Each pair of fixed contacts has an ingoing conductor on one side and an outgoing conductor on the other, between which the blade provides electrical continuity. Fig. 4.5 is a photograph of such a switch.

Mains supply switches of the kind which we meet in the X-ray department and elsewhere are composite units of a switch and fuses. The circuit symbol for a double pole switch with fuses (fuseswitch) is shown in Fig. 4.6. Fig. 4.7 is a triple pole fuseswitch.

The enclosure

The case which contains a composite unit of switch and fuses must meet certain requirements, such as those defined in British Standard 2510:1954

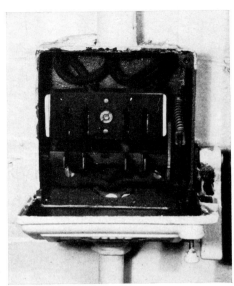

Fig. 4.5 A double pole heavy duty switch.
By courtesy of Picker International Ltd.

which relates to the units in use in industrial systems and domestic circuits: these two categories would include the switches in the X-ray department.

The enclosure must be strong and may be made either of metal or of some insulating material: cast iron is often used. If the case is metal it must be suitably earthed. The operating handle must be insulated from the circuit and if it is metal it, too, must be earthed.

In the composite unit, the fuse carrier should be designed so that during or after its withdrawal accidental contact with live metal is prevented. There should be no openings in the enclosure which would permit live metal to be touched and an interlock should be provided between handle and cover which normally prevents the enclosure being opened unless the switch handle is in the 'off' position. Indicators of the ON and OFF positions should be clear and definite; sometimes these indicators carry a statement of the voltage and current ratings of the unit. Fastening devices on the cover of an enclosure should be designed so that none may be accidentally omitted or readily lost or broken.

The performance of the switch should be to give a quick make and break operation, independently of the speed of action of the user. This is achieved by spring loading the handle. It should not normally be possible for the operator of the switch to leave the handle in such a position that the blades are partially engaged with their contacts. The phrase 'all or nothing' might well have been devised to describe mains supply switches or others of this kind.

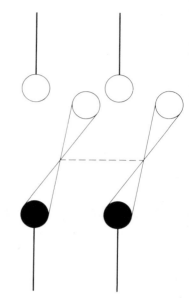

Fig. 4.6

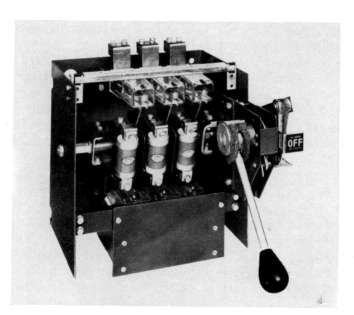

Fig. 4.7 A triple pole fuseswitch. *By courtesy of Picker International Ltd.*

Magnetic relays

A magnetic relay is an electromechanical device which functions as an electrically operated switch. Fig. 4.8(a) is a drawing which illustrates the essential components of a relay. These are:

1 an electromagnet;
2 a movable arm of iron or iron alloy which is known as the armature because it carries a conductor;
3 a pair of opposed contacts, one of which is mounted on the armature.

When the coil of the electromagnet is energized a magnetic field is established which attracts the armature towards the core of the electromagnet. This results in closure of the pair of contacts and a complete circuit across the terminals of the relay at A and B: the relay becomes a closed switch. When the electromagnet is de-energized the armature, which is spring loaded for this purpose, jumps back to its original position: the relay contacts now act as an open switch.

A relay of the kind just described is called a *normally open relay* because the circuit is open unless the coil is energized. It is equally possible for a relay to be *normally closed*, that is the circuit is complete until the electromagnet is energized. This variety is depicted in Fig. 4.8(b).

Relays are extremely useful little gadgets which in certain situations have advantages over manually operated switches. They make it possible for a low tension circuit to control another which carries higher voltage and current. Referring to Fig. 4.8, the circuit carrying the heavy current would be connected across A and B; only a low voltage and current are necessary to operate the electromagnet. In this way a small current such as may be safely manipulated through a handswitch can be employed to switch another

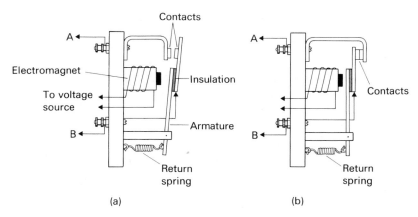

Fig. 4.8   Relays. *Reproduced from Basic Electricity by kind permission of The Technical Press Ltd.*

circuit in which the current is too large to be switched directly by the operator without danger of burns as the result of overloading contacts and causing arcing at the switch. In the next chapter we shall see the application of this principle to the exposure contactor of the X-ray set. Relays are further useful for their ability to switch a circuit, and even several circuits, situated remotely from the operator. Fig. 4.9 depicts a relay with four pairs of contacts: two (A and B) are of the normally closed variety and the others (C and D) are normally open.

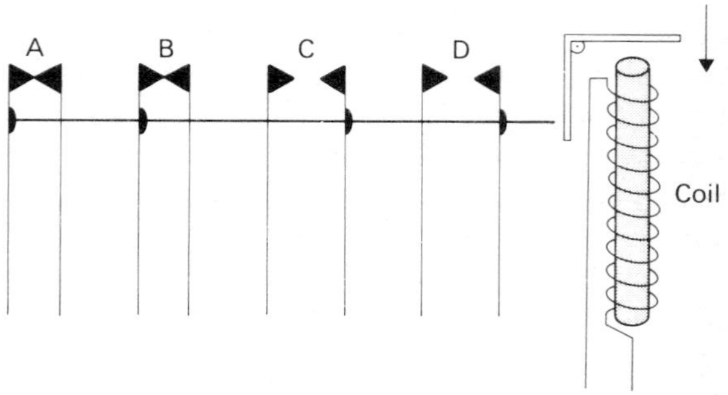

Fig. 4.9 A relay operating four pairs of contacts, two of which are normally open and two normally closed.

Reed switch

A reed switch is an electromagnetic relay of a particular variety. Depicted diagrammatically in Fig. 4.10, the switch consists of a small glass vacuum

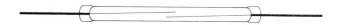

Fig. 4.10

tube, perhaps 20 mm in length and 2 mm in diameter, several sizes being available to meet different needs. A pair of normally open contacts are sealed within the vacuum tube. Their external extensions each provide a lead-in wire by which the relay may be connected in a circuit. When the glass tube is subjected to the influence of a magnetic field, the contacts are observed to close and will open again when the magnetic field is removed. A permanent magnet placed close to it is capable of operating the relay.

Employed like this, one application of such a relay might be in protecting the undertable tube or other part of a tilting table from hazards due to its mobility. (Circumstances are not beyond conjecture in which someone may attempt to operate the table who is not fully trained in its use.) For this purpose, the tube carriage or serial changer would carry a suitable magnet.

In any dangerous relationship of the tube and table (for example, when the tube is at the end of the table and the latter adversely tilted towards the floor) this magnet is in such a position as to influence a suitably placed reed relay. Operation of the relay, that is, completion of the circuit including it, can be used to arrest the table's motion, or slide the table-top upwards as appropriate, and thus prevent the occurrence of expensive damage.

Equally well, the magnetic field may be provided by a coil of wire wound over the vacuum tube and in this case the relay contacts will close when the coil is energized. A magnet placed adjacently may be used to hold the reed switch closed, once the coil has activated it.

Reed switches operate much more quickly than other forms of electromagnetic relay. Their operating time is 1·5 milliseconds, compared with 10 milliseconds for a small relay and 20 milliseconds for a large relay of standard types.

As opposed to electronic methods of switching which are considered in the next chapter, electromechanical magnetic relays are prone to 'bounce'; on closure the contacts may rebound, thus momentarily interrupting the circuit. Reed switches are no exception in this respect but have the advantage that the 'bouncing' time is very short. It is only 0·5 milliseconds, compared with a period which may be as long as 10 milliseconds in the case of other electromagnetic relays.

Another good feature of the reed relay is that the vacuum tube keeps the contacts free of dust. Electrically, dust is a notorious *agent provocateur*, producing conditions favourable to sparking and burning.

Circuit breakers

Thermal relay

Like a fuse, a thermal relay is a device which:
1 protects electrical equipment from overload;
2 uses the heating effect of an electric current to do so.

However, while a fuse acts instantaneously—or nearly so—in the case of a thermal relay the excessive current must flow for a time before the relay operates. This makes it appropriate for equipment which is normally expected to carry high current for a short period, for example the starting current in an electric motor.

In the X-ray department—or rather out of it—thermal contactors are used for overload protection in some portable and mobile units (*not* overload of the X-ray tube: they would be too slow). These contactors are applicable particularly to the system of tank construction (see page 97) in which the X-ray tube and its high tension generator are enclosed together in a single oil-filled unit. The student will remember that within the shield of an X-ray tube a flexible diaphragm is normally fitted which permits expansion of the contained oil as use of the X-ray tube raises its temperature (see page 245). This construction is less efficient in a tube-head containing, not only the X-ray tube, but the high tension and filament transformers which add their own contributions to the rising temperature of an associated larger volume of oil. In the United Kingdom, the Department of Health prefers such equipment to be provided additionally with a thermal cut-out.

A thermal contactor often depends on the different rates of expansion of various metals when heated. Two metals are welded together in a bi-metal strip. Because the component metals have different rates of expansion the bi-metal strip will bend when it becomes hot. In a thermal contactor a bi-metal strip is mounted so that:

1   one end is fixed and the other free to move;
2   the strip carries the significant current or is close to a heating element which does so.

When the value of the current in the circuit remains above some selected level for a sufficient length of time, the temperature of the bi-metal strip becomes great enough to cause its free end to bend. This movement either opens a pair of contacts directly or trips a spring loaded switch.

A thermal contactor, once it has operated, continues to keep the circuit open until it is manually reset, that is, restored to its original position by triggering a latch. This cannot be done until the bi-metal has had a moment or two to cool and has resumed its normal shape.

Magnetic circuit breaker

Circuit breakers of the electromagnetic kind are contactors designed to protect circuits from overload: they are overload switches and have the same purpose as a fuse. A magnetic circuit breaker possesses the advantages of a relay, being capable of rapid action and susceptible to remote control. Although, like the thermal relay, once it has tripped a magnetic circuit breaker must be manually reset, this can be done immediately.

The main ON/OFF switch of an X-ray generator often includes a circuit breaker for overload control. Such a circuit is depicted diagrammatically in Fig. 4.11.

In the circuit in Fig. 4.11 are seen:

A   the mains switchfuse
B   fuses in the generator
C   push button switches for ON/OFF control of the generator;
D   a relay coil which operates 3 sets of normally open contacts, E1, E2 and E3.

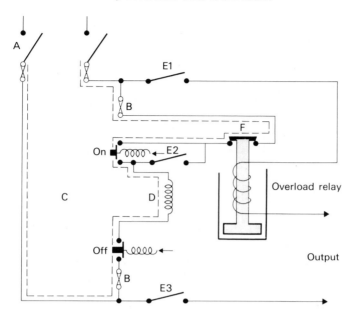

Fig. 4.11

Closing the mains ON switch (C) completes a circuit through D as indicated by the broken line. When D is energized E1, E2 and E3 all close. The output voltage which is fed across the autotransformer is obtained along the route provided by E1, the overload relay coil and E3. E2 maintains a voltage on the coil D; these contacts are called the hold-on contacts.

The overload relay has a special construction. Its armature is the plunger of a small adjustable oil dashpot, similar to those found in some bucky mechanisms (see Chapter 8); the movement of the plunger in the cylinder is impeded by the surrounding oil. If the current in the principal circuit (which passes through the relay coil) rises above some pre-set value, for example 100 amperes, the associated magnetic field becomes strong enough to operate the armature and open the normally closed contacts F. Opening these contacts breaks the circuit which is maintaining voltage across the coil D. This relay is thus de-energized and the contacts E1 and E3 fall open, so breaking the main circuit to the autotransformer: E2 is opened at the same time.

The purpose of the oil dashpot is to prevent the overload relay from operating quickly in response to a merely momentary rise in current. A sustained rise is required to overcome the resistance offered by the oil to the movement of the armature. Under normal conditions in the circuit the overload relay remains closed because—although there is current through its coil—the accompanying magnetic field is too weak to affect the armature. Operation of the mains OFF switch can be seen from the diagram to break the circuit energizing D in ordinary use of the X-ray unit.

The high tension switch

Many X-ray generators must supply power to more than one X-ray tube. This is necessary in the majority of X-ray departments: for instance, the fluoroscopy room will have an overtable tube as well as an undertable tube; the tomography room, in addition to its specialized equipment, may include a tubestand for radiography of the chest; the room which contains a skull-table may house also a plain bucky table for other work or an angiographic table (see Fig. 4.12). Student radiographers no doubt will find in their departments, if the rooms are large enough and the equipment extensive, other examples of generators which supply not only two but perhaps three tubes, each tube being associated with a particular piece of apparatus for a certain category of work.

It is consequently important for any major X-ray generator to include a switch which allows the user normally to operate one from at least two X-ray tubes. This switch is often called the *high tension switch*, although more exactly it is a tube selector switch. It must not be confused with the vacuum triode valves which can switch high tension in the secondary circuit of the high tension transformer in order to initiate or terminate the radiographic exposure (see Chapter 5). The high tension switch has no role whatsoever in exposure switching. Its function is merely to connect the source of high tension to one or another X-ray tube as the user requires; it does not switch high voltages on and off, although it must carry such voltages when it is closed.

Because it carries high voltage, the high tension switch is not manually operated. It is oil immersed in the tank containing the high tension transformer and the filament transformers, the rectifiers (and the valve transformers, if any) and it is remotely controlled. This is consequently an electromagnetic switch functioning on the same principle as a relay but it is many times larger.

Construction

As it is in the transformer tank, radiographers seldom have the opportunity of seeing a high tension switch. Fig. 4.13(a) shows the appearance of one. Each switch consists of:

1 a pair of receptacles or pots for each X-ray tube, one pot for each high

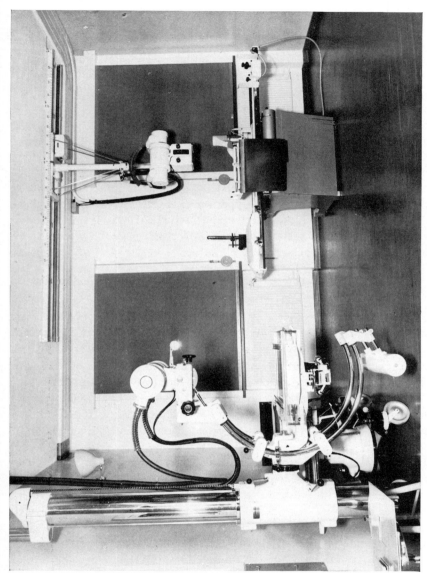

Fig. 4.12 A skull table and an angiographic table in a radiodiagnostic room. *By courtesy of Elema-Schonander.*

tension cable (that is, one carries the cathode cable and the other the anode cable);

2   a contact or contacts at the lower end of each pot (the fixed contacts of the switch);

3   two contacts which oppose the other set and are mounted one at each end of an insulated actuating bar (the moving contacts of the switch);

4   a large electromagnet which can attract a vertical limb of the actuating bar so that the moving contacts are held against the fixed ones;

5   leads from the moving contacts for connection to the high tension and filament transformers.

One switch like this is necessary for each X-ray tube to which the generator is to supply power. The transformer tank contains certainly two, and often three, switches side by side. They are mounted above the transformers, the cable pots being uppermost (as seen in Fig. 4.13(a)), and this means that the moving contacts are normally held away from the fixed contacts by the force of gravity. Fig. 2.3 shows high tension switches in a transformer tank.

The contacts and leads

Fig. 4.13(b) gives a better view of the fixed contacts on the pots which we now see *en face*; the moving contacts are similar to these in arrangement. It is to be noticed that the two in the photograph are not identical: one has an unbroken conducting surface and the other bears a trio of circular prominences. The contact which has a plain face provides connection for the single conductor from the anode of the X-ray tube. The triple sets of contacts, on the other hand, are necessary for the three conductors from the cathode of a dual focus X-ray tube—the broad, common and fine connections (see page 232).

In the high tension switch the anode contacts carry a single lead to one end of the secondary of the high tension transformer; the cathode contacts carry three leads to the other end of the secondary of the high tension transformer and to the secondary of the filament transformers. In this way the anode and cathode of the X-ray tube are each connected via a high tension cable and the high tension switch to the source of voltage.

The contacts in the high tension switch do not have to make and break heavy currents. The X-ray tube is selected before the exposure is made and in normal practice the switch is not again operated until the radiographer is preparing for another procedure. Though they are large, the contacts are lighter in construction than might be expected. They are made of copper which is usually thinly coated with silver.

Assuming there are two or more high tension switches in the one

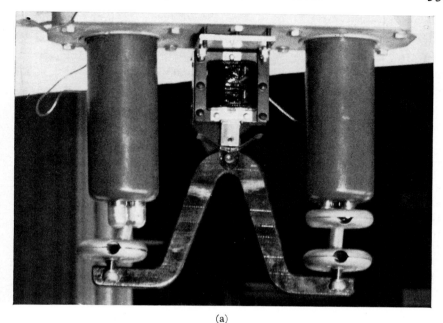

(a)

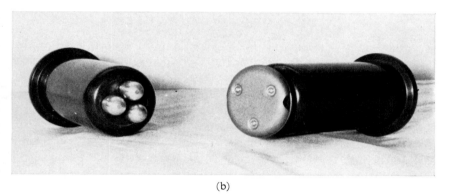

(b)

Fig. 4.13 A high tension (tube selector) switch. *By courtesy of Picker International Ltd.*

transformer tank, when the high tension circuit becomes energized by the exposure switching system voltage is applied across each set of moving contacts and not merely between those which relate to one tube: high tension is present on each switch simultaneously but is not utilized unless the switch has been closed. The feature makes simultaneous bi-plane angiography practicable from a single generator; during this two switches are closed at one time.

The electromagnet

The electromagnet which moves the actuating bar in a high tension switch is a strong one. It must be so if it is successfully to pull the moving contacts upwards against the force of gravity. It is the only part of the switch which is at low tension.

From each end of the magnet's large coil a lead is taken to the top of the generator and then to a rotary selector switch on the control table or a series of press button switches. These—whether a single rotary switch or a number of press buttons—are marked to indicate the appropriate X-ray tube and when any one is operated by the radiographer an energizing voltage is put across the corresponding electromagnet in the high tension switch. The armature and contacts in the high tension switch can be heard to move as the radiographer changes from one X-ray tube to another; radiographers may not normally see high tension switches but they can hear them in action if the set is already switched on when the tube is selected.

This switch or series of switches on the control table may combine three functions:

1   selection of the X-ray tube;
2   selection of the focus (see Chapter 7);
3   selection of milliamperage (see Chapter 2).

INTERLOCKING CIRCUITS

As we have seen, the purpose of fuses and circuit breakers is to protect circuits and their electrical components from damagingly high abnormal currents. However, such measures do not go far enough in protecting the X-ray tube from overload during ordinary use.

In Chapter 7 we consider the load upon the X-ray tube during a radiographic exposure: this load depends upon the combination of kilovoltage, tube current and time. Even in normal practice the heating effect of the load upon the tube target may be great enough to damage it when high tube currents and high kilovoltages are employed together for too long an exposure interval.

Interlocks, or rather interlocking circuits have many applications electrically. To the radiographer the term means often those devices which are intended to save the X-ray tube: they prevent an exposure from being made in circumstances which would result in overheating of the target and in its permanent injury. Some of these devices we shall now consider.

Interlock in the tube stator circuit

A radiographic exposure made on an anode which should be rotating but in fact is stationary will severely damage the X-ray tube (see Chapter 7).

Fig. 4.14 illustrates a simple circuit which will not allow the exposure to occur if a fault in the stator circuit prevents the tube anode from rotating.

The X-ray tube has two stator windings, marked in the diagram as stator 1 and stator 2. Stator 1 is known as the starting winding and operates at a higher voltage than stator 2 which is the running winding: this is because once the anode has been given initial impetus by stator 1, a smaller voltage is all that is required to maintain its speed. A capacitor is shown in the stator circuit but it is not relevant to the function of the interlock: its purpose is to put the stators 90 degrees out of phase with each other and promote smoother running of the anode.

Each stator winding is in series with a relay coil; these are A and B respectively which operate the normally open contacts S1 and S2 in series in the circuit controlling the exposure contactor. Exposure contactors are discussed in Chapter 5: at this stage we need say of the exposure contactor only that it must be energized to obtain the radiographic exposure.

In Fig. 4.14, P and E indicate the customary two-position exposure switch which:

1 completes the circuit to the stators and thus initiates rotation of the anode;

2 completes the supply to the exposure control thus allowing the radiographic exposure to proceed.

It can be seen from the diagram that when P is operated the relay coils A and B are energized and the relays S1 and S2 thereby closed. This allows the

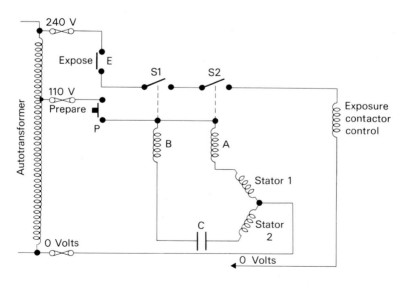

Fig. 4.14

circuit containing S1 and S2 and the exposure contactor control to be completed at E as the radiographer continues the pressure on the exposure switch. However, should there be a defect in either stator winding which results in an open-circuit condition the appropriate relay coil is not energized and S1 or S2 remains open. These relays have their contacts in series and if either is open the circuit to the exposure contactor control cannot be completed even when E is closed by the radiographer. Consequently the radiographic exposure is prevented from occurring.

Delay circuit with the tube stator

The interlocking circuit described in the previous section is concerned with failure of the tube anode to rotate. It is hardly less important to ensure that the radiographic exposure is made only when the anode has reached its maximum speed. If the anode is subjected to the full load while it is accelerating it may overheat nearly as harmfully as if it were stationary, especially if this occurs on more than one occasion over a period of time.

The standard rate of rotation of the anode of an X-ray tube is about 3,500 revolutions per minute and an interval of 0·8 second is required for it to reach this speed. If the tube has a high speed anode (see Chapter 7) a longer period is necessary (up to 2 seconds). Radiographers are usually aware of the need to allow time for the anode to reach its correct running speed and normally hold the exposure switch in the 'prepare' position long enough to permit this to happen. Nevertheless situations occur in which immediacy in obtaining the radiograph may become the dominant consideration; for example when the patient is restless or unco-operative or during filming of rapidly transient fluoroscopic appearances. Under this kind of pressure the operator might easily use the exposure switch prematurely and damage the tube.

To avoid harm occurring in this manner it is usual to employ a circuit which introduces an automatic delay between the 'prepare' and 'expose' positions, so that even if the operator goes straight through from one to the other the exposure does not actually begin for a period which is variable between 0·8 and 2 seconds. A simple circuit for doing this by means of a slugged relay is shown in Fig. 4.15.

In Fig. 4.15 we see the slugged relay S of which the contacts are in series with the exposure contactor control. There are three things to notice about it.

1   The relay is normally open and until it is closed no exposure can take place, even though the circuit to the exposure contactor control had been completed through the exposure switch by a radiographer in a hurry. For simplicity's sake the exposure station has not been included in the diagram.

2   The small circuit which includes the relay coil is completed at the same time as the stator circuit when the exposure switch is put at prepare. Again for reasons of simplicity the stator circuit is not included in the diagram. (It appears in Fig. 4.14.)

3   There is a capacitor C connected in parallel with the relay coil.

In this circuit the voltage across the relay coil is virtually the same as that across the capacitor. When the circuit is first completed, however, the capacitor draws a heavy current and for a short time very little current passes through the relay coil.

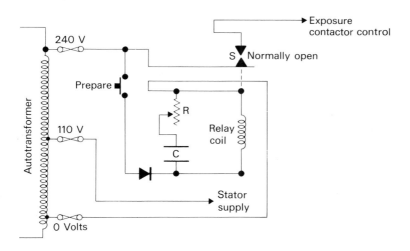

Fig. 4.15

We may make a simple domestic comparison here by thinking of the relay coil as a garden hose which someone is trying to use while another person has the kitchen taps fully running in order to fill a washing machine (the capacitor). Until the washing machine is full the supply to the hose is rather poor but it will immediately increase as soon as the demands of the washing machine are met. Similarly, when the capacitor has been charged to its full potential the current through the relay coil then rises and operates the relay; S will close and the radiographic exposure may begin.

The length of the delay imposed by the inclusion of the capacitor in the circuit depends upon characteristics of the capacitor itself and upon the value of the charging resistor: in this case the required period is 0·8–2 seconds. The circuit diagram shows that the series resistor R is variable and this feature facilitates adjustments in the duration of the interval.

Overload interlocks

Apart from the possibility in a rotating anode tube that the anode is not operating correctly or at the proper speed, any X-ray tube may be overloaded in normal practice if the selected exposure factors are too high (see Chapter 7). X-ray generators commonly include interlocking circuits which prevent the radiographic exposure from occurring in these circumstances.

There are several ways in which such an overload interlock may operate. The methods at present employed are electronic. Below is described the use of an analogue circuit to provide protection of the X-ray tube against a single exposure which will overload it.

An analogue circuit

An analogue circuit is one which performs an electronic addition sum. The circuit in Fig. 4.16 is an example which is used to provide overload control for the X-ray tube. In effect this circuit adds together voltages which are each representative of one of the factors comprising the tube load (kilovoltage, milliamperes and exposure time).

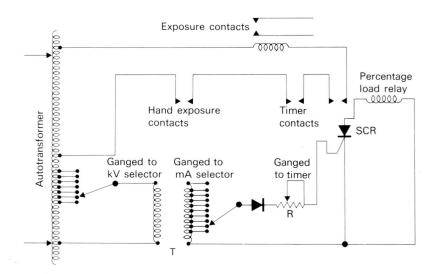

Fig. 4.16

In Fig. 4.16, T is a special transformer. The voltage across its primary winding is obtained from the autotransformer by means of a sliding contact which is ganged to the kilovoltage selector; the higher is the chosen kilovoltage, the higher is the input voltage to this transformer.

The secondary winding of the transformer is itself tapped by another sliding contact, this one being linked to the milliamperes selector as illustrated in the circuit diagram. Thus, the output voltage from the transformer is subject to two independent quantities:

1   the selected kilovoltage;
2   the selected tube current.

Alteration in either of these factors will correspondingly raise or lower the output from the transformer.

The output voltage from T is rectified as shown in Fig. 4.16 and fed, by way of a series resistor R, to become the gate voltage on a thyristor or SCR (see page 166). R is a variable resistor and has a sliding contact which is ganged to the timer in such a way that when the timer is set for longer intervals of exposure the resistance in the circuit is progressively diminished.

As R decreases in value the voltage drop across it becomes less. In this way the ultimate voltage applied to the gate of the thyristor is an aggregate of:

the selected kilovoltage;
the selected milliamperes;
the selected exposure time.

The gate voltage is raised or lowered whenever any of these factors is raised or lowered.

The thyristor is conductive until the gate voltage mounts to some predetermined value. When this critical point is reached the thyristor becomes at once non-conductive, that is it will act as an open switch in the part of the circuit which contains it.

As Fig. 4.16 indicates, the current through the thyristor passes also through the coil of a normally open relay (the percentage load relay) which has its contacts in series with the exposure contactor gate. So long as the thyristor is conducting the percentage load relay is closed. The circuit to the exposure contactor coil can be completed through the handswitch and timer contacts and the radiographic exposure can be made. However, once the thyristor is non-conductive the relay coil is no longer energized, the percentage load relay opens and the occurrence of the radiographic exposure is prevented.

This form of overload interlock allows the radiographer a free choice of kilovoltage, tube current and time independently. If the aggregate voltage in the analogue circuit is too high, a reduction in any of the tube factors is effective.

It should be emphasized that there is only one kind of overload of the X-ray tube from which an exposure interlocking circuit or device, such as that described, can give protection: this is the overload which may arise during a single exposure. Perhaps radiographers have learned to rely on these interlocks too well and do not now make such regular use of tube rating charts as once they must. The appropriate rating chart (see Chapter 7) should be consulted whenever it is intended to make a rapid repetition of radiographic exposures, for example during angiography. A tube load which is permissible in itself may not be so when it is frequently recurrent.

Chapter 5
Exposure Switches and Exposure Timers

Control of the duration of an X-ray exposure has some of the elements found in control of the length of time it takes to boil an egg—is it to be 3 minutes for a 'soft-boiled egg' or 6 minutes for a 'hard-boiled egg'? Is the X-ray exposure to be 0·02 second for a projection of the chest or 1·5 seconds for a projection of the pelvis?

In both cases there are these three elements to be considered:

1 a process must be started;
2 a process must be timed;
3 a process must be stopped.

For precise control, the timing must begin *as soon as* the process starts and the process must stop *as soon as* the selected period of time has elapsed. If the reader thinks of the actions taken in the cooking of an egg, it will be realized that (a) starting and stopping the procedure and (b) timing the procedure are separate matters. So are they also separate matters in controlling the duration of an X-ray exposure.

In the case of the radiographic exposure, what is the process that must be started and stopped and timed in between? Clearly the process is the X-ray tube producing X-rays, and it does this when electric current flows in the secondary circuit of the high tension transformer and through the X-ray tube. So the process that is to be started and stopped is the flow of current in the secondary circuit of the high tension generator.

One way to start and stop this current is to put devices in the secondary circuit which will (i) close the circuit (i.e. provide a continuous pathway for the flow of current) at the start of the exposure; and (ii) open the circuit (i.e. break the continuity of the pathway) at the end of the exposure. This is called secondary switching and it involves switching a low current (the X-ray tube current) at a very high voltage (the X-ray tube voltage). Fig. 5.1 is a block diagram to depict such secondary switching.

Because of the high voltage, there have been problems in switching the secondary circuit and this method was not used for X-ray circuits until modern electronics found some answers and enabled secondary switching to be incorporated in X-ray equipment. However, since X rays were discovered in 1895 an enormous number of exposures has been started and stopped

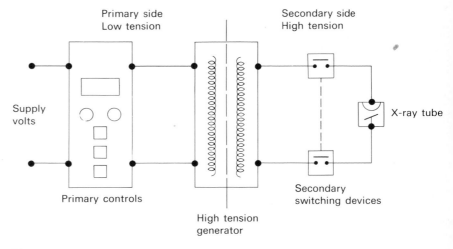

Primary side
Low tension

Secondary side
High tension

Supply
volts

X-ray tube

Primary controls

Secondary
switching devices

High tension
generator

Fig. 5.1

prior to present-day electronic developments. So obviously a method must have been used which did not involve putting switches directly into the secondary circuit to make and break current which was flowing at high tension.

Between the input of the mains supply and the secondary high tension circuit is the primary circuit. When there is a continuous pathway in the primary circuit which allows current to flow through the primary winding of the high tension transformer, then current flows in the secondary circuit if that too has a continuous pathway, for the two circuits are linked by electromagnetic induction in the high tension transformer. If there is no continuous pathway in the primary circuit, no current will flow through the primary winding of the high tension transformer and therefore there will be no current in the secondary circuit. So current flowing in the secondary circuit (and the production of X rays by the X-ray tube) can be stopped and started by switching the primary circuit and leaving the secondary circuit intact. Fig. 5.2 is a block diagram to depict such primary switching.

This is the method that has been used from the early days and it is still in common use in modern X-ray equipment. Primary switching involves making and breaking currents at voltages which have not been stepped up from the mains voltage to the kilovoltages necessary for operation of the X-ray tube; but these currents may be very big ones of several hundred amperes for modern X-ray sets of high output. So primary switching involves the switching of high currents at mains voltage.

The switching devices put on the primary side of the high tension generator in the past were mechanical contactor switches operated

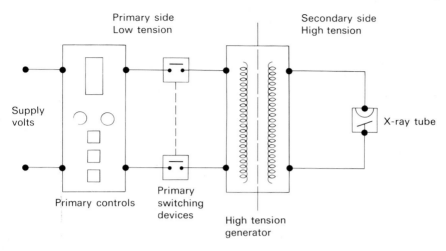

Fig. 5.2

electromagnetically. These switches have moving parts: these are metal contact pieces which come together to close a circuit and spring away from each other to open it. The modern switching devices used are electronic and the *closed* state or the *open* state for a circuit is achieved by variations in certain electrical characteristics as explained later in this chapter. There are no moving parts at all.

In conjunction with switching, periods of exposure must be timed and for this a timing system must be used. Timers are discussed in more detail later.

It is important to realize the following points.

1 If the switching system is slow to operate in starting and in stopping the exposure, a timer which is accurate for very short intervals is no advantage: the switching system will introduce errors by not starting the exposure soon enough or by causing it to last too long.

2 If the X-ray set is a low-powered one very short exposures (say less than 0·5 second) will not be used. Small errors in timing which arise from the timing system or the switching system or both will be only a small percentage of the selected exposure time and therefore not significant. Low-powered X-ray sets draw small currents (as low as 10 A) from the mains, so the current to be switched is relatively small. For these reasons, the timing and switching systems used in low-powered X-ray sets can be simple.

3 X-ray sets of medium and high power give outputs which allow short exposures to be used—down to 0·01 second and below this. A small error from the timer or the switching system or both can be a big percentage error in relation to a selected short exposure time and is unacceptable.

Furthermore, when X-ray sets with high output are used it may be necessary to repeat exposures quickly (as in angiographic examinations), so the timing and switching systems must be capable of functioning quickly, accurately and repeatedly. When high X-ray outputs are used large primary currents (up to 250 A) flow, so it is necessary to switch high currents in the primary circuit. For these reasons the timing and switching systems in medium and high powered X-ray sets must be more sophisticated.

An important feature of the exposure switching system is an arrangement so that the circuit is closed for the start of the exposure and opened at the end of the exposure time only at points of zero voltage in the cycle of the mains supply: that is, the exposure begins and ends at the points marked X in the sine waveform shown in Fig. 5.3. This is called *phased switching, synchronous switching, synchronous exposure*: all these terms mean the same thing and refer to the fact that the initiation and subsequent duration of the exposure are related synchronously to the mains frequency.

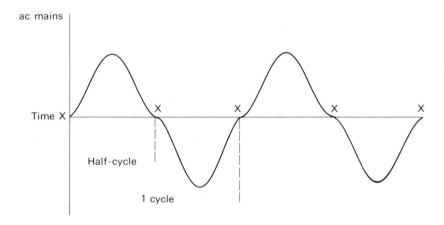

Fig. 5.3

The usefulness of phased switching is (i) that it avoids surges of voltage and arcing as a circuit opens and closes; and (ii) that it makes radiographic exposures consistent at short exposure times. Disadvantages arise in such special applications as cine filming and angiography when it is necessary to use very short exposures and to repeat them at rapid rates. A duration and a repetition rate tied to the mains frequency are then unsuitable because of the limitations which are implied.

A term that may prove baffling to the insufficiently initiated when it is seen in manufacturer's catalogues is the *interrogation time* of a modern generator: another version is *phase-in time*. It is simply explained as the time which it takes for the generator to 'get the message' or to react or, if you like, to begin or to stop some action in accordance with signals received from the controls. For exposure switching, interrogation time is the time that elapses between the instant when the radiographer presses closed the exposure button and the instant when the X-ray tube starts to pass current. At the end of the exposure, interrogation time is the period that elapses between the instant when the timing circuit signals the end of the exposure and the instant when the flow of current through the X-ray tube actually stops.

With a conventional single-phase generator operating on a 50 hertz mains supply, synchronous exposure switching gives the generator a minimum interrogation time which is the period between two zero points in the cycle of alternation: that is, 0·01 second or 10 milliseconds. With a three-phase generator operating on a 50 hertz mains supply, if it is of the 6 pulse type the interrogation time is 3·3 milliseconds and if the generator is providing 12 pulses for each cycle of mains alternation the interrogation time is further reduced to 1·6 milliseconds.

A generator which provides constant potential with the exposure switching on the secondary side of the high tension transformer can achieve an interrogation time which is close to the zero value. X-ray generators which are to be used for the purposes of angiography when a rapid physiological cycle is to be recorded and for cine filming must be able to switch for very short exposure times and repeat these at rapid rates. For such equipment a long interrogation time is unacceptable and the closer it is to zero the better.

SWITCHING SYSTEMS

Switching in the primary circuit

Mechanical contactors

A long-established form of switching consists of electromagnetic mechanical contactors which are put in the primary circuit of the X-ray set: that is, between the autotransformer (marked Primary Controls in Fig. 5.2) and the primary winding of the high tension transformer (marked High tension generator in Fig. 5.2). The problems of such contactors in modern X-ray sets relate to the facts that X-ray equipment today can be used with very short exposures (a few milliseconds) and that in certain procedures the very short exposure intervals must be repeated at rapid rates. So the exposure switching systems must (i) function quickly and precisely and (ii) be suitable for rapid repetition.

Electromagnetic mechanical contactors require the following properties.
1   They must be spring-loaded so that they close firmly and without
bounce, the spring acting strongly to keep the contact pieces together. If an
exposure contactor bounces, electrical connection for the primary circuit is
momentarily broken and the X-ray exposure is momentarily interrupted.
This effect can be important on very short exposure times.
2   The spring which pulls the contact pieces apart when they are opening
the circuit must be strong so that they open quickly and consistently.
3   Since the contactor operates through moving parts there will be some
inertia associated with it. This means that there will be a small delay before
the contactor can close for the start of the exposure. Similarly there will be a
small delay at the end of the exposure before the contacts actually open the
primary circuit of the high tension transformer. These periods of delay must
be as small as possible. The inertia will be least if the moving parts of the
contactor are small in mass; set against this is the fact that a contactor to
carry a large current cannot be very small and high-powered X-ray sets
which use short times and therefore have the greatest need of least delay in
the operation of exposure contactors are the ones which are the least able to
use contactors which are small in mass. They need contactors which are
robust with large areas of contact.
4   The copper contacts which close to complete the circuit and open to
break it must be strong enough not to become distorted by the continual
positive closure.
5   The contact pieces must be able to withstand high temperatures. They
become hot because they carry current when they are closed and because
when they are slightly apart electric arc discharges (large and sustained
sparks) may pass between them. These arcs can make the contact pieces
very hot indeed. These contacts may be made of a tungsten alloy so that they
are less affected by the arcing which occurs.

It can be seen from the above requirements that these electromagnetic
contactors must be carefully designed and constructed so that some
conflicting requirements are reconciled: the needs for strong springs and
massive parts to be reconciled as satisfactorily as is possible with the needs
for near-instantaneous action and a high repetition rate. These contactors
are today replaced by electronic switches which are without moving parts as
explained below.

Electronic primary switching

An electronic switch widely used as the exposure contactor in the primary
circuits of X-ray sets is of a type which is called a thyristor or silicon-
controlled rectifier (SCR). Thyristors are suitable for switching very big

currents: for example, they can be made to switch 250 A at 500 V and so they can be used in the primary circuits of the 1000 mA and high kilovoltage X-ray generators which are available in diagnostic departments today.

Such switching may sometimes appear in manufacturers' descriptions as 'solid state primary switching' and the manufacturer will certainly point out (with truth) that this form of switching allows very short exposure times to be precisely switched and to be rapidly repeated. The term *solid state* is used in the description because in these switches electrons flow through solid materials as opposed to the flow through gas-filled or evacuated spaces which takes place in triode valves.

Materials used to construct thyristors are the semi-conductors mentioned in Chapter 3 for barrier layer rectifiers. We there concerned ourselves with the following:

1   N-type semi-conductor material in which conductivity is increased by increasing the number of free electrons;

2   P-type semi-conductor material in which conductivity is increased by increasing the number of vacancies or holes where electrons should be;

3   the fact that a device constructed with a layer of N-type material and a layer of P-type material laid together has a barrier at the P–N interface which stops electron flow in the P to N direction, the device being connected to a voltage source so that the N-type layer is positive in regard to the P-type layer; if the connection is the other way round so that the P-type material is positive in regard to the N-type material, then the barrier breaks and electrons flow from the N layer to the P layer. It is the barrier at the P–N interface which makes the device act as a rectifier.

For the barrier–layer rectifiers discussed in Chapter 3, the construction is of two layers. There is one N-type layer and one P-type layer. The thyristor is a more elaborate construction and has four layers: these are two N layers and two P layers.

The four layers of construction are depicted in Fig. 5.4 and, as the diagram shows, the arrangement can be p n p n or n p n p. A circuit symbol for a thyristor is shown in the diagram beside the sketches of the construction. In this circuit symbol, electrons can be considered to flow into the point of the arrow from the barrier layer drawn below it.

Since thyristors are made up of four layers, a thyristor has three interfaces or barrier layers; this may be contrasted with the one interface of the junction diode. We must consider how electrons may be made to pass through a thyristor, and let us take the n p n p thyristor first.

In Fig. 5.4(a) electrons can move from the left of the diagram and travel from n layer to p layer; but they are prevented from passing through the thyristor from one end to the other by the barrier at the pn interface. They can, however, be made to flow by injecting 'holes' or positive charge into

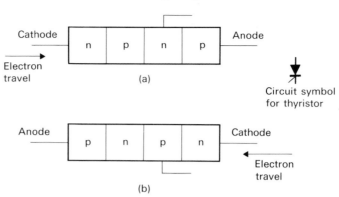

Fig. 5.4

the n zone—the third zone from the left in the diagram we have depicted in Fig. 5.4(a). Because the polarity of this third section operates to let electrons through or not to let them through, it is called appropriately enough a gate.

Similarly with the pnpn thyristor in Fig. 5.4(b) electrons can move from the right of the diagram and travel from n layer to p layer; but they cannot pass through the thyristor from end to end by reason of the barrier at the pn interface. They can be made to flow by injecting electrons into the p zone or gate—again the third zone from the left in Fig. 5.4(b).

Thus for both these sorts of thyristor it is possible to initiate current flow by passing another current into an intermediate zone called the gate. So a thyristor can be changed from an open switch to a closed switch very easily and extremely quickly by passing current into the gate region.

Fig. 5.5 is a block diagram to indicate arrangements for thyristors acting as exposure switches. It shows the location of the thyristors on the primary side of the high tension generator. Since a thyristor, when it can pass current, must pass it in one direction only and the ac mains and auto-transformer voltages are of course alternating, the requirement is a pair of thyristors connected back to back as in Fig. 5.6 or a similar device called a triac which can pass current in both directions.

From the block diagram in Fig. 5.5 it can be seen that if the thyristors are on 'open circuit' (that is, with the barriers at pn interfaces existing to block electron flow) no current will flow in the primary circuit of the high tension generator and the exposure cannot start. The diagram in Fig. 5.5 indicates links between the exposure pushbutton, the timer circuit and the gate circuits of the thyristors. When the exposure pushbutton is pushed through to 'Expose', there is almost instantaneous response in the gate circuits of the thyristors: the delay is about 1 millisecond. Through this

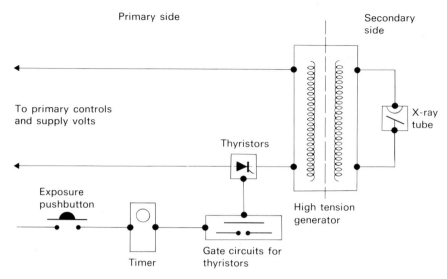

Fig. 5.5

response of the gate circuits, the barriers at pn interfaces are broken and electrons at once can flow through the thyristors from one end to the other. The thyristors then are acting as closed switches and the exposure begins.

Towards the end of the required exposure time, the timer circuit operates to achieve, through the gate circuits, another response: the opposite response which makes the thyristors return to the open circuit state and the exposure stops.

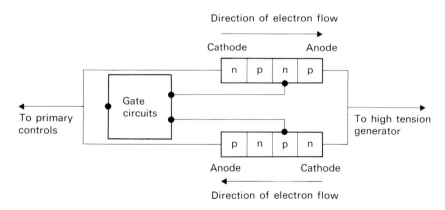

Fig. 5.6

Thyristors in phased switching

The requirements for phased switching are that the exposure must start (thyristors become conductive and pass current) and the exposure must stop (thyristors become nonconductive and block current-flow) only at zero voltage points in the mains cycle of alternation. It is arranged to phase the beginning of the exposure to a zero voltage point by feeding current to the thyristor gates from a special pulsing transformer which provides an output voltage only at the start of each half-cycle.

The sequence is indicated in Fig. 5.7. When the exposure pushbutton is pressed (at whatever point in the cycle-time of the mains) at the *next* point of zero voltage the pulsing transformer provides voltage and current for the gate circuits of the thyristors and the thyristors instantaneously become closed switches. The exposure begins.

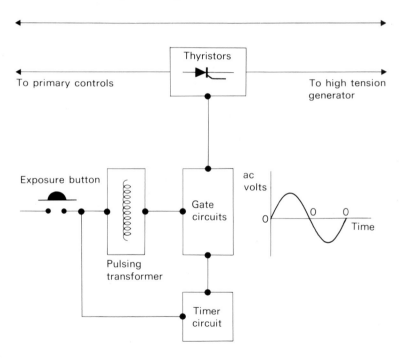

Fig. 5.7

Once current is flowing through the thyristors, it cannot be stopped by re-imposing the barriers of pn interfaces. It *can* be stopped by (i) bringing the anode voltages down to zero or (ii) opening the anode circuits. In the X-ray equipment which we are considering, the alternations of the ac mains bring the thyristor anode voltages down to zero at the end of every half-cycle and this fact is used to stop the exposure. The sequence of events is as follows.

Just before the end of the exposure time, the supply to the gate circuits of the thyristors is removed through the timer circuit. Whichever of the back-to-back thyristors is passing current continues to do so until, at the next zero point in the cycle, its anode voltage becomes zero. At that instant it ceases to conduct and becomes an open switch. The exposure stops.

Thyristors in unsynchronized switching

In the immediately preceding paragraphs we have described how the exposure may be controlled by means of thyristors which have their actions synchronized so that they occur at zero voltage points in the voltage waveform of the mains supply. Such systems imply that the repetition rates and the duration of exposures must be related to the mains frequency.

Modern equipment features methods by which the exposure may be initiated and terminated at instants which are unrelated to the mains cycle of change and may be at any points in the voltage waveform. Such a divorce, which frees the exposure time from the limits imposed by its marriage to the mains frequency, must allow more choice of exposure times at the short-time end of the range. This is most advantageous and in some applications essential if the equipment is to be used for the following: angiography with rapid serial film changers; serial filming from an image intensifier; use of automatic exposure controls; use of fast recording systems such as rare earth screens and films with high speed.

The technique used to make the exposure *begin without waiting* for the point of zero voltage in the mains cycle is called *pulsed commutation* (or rectification) *plus high speed electronic precontacting*. The technique used to make the exposure *end without waiting* for the point of zero voltage in the mains cycle is called *forced extinction*. It is not important that radiographers should remember these terms. It *is* important that, as knowledgeable operators of the equipment, they should know the following facts:

1   that thyristors can be made capable of unsynchronized switching;

2   that unsynchronized switching can reduce interrogation time down to 1 to 2 milliseconds for the beginning of the exposure and to almost the zero value for the exposure's end;

3   that unsynchronized switching allows the shortest available exposure times to be down to 1 to 2 milliseconds;

4   that unsynchronized switching allows repetition rates to be unrelated to the mains frequency.

Switching in the secondary high tension circuit

Exposure-switching devices inserted directly in the high tension circuit must be wholly electronic and they must be vacuum valve devices. Other methods for switching currents at very high voltages are not available.

Triode valves as switches

A method used for secondary-side switching is the placing of special triode valves in the circuit of the X-ray tube as indicated in Fig. 5.8. These triode valves are particularly designed to act as electronic switches operating at high kilovoltages (say, up to 150 kV) and they directly close at the start of the exposure and open at the end of the exposure the circuit of the X-ray tube itself: thus the electrons flowing through the X-ray tube are provided with a continuous pathway in the high tension circuit for the duration of the exposure and at the end of the required exposure-time the continuity is broken and the current-flow stops.

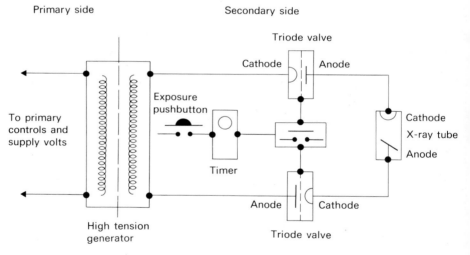

Fig. 5.8

A triode valve of this type has a cathode which is an electron source by thermionic emission (exactly comparable with the function of the filament of an X-ray tube); an anode which is a receiver of the electron stream from the cathode (as is the anode of an X-ray tube); an interior vacuum (as an X-ray tube has); a third electrode, called a grid, which takes the form of a wire situated close to the cathode and functions to control the operation of the triode valve.

The source of the control is the voltage on the grid. When this voltage (called the grid bias voltage) is sufficiently negative with respect to the cathode, no electrons can pass through the grid and the triode valve is nonconductive: it is an open or OFF switch. If the negative grid bias voltage is reduced, a point is reached at which the restraint of the grid ceases and the triode valve becomes instantly conductive: it is a closed or ON switch. Thus the triode valves can be made to function as switches and are controlled through electrical characteristics of their grid circuits: this functioning is comparable with the control of thyristors through their gate circuits as earlier described.

For the triode valves an important point is that they can do more than just act as switches opened and closed; they can be used to absorb different values of voltage by alteration to their grid voltages; thus they can be used as voltage-stabilizing devices. These triodes may therefore be used in high tension circuits in which they have more than one function to perform— that is they (a) switch the circuit and (b) may act also to stabilize kilovoltage. This is described in more detail on page 123. Here it may be said in general terms that control valves in the secondary circuit of the high tension transformer may be used:

1   just as switches to apply to the X-ray tube one or more half-waves of rectified high voltage, or a fraction of one half-wave;
2   as switches and as voltage-stabilizing devices so that the kilovoltage applied to the X-ray tube is stabilized by the control valves which also switch the high tension circuit.

Triode valves acting as switches in the high tension circuit and as stabilizers for the tube voltage may be used in a twelve-pulse three-phase generator (Chapter 3, pages 121–124). Very short exposures become possible with such an arrangement, and they can be as short as a fraction of a millisecond.

Grid controlled X-ray tube

In the previous section some features of the high tension triode valve were likened to those of an X-ray tube: the cathode, the anode, the vacuum. So it is not entirely surprising to learn that an X-ray tube can be converted to a triode by the insertion of a control grid: this is mentioned in Chapter 7 on page 270. When this is done, the X-ray tube is itself acting as a switch. At the beginning of the exposure it provides a continuous pathway for its own flow of electrons (that is, it closes the high tension circuit as if it were a switch turned ON) by becoming conductive through change in the negative bias voltage on its grid: at the end of the exposure it becomes non-conductive, again through the grid bias voltage, and it instantaneously opens the high tension circuit (as if it were a switch turned OFF) and the exposure stops.

It is a method of exposure switching that gives precise control for very short exposures of a few milliseconds only. Fig. 5.9 is a block diagram to indicate arrangements.

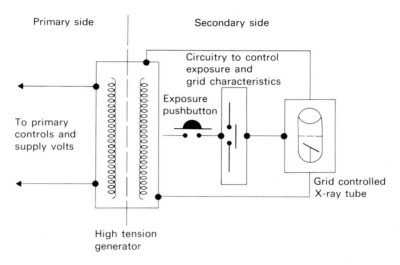

Fig. 5.9

TIMING SYSTEMS

There are many timing devices applied to many procedures in industry, science and ordinary domestic and social life. They range from an item as simple as a sand-glass for use in the kitchen to instruments as sophisticated as a navigator's chronometer for use at sea or an electronic clock.

Choice of timing devices for any particular task takes account of the accuracy which is required. If it is unnecessary for a timer to be extremely accurate, then a simple device will do; if a high degree of accuracy is needed then the timing device must be more complex and of course also more expensive. As already explained, a timing device for control of the duration of X-ray exposures is chosen with regard to the type of X-ray set in which it is to be used. With low-powered X-ray sets, radiographers will employ exposure times of which many will be over 1·0 second. Small inaccuracies will not be a significant proportion of these intervals, so the timing mechanism is a simple one. With medium and high powered X-ray sets radiographers can use exposure times which are very short and minimum time intervals will be down to 0·01 second and to a millisecond or less in some cases. The timer used for these intervals must have a high degree of accuracy, for small errors are too great a proportion of the exposure period; an error of 0·01 second is 100 per cent of an exposure time of 0·01 second. So high-powered X-ray sets have more precise timers.

In older X-ray equipment were types of timer which are now ceasing to be used. Small portable and dental sets had clockwork timers in which a spring provided the motive power for the timer movement. Major X-ray sets had timers capable of more accurate timing than the simple clockwork mechanism could provide. These were worked by electromagnetic devices, the drive for moving parts being provided by an electric motor running in synchronization with the mains supply.

Student radiographers studying modern X-ray equipment need not concern themselves with the older types of timer since new apparatus is fitted with electronic timing circuits which are to be described.

Electronic timers

The basis of nearly all electronic timers is the charging and discharging of a capacitor. If a capacitor is charged from a dc source, the time taken for it to become fully charged depends on the resistance in the charging circuit; by varying this resistance the charging time can be altered. Little resistance implies a short charging time; higher resistance makes the charging time longer.

Similarly, if a previously charged capacitor is put into a circuit through which it discharges, the time taken for the discharge depends on the resistance of the circuit. Low resistance results in a rapid discharge and higher resistance increases the time that discharge takes.

These facts allow a time interval to be altered by selecting different values of resistance for a circuit which has in it a capacitor. So it is easy to see that such arrangements might be used to make a timer for the X-ray exposure. A radiographer selecting a time-interval on an electronic timer is in fact selecting a value of resistance in a circuit through which to charge or discharge a capacitor.

Fig. 5.10 is a block diagram which shows the following items related to each other:

1 capacitor circuitry;
2 timer resistance circuitry;
3 an exposure pushbutton.

A charging capacitor

If a timer is to operate through the charging of a capacitor, the important sequential points are as below:

1 the capacitor is fully discharged before the exposure;

2 pressing the pushbutton through to EXPOSE achieves simultaneously (a) closure of the exposure switching circuit (in Fig. 5.10 thyristors through their gates) so that the X-ray tube is energized and the exposure begins and (b) connection of the capacitor to its charging source through the selected resistance;

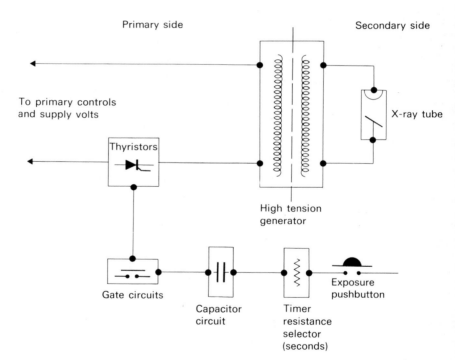

Fig. 5.10

3 from the instant of its connection to its charging source, the capacitor has increasing charge and a rising voltage;

4 when the voltage has risen to a specific value, the exposure stops;

5 the time that elapses before this specific value is reached is altered through the selected resistance. If the resistance is low the capacitor charges to the required level in a shorter time.

A discharging capacitor

If a timer operates through the discharge of a capacitor, the important sequential points are as below:

1   the capacitor is fully charged before the exposure;
2   pressing the pushbutton through to EXPOSE achieves simultaneously (a) closure of the exposure switching circuit (in Fig. 5.10 thyristors through their gates) so that the X-ray tube is energized and the exposure begins and (b) connection of the charged capacitor to the selected resistance through which it begins to discharge;
3   from the instant of its connection to the resistance, the capacitor is losing charge and has a falling voltage;
4   when the voltage has fallen to a specific value, the exposure stops;
5   the time that elapses before this specific value is reached is altered through the selected resistance. If the resistance is low the capacitor discharges to the required level in a shorter time.

Terminating the exposure

The block diagrams in Figs 5.5 and 5.7 show an exposure switching system which consists of thyristors on the primary side of the high tension generator which are controlled through their gate circuits. The exposure begins after pressure on the pushbutton energizes the gate circuits and the thyristors become conductive: that is, they act as closed or ON switches.

In order to make voltage on a capacitor terminate the exposure, the circuitry is arranged so that a specific voltage across the capacitor circuit at once cuts off the supply to the gate circuits. The specific value of voltage required can be achieved, as we have seen, through a process either of a rising voltage as a capacitor charges or of a falling voltage as a capacitor discharges.

With the supply to the gate circuits cut off, the thyristors cease to pass current at the next zero point in the ac mains cycle since this brings their anode voltages also to zero (as we described for phased thyristor switching on page 170). Nonconductive thyristors are effectively open or OFF switches and the exposure stops.

Automatic timers

The timing so far considered ensures that the X-ray exposure is terminated after a given period of time. Automatic timers which are to be described now are quite different in that their use terminates the exposure after a given amount of radiation has reached the film—that is when the film has received a certain dose. Radiographers controlling the electrical factors of the X-ray exposure are not in fact controlling the exposure dose to the film: they *are* controlling the radiation emitted from the X-ray tube, but they cannot control the dose which the film receives because they cannot measure or control the absorptive effect of the interposed patient.

Concerning this very important factor of absorption in the patient, radiographers can only make an inspired guess backed by their knowledge and previous experience. Various systems to aid guess-work have been used—such as measuring the thickness of the part to be radiographed or taking the patient's body-weight as a guide in estimating capacity for absorbing X rays. But a well-developed child and an old man might be the same weight and their limbs might be the same size; but they would be very different as absorbers of X rays. Twins might have the same chest measurements and be the same weight, but one could have a dense hemithorax from the presence of fluid arising from injury or disease; they would look very different to a beam of X rays even if alike to the observer. The radiographer might be sufficiently informed to be able to predict the presence of the fluid but could make only a subjective estimate as to its probable absorptive effect. So in the end these systems can do no better than reduce the amount of guesswork which is necessary; they cannot eliminate it entirely.

An automatic timer overcomes the difficulties of varying absorption in the patient because the exposure is terminated only when the film has received that dose of radiation necessary to give it the required range of densities after processing. If the timer is properly used and is functioning correctly, all radiographs should receive standardized exposure and be 'correctly exposed'.

Together with automatic processing, automatic timing devices are a valuable aid to maintaining a radiographic standard which is consistently high, particularly in busy departments staffed by many radiographers with different amounts of experience. Automatic timers were first applied many years ago in chest surveys by fluorography (mass miniature radiography) and they are now being used in general departments.

Radiographs are repeated because of dissatisfaction attributable to the following:
1   faulty or incorrectly used equipment;
2   poor positioning of the patient;
3   movement of the subject;
4   over- or under-exposure;
5   film artefacts;
6   processing errors.

Malpositioning and misjudgements on the exposure are the common causes for repeat radiographs. The misjudgements may be eliminated by the use of the automatic control of exposure which is given by automatic timers (autotimers).

Automatic timers all employ similar principles. Their essential components are indicated in a block diagram in Fig. 5.11 and are as follows.

1   A device to monitor the amount of radiation which reaches the film during the X-ray exposure.

2   An arrangement by which the magnitude of a small current flowing in a circuit can be made proportional to the intensity of radiation which reaches the film during the X-ray exposure.

3   An arrangement by which a predetermined charge (milliampereseconds) which passes by reason of this small current can be related to an exposure dose to the film such that the radiograph, having received this

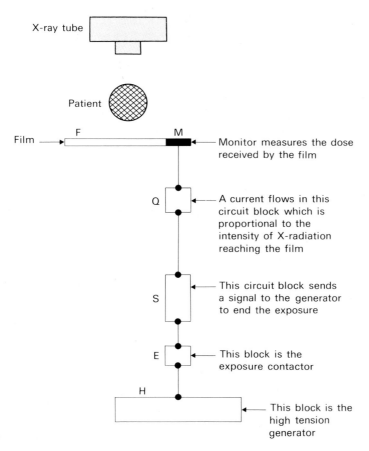

Fig. 5.11

dose, is 'correctly exposed'. 'Correct exposure' means that all the densities in the radiograph are within the useful density range of the diagnostic radiographic image.

4   A circuit arrangement which, once the predetermined value of charge has passed, sends a signal to the exposure contactor of the generator so that the exposure is ended.

In Fig. 5.11, the X-ray tube and the patient are seen at the top of the diagram. Beneath the patient is the film which is to receive an image and also a monitor or detector is there to measure the intensity of the X radiation which reaches the film. In the diagram the film and the detector are shown in the same plane. In practice this is not so: the detectors may be just in front of the film, in which case they are called entrance type detectors because they monitor the radiation on its way to the film; or they may be just at the back of the film, in which case they are called exit types because they monitor the radiation after it has passed through the film. By putting the detectors and the film in the same plane in the diagram we hoped to make it stand for both entrances and exits.

In Fig. 5.11 block Q indicates a circuit where a small current flows which is proportional to the intensity of the radiation reaching the film: so a certain charge is passed. We call this charge Q millicoulombs in this explanation, or Q milliampereseconds since they are equivalent quantities. If the intensity of the radiation reaching the film is low, the current flowing in the circuit is very small and it will take a longer time before a charge of Q millicoulombs is achieved. If the intensity of the radiation reaching the film is higher, the current flowing in the circuit is greater in value and a charge of Q millicoulombs is reached in a shorter time.

The arrangements are set up so that the dose which the film must receive for correct exposure is equated with the charge of Q millicoulombs passed in the block marked Q in fig. 5.11. This means that at the instant when the charge of Q millicoulombs is achieved, the film has received just that amount of energy from the irradiating X-ray beam as is necessary to produce an image with the required range of densities after processing. As soon as Q millicoulombs are achieved, there is a reaction in the circuit block marked S in Fig. 5.11. A signal is sent to the exposure contactor (exposure switch) of the high tension generator and the exposure terminates.

So automatic control of the exposure is achieved. If there is high absorption of X rays in the subject, there is low intensity of radiation received by the detector; the resultant current passed is low in value; the exposure time is extended longer before the predetermined charge (which will stop the exposure) is achieved. If there is low absorption of X rays in the subject, there is higher intensity of radiation received by the detector; the resultant current passed is higher in value; the exposure time required for the predetermined charge to pass is shorter and the exposure stops at the end of a briefer interval. Thus the duration of the exposure in time is adjusted automatically to different types of subject and the radiographs receive the same exposure dose: this is the dose equated with a predetermined charge of millicoulombs in the circuitry of the automatic control.

From the foregoing explanation it can be seen that very important elements in automatic timers are those devices which detect the radiation and as a result can send a small current flowing in a circuit. These devices are of two basic types as follows:

1   those which essentially are ionization chambers and pass a small current between their electrodes when they are irradiated by an X-ray beam (these may be described as the ionization types of automatic timers);

2   those which are based on a response to light-intensity (these may be described as photo-timers). The method used is to allow the X-ray beam to irradiate a fluorescent material and then to feed the light which is produced to a photoelectric device which measures the intensity of the light. This device passes a current which is proportional to the intensity of the light (itself proportional to the intensity of the X rays irradiating the fluorescent material).

In the past automatic timers using ionization chambers have been able to provide shorter times of exposure than could the photoelectric type but some modern phototimers have been developed which give very short exposure periods. Other developments in automatic timing are:

1   the use of specially shaped detector fields for mammography;

2   equipment suitable for mobile sets;

3   automatic timing applied to tomography.

An ionization timer

Automatic timers which make use of an ionization current are being used in equipment for general diagnostic radiography. In such timers, the X radiation reaching the film passes through an ionization chamber; the action of the X rays is of course to ionize the air contained within the chamber.

If a potential difference is maintained between the electrodes of the ionization chamber by connecting them to a source of voltage, and if the ionization chamber forms part of a complete circuit, then when the air in the chamber is ionized by exposure to X rays an ionization current flows in the circuit associated with the chamber. As any radiographer should know, the magnitude of this ionization current is dependent on the intensity of the radiation reaching the ionization chamber.

So it is possible to set up a circuit in which a small current varies with the effective intensity of the radiation reaching a film. The ionization chambers used are very thin, the construction of the detector fields being of aluminium foil or lead foil. They are put in front of the film as shown in Fig. 5.12 so that the dose received by the chamber and the dose received by the film are nearly enough the same. That they are not exactly the same does not really matter, for the film dose is proportional to the chamber dose.

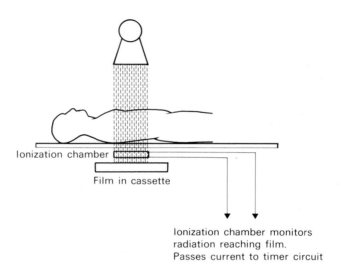

Ionization chamber

Film in cassette

Ionization chamber monitors radiation reaching film. Passes current to timer circuit

Fig. 5.12

The very small current passed by the ionization chamber is amplified and can be used to send a signal to the generator to stop the exposure. A block diagram is shown in Fig. 5.13. The ionization chambers have low absorption and they monitor the film area. In an X-ray table they are mounted in the bucky assembly as entrance-type detectors: they are being reached by radiation as it passes towards the film.

They must not be very thick since the installation of large chambers would keep the patient–film distance too great. The chambers must also not impose any shadow on the X-ray film. Upright bucky stands and stands for chest radiography can equally well be fitted with ionization chambers if the X-ray department uses this type of timer for the whole range of its work. Tube to film distances used should be at least 1 metre (40 inches) to compensate for the increased patient-film distance.

The type of ionization chamber which will be encountered has a thin aluminium outer wall and has three detector fields—that is three areas where

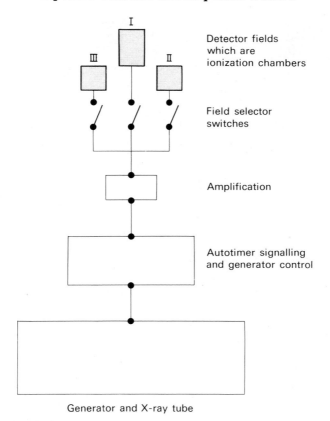

Fig. 5.13

the dose is measured. These are arranged as one central and two lateral fields as seen in Fig. 5.14. The fields are all of the same surface area, which is about 50 cm², but they are not of the same dimensions, the central one being longer and narrower than the other two.

Push buttons on the control panel (Fig. 5.15) of the timer enable the radiographer to select which of the three detector fields is to be used; choice will be determined by the particular X-ray examination which is being undertaken.

Upright buckys or chest stands have the situation of the three fields marked upon their front covers. For the X-ray table the position of the fields can be indicated by the insertion of a plastic plate in the beam from the light-beam diaphragm. This plate is inscribed so that when the tube-column and the bucky are coupled together and the light-beam is switched on, the location of the measuring fields is projected on to the patient's body surface

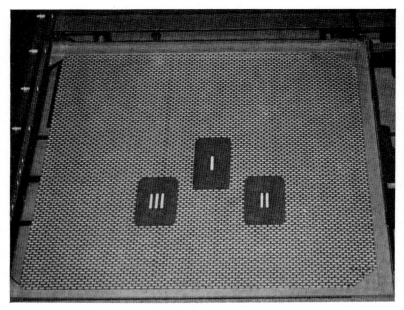

Fig. 5.14 Detector fields in an automatic timer of the ionization type. *Illustration by courtesy of* Radiography, *The Journal of the College of Radiographers.*

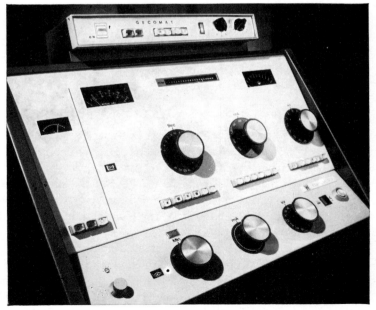

Fig. 5.15 The controls for an automatic timer are here seen on a small panel across the top of the console. *By courtesy of Picker International Ltd.*

which is uppermost to the light. The patient must be very carefully positioned in relation to the field used. Once the detector chamber is selected and the patient positioned relative to it, the bucky tray must not be moved. The film may be moved up and down in the tray. It is not essential for the central X-ray beam to be over the detector chamber which is being used.

A photomultiplier phototimer

The basis of a phototimer is a system which responds to the intensity of a light which reaches it and allows the light to be coupled to a photomultiplier tube which can convert the light signal to an electrical signal. In a photomultiplier tube the energy of the light photons is transferred as energy given to electrons and an electric current is passed.

The photomultiplier tube is a vacuum tube with a glass envelope and it contains several electrodes, the first being a photoemissive cathode. Other electrodes (called dynodes) emit electrons when they are bombarded by electrons; there may be 9 or 10 of these dynodes in the tube. The first dynode is positive in relation to the photoemissive cathode and each succeeding dynode is at a higher positive potential than its immediate predecessor. The last electrode is the anode.

The photomultiplier functions in this way. Electrons emitted by the photo-emissive cathode as a result of the action of light are accelerated by the electrostatic field within the envelope, and they impinge on the first dynode. For every electron which the first dynode receives, a specific multiple of electrons is emitted—say × 8. The electrons emitted by the first dynode are accelerated to the second dynode, and again a specific multiple of electrons is emitted for every electron received. This process continues as the electrons travel from dynode to dynode, and the repeated multiplications result in a number of electrons arriving at the last electrode (the anode) which is much bigger than the number emitted by the cathode in the first place. So the final current from the anode can be a few milliamperes when the original emission at the first cathode was such as to be only a minute fraction of a microampere. The total multiplication factor is obviously related to the emission factor of each dynode and to the number of dynodes and it may be of the order of 1000 million.

Phototimers in fluorography

A photomultiplier tube such as is described above can be used to give automatic exposure control for radiographic systems in which the film is recording solely a visible light image: that is to say, in fluorographic systems. Fluorographic systems in X-ray departments today are in two categories as follows: (i) those in which the film to be exposed is receiving an image from an X-ray image intensifier used for fluoroscopy; (ii) those in which the film to be exposed is receiving an image which is focused by means of a mirror lens in a fluorographic camera unit.

Fig. 5.16 is a block diagram to show the sequence in fluorography with an image intensifier. When the X-ray tube is energized the emission from the image intensifier is a visible light image displayed by the output phosphor. This visible image is received by an image distributor which splits the light, so that part goes to a television pick-up tube for subsequent display on its associated monitor; and part goes to a spot-film camera which has an optical system and a film to which the image is focused. In Fig. 5.16 a photomultiplier tube is shown just in front of the camera. It is an entrance-type detector since it measures the intensity of the light which is passing to the film. The photomultiplier tube responds to the intensity of the light which is coming from the image intensifier. When the film has received sufficient light-energy to ensure that it is correctly exposed, the photomultiplier tube signals to the generator-control and the exposure stops.

Fig. 5.17 shows the arrangement in a mirror camera unit which is being used for chest radiography. When the X-ray tube is energized a visible

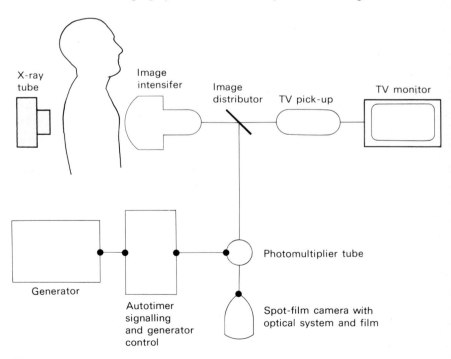

Fig. 5.16

image is produced on the fluorescent screen. This light-image is focused by the mirror lens of the camera to a film held in the focal plane. The diagram shows a photomultiplier tube located where it can monitor the intensity of the light emitted by the fluorescent screen. The photomultiplier tube is an entrance-type detector since it measures the intensity of the light which has yet to reach the film. The light coming from the fluorescent screen can of course be equated with the intensity of the light which is reaching the film since the two intensities are effectively the same and in fact close to each other in value. When the film has received sufficient light-energy to ensure that it is correctly exposed, the photomultiplier tube sends the signal which is transmitted to the generator and the exposure stops.

Phototimers in direct radiography

Phototimers can be used in conventional systems for direct radiography: that is, with the use of X-ray films held in cassettes with intensifying screens

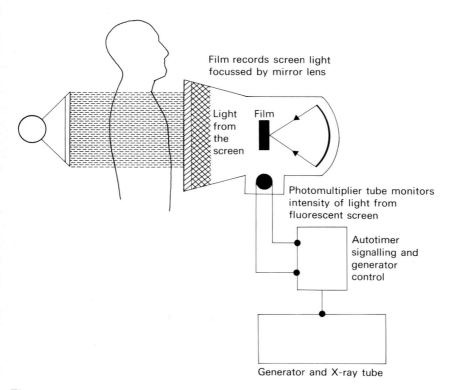

Fig. 5.17

in the standard practice. For such an application, the detectors used with photomultiplier tubes may be exit-type detectors which receive radiation *after* it has reached and has energized the film. This arrangement implies the need to control the radioabsorptiveness of the backs of cassettes since it is a prime requirement that the radiation energy which is reaching the film during the exposure must be in practice equatable with the radiation energy which is reaching the detector field located behind the cassette.

Alternatively the detectors may be the entrance-type and thus any problem connected with the control of absorption in the back of the cassette is evaded.

The detectors are often made of lucite, which is a material capable of transmitting light as can a fibre-optic bundle: the sheets of lucite used are known as lucite paddles. The lucite is covered in black paper except for any area which is to be used as a detector field for the X rays. So that it may function as a detector of radiation, the lucite in these areas is coated with a phosphor which will emit light when it is irradiated with X rays. The intensity of the emitted light is of course proportional to the intensity of X radiation which is reaching the phosphor coat of the lucite paddle.

The lucite transmits the light to an output region which is called (reasonably enough) a light gate. This light gate leads to a photomultiplier tube which measures the intensity of the light coming from the phosphor of the detector field and converts the received light-energy to a usable electric signal. The sequence is given in Fig. 5.18 which includes a link between the photomultiplier tube and the generator control which functions to stop the exposure. Fig. 5.18 has a single detector field and light gate: in practice when the phototimer is of the entrance-type, three detector fields are usually present (as is indicated in Fig. 5.19) each field being about 1000 square millimetres. The fields each have individual light gates to which the lucite transmits the light from the phosphor coat on the detector area.

Using switches on the control console, the radiographer can select fields in arrangements up to a total of seven. Referring to Fig. 5.19, the possibilities are as follows:

1   A only;
2   B only;
3   C only;
4   A and B;
5   B and C;
6   A and C;
7   A and B and C.

If the radiographer has choices over such a range, there is obviously also a greater scope for suitable positioning of the patient and of the area under examination relative to the operating detector fields.

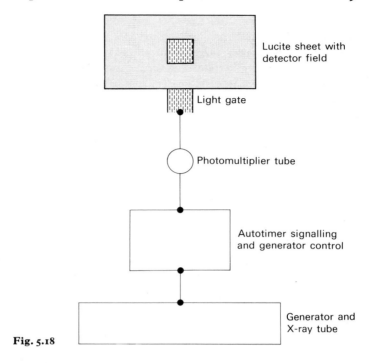

Lucite sheet with detector field

Light gate

Photomultiplier tube

Autotimer signalling and generator control

Generator and X-ray tube

Fig. 5.18

Missing from Fig. 5.19 is any photomultiplier tube to be a sensor of the light from the light gates. In practice there may be only one photomultiplier tube receiving light from all three gates or each gate may have assigned to it an individual photomultiplier tube. A single photomultiplier tube is electronically less troublesome than three tubes, for each is sensitive to changes in its power supply and clearly it takes more time and trouble to get three such tubes functioning precisely than to maintain one only in the required consistent performance. If a single photomultiplier tube is used for

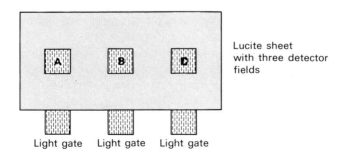

Lucite sheet with three detector fields

Light gate   Light gate   Light gate

Fig. 5.19

three gates, however, there are other problems associated with mechanical difficulties in connecting three light gates to one photomultiplier tube. So there is no 'right answer' to the question: is it better to have three tubes or one? If there are three tubes and three gates there is electronic multiplicity to give problems; if there is one tube and three gates there are mechanical problems. This is why we stopped Fig. 5.19 short at the light gates!

Phototimers which are of the exit-type usually have one (larger) detector field, one light gate and of course one photomultiplier tube. Not unexpectedly, such singleness in the components makes the equipment less costly to buy and simpler to maintain. But obviously the use of a single field makes demands more exacting on the radiographer's skill in positioning if the automatic control of exposure is to give consistent and acceptable results.

Practical considerations in automatic timers

Any automatic timer (automatic exposure control) is intended to provide radiographs which are 'correctly' exposed and show a range of densities which are all diagnostically useful. When such timers are operating correctly and are properly used, they can be expected to achieve the required results repeatedly. In considering the performance of an automatic timer, the question asked is 'Are the radiographs correctly exposed?' and so the standard set for the timer's performance may be expressed in terms of reproducible image densities.

Testing an automatic timer

Performance of an automatic timer might be tested by radiographing a stepwedge as follows.

1   Use a stepwedge large enough to cover the detector field which is selected and place it over the detector.
2   Choose settings of kilovoltage and milliamperes which will give a short exposure time: for example, 0·05 second.
3   Make five radiographic exposures for the stepwedge with the settings unchanged, so that five separate images are obtained.
4   Process and compare the images which result. The five should match in density step for step. Variation can be accepted if it is not more than a plus/minus 10 per cent change in density; or a variation which is not greater than one step of density on the stepwedge images.

An automatic exposure control should of course provide consistent results whether the exposure time is long or short. The previous test can be used just as well for long exposures if the settings are adjusted to give a time which is about 1 second.

The use of automatic control of exposure

There are a number of important technical factors to be considered when an automatic exposure control is used. If these are not fully appreciated there may be dissatisfaction with the results obtained and the timer may be falsely accused of incorrect operation. We enumerate the main considerations below.

1   Any radiograph has a dominant area and if that is 'correctly exposed' the rest will be satisfactory too. So the dominant area should be the one monitored by the detector field.

2   If three fields are provided, the following considerations apply:

(a) for paired structures such as kidneys, hips, lungs, select a lateral field;

(b) for the spine and skull, choose the central field;

(c) for the chest, choice of the central field gives a radiograph correctly exposed for the mediastinal region; choice of one of the lateral fields (preferably that on the patient's right to avoid the heart shadow) results in correct exposure for the lung fields; if there is a lesion on one side which is so radioabsorptive as to show an undifferentiated white shadow in a conventionally exposed radiograph, then selection of the central detector field or a lateral one positioned in relation to the lesion should give adequate exposure for a study of the lesion.

3   If only one field is provided, the patient must be positioned in relation to it with the above considerations in mind.

4   The region of interest must be placed over the detector field which is used. If a lateral projection of the thorax is for the lung fields, then that part of the patient's trunk must be over the detector area; if it is for the thoracic spine, then the patient must be placed so that the vertebral bodies cover the detector field.

5   Scattered radiation reaching the detector field must be a minimum. The detectors find no difference between scattered radiation and useful, image-forming rays and the exposure will stop when a certain dose has reached the film. If only a small proportion of this dose is image-forming, the radiograph will be lacking in detail.

6   If the detector field is not completely covered by the part of the patient under examination, some direct radiation may reach the measuring area. This will increase the dose to the measuring area while not assisting to produce the image. The exposure will end before the area of diagnostic interest in the radiograph is fully exposed.

7   If a feature which absorbs X rays very heavily is over the detector, the dose to the measuring field will be diminished and this can result in the exposure lasting too long so that other areas in the radiograph will be over-

exposed. Examples of heavily absorptive features are: a hollow organ filled with barium sulphate; a metal replacement for a femoral head; a metal plate in a bone.

8   The X-ray beam must cover an area which is larger than the detector.

9   Screens, films and cassettes must be carefully matched so that the automatic exposure control operates for a consistently standardized recording system.

10   If the detectors used are of the exit-type, the absorption characteristics of the backs of cassettes become especially important.

11   If automatic exposure control is to be used for a wide range of examinations, equipment which provides three detector fields of the entrance-type is the best choice, whether the detection is by ionization chambers or photomultiplier tubes. A single-field photomultiplier timer (this will be of the exit-type) can serve well in a bucky table with its use restricted to skeletal radiography. For a camera unit used for chest radiography, a single-field photomultiplier tube is an obvious choice.

EXPOSURE-SWITCHING AND ITS RADIOGRAPHIC APPLICATIONS

It may be of help to the student if we end this chapter with a brief summary of the methods of exposure switching and exposure timing which have been discussed. To the practising radiographer it may seem unimportant to know how the timing and switching are done; but the fact remains that the different systems have limitations in their radiographic usefulness, and well-informed radiographers should certainly know about these aspects. So we include here some reference to the applications of the different methods.

Exposure contactors can operate:

1   in the primary circuit of the X-ray generator in the forms of

(a) mechanical electromagnetic contactors, which are virtually obsolete;

(b) electronic contactors which are thyristors (silicon controlled rectifiers);

2   in the secondary circuit (X-ray tube circuit) of the generator in the forms of

(a) vacuum triode valves (high tension);

(b) grid-control in X-ray tubes.

Exposure contactors may be:

1   synchronized to the mains frequency (phased) in which case the minimum periods of time and the fastest repetition rates available must be related to the mains frequency;

2   not synchronized and so unrelated to the mains frequency, in which case the minimum periods of time available can be very short and the repetition

rates very high. For angiography with rapid serial film changers which use repetition rates up to 12 per second and in pulsed cine filming with exposure rates up to 80 per second (or more), unsynchronized exposures are essential.

Exposure control (timing) may be done by means of:

1   an electronic timer;
2   an automatic exposure control which may be
    (a) a phototimer with photomultiplier tube(s);
    (b) an ionization type of timer.

Chapter 6
Logics

In many respects, diagnostic X-ray equipment has moved away from electro-mechanical engineering and now—very much to the advantage of those who use it—depends increasingly upon electronic technology. On the control desk, the digital display replaces the less emphatic statement of the milliampere-seconds meter. Within the console, logic circuits perform the functions of electromagnetic relays many times faster and more efficiently.

These advances in the equipment which they use do not mean that radiographers are obliged to become computer chiefs and experts in electronics. Nevertheless, in a book which professes to help radiographers understand diagnostic X-ray equipment some reference to these matters is necessary. To this end, as a first step we have to explain the title of this chapter.

One of the troubles besetting such seekers of acquaintance with computers is a language barrier, which the very familiarity of the words themselves does little to breech. Simple well-known words—or words very like them—are used with particular, highly esoteric and unknown sense in a convenient shorthand. The jargon puzzles us the more by its overlay of commonplace associations. An example is the word which appears at the head of this chapter.

For the present we are to forget that 'logic' is the broad science of thought and reasoning. These things are not the immediate concern of this book. In this context of electronic data-processing 'logic' is associated with the design of a computer system or unit and refers particularly to the relationships between components of the unit. A *logic* (or *logical*) *element* is a device which will perform a particular operation (a *logical function*) in a computer and is equivalent to a *gate* (see page 207). It is in effect an electronic switch, capable of directing a circuit. Thus, the substance of this chapter is concerned with electronic counting and switching, both being significant processes for diagnostic X-ray equipment.

THE BINARY COUNTING SYSTEM

Electronic counting employs a method of numbering which is called the binary system or binary notation system. In order to understand this we need to remind ourselves of the structure of the decimal system, which is so familiar to us that perhaps only teachers of mathematics are continuously aware of it.

In the representation of a number, the position—as well as the value—of a particular digit is commonly significant. The mathematical term *radix* (root) is used for the basis of such positional representation: the decimal system uses a radix of 10. By this we mean that a change in the position of a digit from one place to the next on the left represents an increase by a factor of 10. When we write a number such as 111, we understand that there is a difference between the weights of successive digits, though each appears the same in value, and that this difference is that the first is 10 times greater than the second and the second is 10 times greater than the third, as we read the number from left to right.

In binary notation the radix is two: the displacement of a digit to the next place on the left indicates that the digit is multiplied by two. Thus, for nine places to the left of the radix point (in the decimal system the radix point is the decimal point), successive positions are as follows:

256   128   64   32   16   8   4   2   1.

The binary numbering system has a further characteristic: it uses only two digits. These are 0 and 1. In binary notation two is written as 10, four as 100 and eight as 1000. This will be the easier to understand if the reader will study the table on p. 196, in which the numbers one to ten in the decimal system are expressed first in binary notation and then in a 'longhand' version for translation purposes.

Taking some random examples from Table 6.1, the binary notation for six is seen to be derived from its consideration as $4 + 2$; seven as $4 + 2 + 1$; and nine as $8 + 1$ (8, 4, 2 and 1 all being values capable of expression by their digital positions within the binary system). It will be appreciated—from study, for example, of the binary notation for twenty—that a nought indicates a binary digital position which is not utilized. In expressing any particular number, all 'empty' positions must be completed with a nought in this way, just as they are in the decimal system. (Consider the significance of the nought when twenty is written as 20.) Any number can be expressed in the binary system by a sufficient implementation of 0s and 1s. In the language of computers each 0 and 1 is called a *bit*, this being a contraction of binary digit.

Because we are so accustomed to the decimal system the human brain may not easily recognize numbers recorded in binary notation but a computer does so very readily. Effectively, each 'bit' is expressing a 'yes' (1) or a 'no' (0) situation. When we write twenty as 10100, we really say, 'Yes,

Table 6.1

Decimal	Binary	64	32	16	8	4	2	1
1	1							★
2	10						★	
3	11						★	★
4	100					★		
5	101					★		★
6	110					★	★	
7	111					★	★	★
8	1000				★			
9	1001				★			★
10	1010				★		★	
11	1011				★		★	★
11	1100				★	★		
13	1101				★	★		★
14	1110				★	★	★	
15	1111				★	★	★	★
16	10000			★				
17	10001			★				★
18	10010			★			★	
19	10011			★			★	★
20	10100			★		★		
100	1100100	★	★			★		

we are using a certain two digital positions' and 'No, we do not need to use three others'.

The simplicity of this yes-no situation makes binary numbering particularly appropriate for electronic counting systems. It is very easy to construct reliable electronic circuits which can be set in one of two states: 'yes or no'; high voltage or low voltage; open circuit or closed circuit.

LOGIC ELEMENTS

The binary symbols 0 and 1 have several electrical counterparts, as follows.

Lights	Off = 0	On = 1
Switches	Open = 0	Closed = 1
Current	Not flowing = 0	Flowing = 1
Voltage	Low = 0	High = 1

Logic circuits, that is those associated with binary functions, are essential to the operation of digital computers but this is not their only application. Our present interest in them is in relation to their use in contemporary diagnostic X-ray equipment.

Logic circuits employ two fixed voltages. Although these are called a high voltage (1) and a low voltage (0), it is to be understood that the terms are entirely relative. The high voltage in question is 2·5–5 volts and the low voltage is 0·4 volts. Logic circuits depend on the operations of various kinds of logic element or gate, of which some examples are described below and which perform the same functions as relays in the electro-mechanical switching of circuits.

And gate

An *and gate* is a logic element which provides an output signal (a voltage) from two input signals or voltages, in accordance with certain fixed rules. Its circuit symbol is depicted in Fig. 6.1.

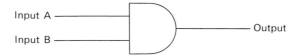

Fig. 6.1.

To obtain a high voltage output-signal from an and gate, both A and B must each be at high voltage (binary function 1). If A and B are dissimilar or if both are at low voltage (binary function 0), then the output is a low voltage (binary function 0). These relationships are expressed in Table 6.2.

Table 6.2

A	B	Output
Low	Low	Low
High	Low	Low
Low	High	Low
High	High	High

A table of this kind is called a truth table. Such a table describes a logical function by listing the possible combinations of input values, together with the true output value of each combination.

In a circuit which was electromechanically switched, two electro-magnetic relays in series would be similar to an and gate in purpose but much slower in operation. The relevant part of such a circuit we might represent diagrammatically as shown in Fig. 6.2.

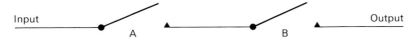

Fig. 6.2

Both relays A and B must close before the circuit can be completed.

The student will recognize elsewhere in this book other examples of electromagnetic relays arranged in series (for example, see Fig. 4.14 on page 155). These are mentioned now only to help the reader appreciate the functions of logical elements by association with their more familiar electromagnetic forerunners in X-ray equipment.

Or gate

An *or gate* is shown diagrammatically in Fig. 6.3.

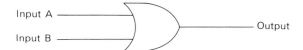

Fig. 6.3

In this case if either A or B is at high voltage a high output signal is obtained. The truth table for an or gate is written as shown in Table 6.3.

Table 6.3.   Truth table for an or gate.

A	B	Output
Low	Low	Low
High	Low	High
Low	High	High
High	High	High

A circuit containing the electromagnetic equivalents of an or gate would have its relevant part drawn as shown in Fig. 6.4. The student will remember

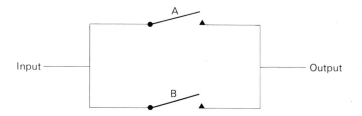

Fig. 6.4.

that, as the relays A and B are connected in parallel, closing either one of them is sufficient to provide a complete electrical circuit.

Inverter

An *inverter* is a device which changes the received signal to its opposite. If the input is a high voltage the output is a low voltage; and conversely. The circuit symbol for an inverter is shown in Fig. 6.5.

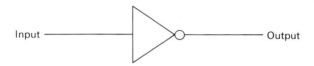

Input ——————————————⊳∘—— Output

Fig. 6.5

The truth table of an inverter is written as in Table 6.4.

Table 6.4   The truth table of an inverter.

Input	Output
High	Low
Low	High

Nor gate

A *nor gate* is a single logical element which combines an or gate with an inverter in series. The circuit symbol for a nor gate is shown in Fig. 6.6.

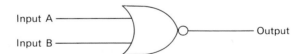

Input A ——————
Input B —————— ——— Output

Fig. 6.6

A nor gate provides a high output signal only when neither of the two input signals is high. The truth table for a nor gate is written as in Table 6.5.

Table 6.5.   The truth table for a nor gate.

A	B	Output
Low	Low	High
High	Low	Low
Low	High	Low
High	High	Low

Nand gate

Nand is a contraction of *not-and*. This is a logical element which combines an and gate with an inverter and is diagrammatically depicted in Fig. 6.7.

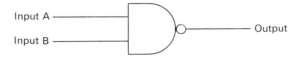

Fig. 6.7

A nand gate produces a high voltage output when either one of its input signals is at low voltage (or when both are at low voltage). The truth table for a nand gate is written as in Table 6.6.

Table 6.6.   The truth table for a nand gate.

A	B	Output
Low	Low	High
High	Low	High
Low	High	High
High	High	Low

APPLICATIONS OF LOGIC CIRCUITS

Logic circuits can be used in X-ray equipment in several applications. In this section of the chapter we propose to describe some of them.

Digital display

The control desks of many contemporary X-ray units use digital displays of the values of various quantities which are significant to the radiographer; for example, milliampereseconds are more easily read in this form, in preference to making an observation from a meter, and any deviation from the correct value is quickly recognized.

For the digital presentation of electrical quantities it is necessary to have a device known as a binary to decimal decoder which would drive one digital display tube, showing any of the decimal digits 0–9. Fig. 6.8 is a schematic representation of such a decoder.

The decimal digits are listed in the last column. They are severally illuminated by means of an output signal (a high voltage) resulting from some appropriate combination of four input voltages. For example, to

Input				Output to
D	C	B	A	digital display
low	low	low	low	0
low	low	low	high	1
low	low	high	low	2
low	low	high	high	3
low	high	low	low	4
low	high	low	high	5
low	high	high	low	6
low	high	high	high	7
high	low	low	low	8
high	low	low	high	9

A = binary 1   C = binary 4
B = binary 2   D = binary 8

Fig. 6.8

illuminate zero the necessary logical operation requires all four inputs to be at low voltage.

The inputs marked A, B, C and D represent respectively the binary positions of one, two, four and eight. A high voltage on any of these inputs is congruous with the binary digit 1 and a low voltage with the binary digit 0 (Compare Fig. 6.8 with Table 6.1.) Thus, decimal 5 is produced from the binary positions for one and four; high voltages at A and C respectively will result in the illumination of this decimal digit.

Similarly, any of the other decimal digits can be shown on the display tube by an appropriate combination of high and low voltages on the individual gates.

Prepare and exposure circuit

Fig. 6.9 depicts a typical circuit which may be found in diagnostic X-ray equipment. It uses electromagnetic relays in series in order to satisfy successive circuit conditions which are essential to making a radiographic exposure. These conditions have been fully discussed elsewhere in this book but at this stage a brief remark on each may be of help in reminding the reader of the several circuits which are interlocked through the operation of the relays in the diagram.

On the left side of Fig. 6.9 is seen the 'prepare' station of the exposure switch which will energize the delay circuit and the prepare relay. However,

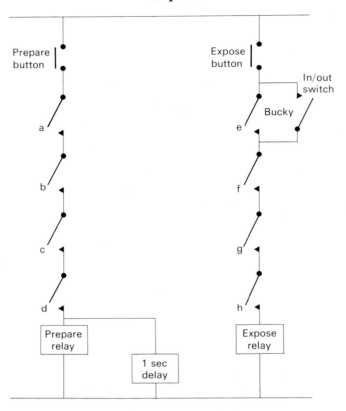

Fig. 6.9

this will not occur until the contacts of four other relays in series have all closed. These relays are linked with the following circuitry:

a closes when the X-ray tube filament is energized at its proper value (page 272);

b is the percentage load relay (see page 159) and is closed unless the selected exposure factors constitute an overload of the X-ray tube;

c is triggered by a thermally-operated circuit breaker (see page 147) and is closed unless the tubehead has become overheated;

d closes to prevent operation of the automatic mains voltage compensator during an exposure (see page 82).

On the right side of Fig. 6.9 we see the 'exposure' station itself which will operate the exposure contactor (energizing the exposure contactor gate, see page 168). Before it can do so, however, the series relays e, f, g and h must all have closed. These relays are severally associated with the following circuitry:

e is the in-out switch for the bucky (page 344);

f is closed when the tube stator windings are energized (page 154);

g and *h* ensure first that the correct interval has elapsed to allow the rotating anode to have reached full speed and secondly that the X-ray tube is finally set ready for the exposure.

An X-ray set may perhaps give to its user a superficial impression that initiation of the exposure requires only two switching operations, the 'prepare' and 'expose' stations of the familiar 2-position switch. The facts are that, in this circuit alone, the number of 'switches' involved before the X-ray tube is energized is of the order of ten. When we know this, we can appreciate a possible difficulty in obtaining a very rapid succession of short exposures.

Let us look now at the organization of an equivalent electronic circuit using logic elements, which—as they are not mechanical relays and have no inertia—will 'switch' the circuit instantaneously. Such a circuit is depicted in Fig. 6.10. Perhaps the first thing to say about Fig. 6.10 is that the block at the top of the diagram which is marked 'clock' represents no conventional timepiece. This is a quartz crystal which oscillates when a voltage is applied to it, the frequency of these oscillations being determined by characteristics of the particular crystal (thickness of section). Very high frequencies of oscillation result; we are concerned here with hundreds of thousands of pulses in a second. If we add a counter capable of counting impulses from the crystal we have an interval-timing system in the circuit.

On the left of Fig. 6.10 is a five-input gate (1) which gives one output signal when five input signals are at high voltage. These five input signals are fed from the various circuits named in the diagram and are analogous to the voltages energizing the relays in Fig. 6.9.

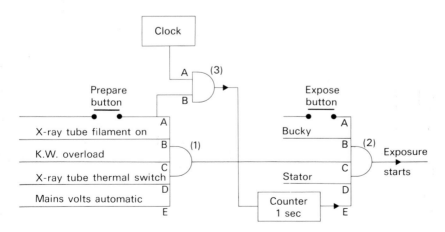

Fig. 6.10

The output signal from this first gate becomes one of the input signals (C) to a similar gate (2) on the right of Fig. 6.10.

Gate 3 is an and gate: it gives an output signal when it receives high voltage signals from A (the clock) and B (the prepare button).

The output signal from gate 3 is fed to gate 2 via a counter which inserts a delay of 1 second in the signal (E). The identities of the other three input signals, A, B and D, are labelled in the diagram. They should be familiar to the reader and require no further explanation here.

Thus, when the five input signals are all at high voltage, the output from gate 2 is the exposure-initiating impulse.

A logic circuit of this kind not only operates much more rapidly than its electro-mechanical predecessor but—utilizing printed circuitry—requires less space in the generator and is readily replaced in the case of a fault.

A radiographic timing and switching circuit

Fig. 6.11 illustrates the organization of logic circuits for timing and switching, in association with the output of a quartz crystal, high-speed oscillator and a divider chain. The emission of the crystal here is 1,000,000 pulses a second. It is clear that at this frequency the loss or gain of a few impulses is totally insignificant and that very accurate timing of short intervals is possible.

The divider chain—as one might expect—arithmetically divides. Each of its stages reduces the pulse-emission by a factor of ten, so that we have available a variety of 'parcels' of impulses/second, more convenient in 'size' for different timing purposes in the equipment. The greater the accuracy needed for any particular application, the higher is the point in the divider chain from which the oscillator's signal is taken.

Thus, in the right lower corner of Fig. 6.11, we see that the run-up delay circuit for the X-ray tube's stator and filament operates from the stage of the divider chain which is emitting 100 pulses per second. The timing function of this circuit is not concerned with any interval which is less than 1 second in duration. A possible 'mis-count' of one or two impulses in a series of 100 is proportionally immaterial to the circuit's purpose, the safeguarding of the X-ray tube.

The delay circuit—as we can see from the diagram—depends on an and gate which receives input signals A from the divider chain and B from the 'prepare' station of the handswitch. The output voltage from the and gate is fed to a counter, which emits one output pulse at the end of a count of 100 pulses: this is the 'exposure ready' signal.

The exposure is timed and terminated through the logic circuit shown in the right upper part of Fig. 6.11. As we may need to measure radiographic

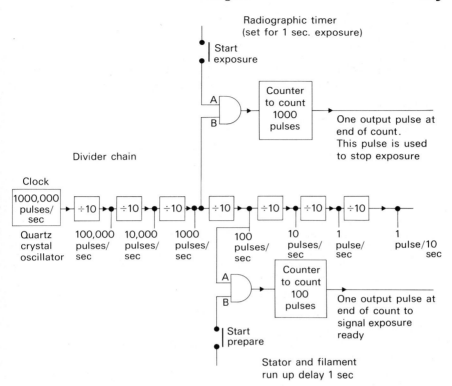

Fig. 6.11

exposures in fractions of a second, the and gate in this circuit takes its input signal B from the stage of the divider chain giving 1000 impulses a second. At that frequency a minimum radiographic exposure of 0·01 second could be timed to a high level of accuracy.

The input A to the and gate is provided from the 'expose' station. With inputs A and B at high voltage the and gate feeds a high voltage output signal to a counter which—we see—counts 1000 pulses when the radiographic timer is set by the radiographer for 1 second. At the end of the count, one output pulse is used to terminate the exposure.

GLOSSARY

This chapter ends with a brief glossary of computer terms. The definitions are taken from *A Dictionary of Computers* (Chandor, Graham and Williamson) which is published by Penguin Books Ltd (1970) and is fascinating reading for anyone with even a superficial interest in comprehending computers.

And circuit (and element) A logic element operating with binary digits which provides one output signal from two input signals according to the rules in Table 6.7.

Table 6.7

Input		Output
1	0	0
1	1	1
0	1	0
0	0	0

Thus a 1 digit is obtained as output only if two 1 digits are present as coincident input signals.

And gate Synonymous with and element.

Binary digit A digit in binary notation; i.e. either 0 or 1. Generally abbreviated as *bit*.

Binary notation A positional notation system for representing numbers in which the radix for each digit position is two. In this system numbers are represented by the two digits 0 and 1. In the same way that in the normal decimal system a displacement of one digit position to the left means that the digit is multiplied by a factor of 10, so in the binary system displacement means multiplication by 2. Thus the binary number '10' represents two, while '100' represents four.

Binary number Any number represented in binary notation.

Binary numeral One of the two digits 0 and 1 used for representing numbers in binary notation.

Bit An abbreviation of binary digit, one of the two digits (0 and 1) used in binary notation.

Computer Any machine which can accept data in a prescribed form, process the data and supply the results of the processing in a specified format as information or as signals to control automatically some further machine or process.

Decode To alter data from one coded format back to an original format. To translate coded characters to a form more intelligible to human beings or for a further stage of processing.

Digital Referring to the use of discrete signals to represent data in the form of numbers or characters. Most forms of digital representation in data processing are based upon the use of binary numbers, sets of binary digits being grouped together to represent numbers in some other radix when required; e.g. binary coded decimal notation.

Electronic switch A switch which makes use of an electronic circuit, enabling the switching action to take place at high speed.

Gate In general, an electronic switch. Used in data processing to refer to an electronic circuit which may have more than one input signal but only one output signal. In this sense used synonymously with logic element.

Impulse An electrical signal the duration of which is short compared with the time scale under consideration.

Logical (logic) element A device used to perform some specific logical operation; e.g. an *and element, or element, nor element* etc.

Nand (not-and) element A logic element operating with binary signals which will produce an output signal representing 1 when any of its corresponding input signals represents zero.

Nor element (nor gate) A logic element operating with binary digits which provides an output signal according to the following rules in Table 6.8 applied to two input signals.

Table 6.8

Input		Output
1	0	0
1	1	0
0	1	0
0	0	1

Thus a 1 digit is obtained only if neither of the two input signals is 1.

Or element A logic element operating with binary digits and providing an output signal according to the following rules in Table 6.9 applied to two input signals.

Table 6.9

Input		Output
1	0	1
1	1	1
0	1	1
0	0	0

Thus a 1 digit is provided as an output if any one (or more) of the input signals are 1.

Pulse A sudden and relatively short electrical disturbance.

Radix The basis of a notation or number system, defining a number representational system by positional representation. In a decimal system the radix is 10, in an octal system the radix is 8 and in a binary system the radix is 2.

Radix point The location of the separation of the integral parts and the fractional part of a number expressed in a radix notation. This location is marked in the decimal system by the decimal point (a dot in English usage, a comma elsewhere).

Chapter 7
X-ray Tubes

GENERAL FEATURES OF THE
X-RAY TUBE

X rays are produced by a process which converts energy from one form into another. Fast-moving electrons possess energy of motion and this becomes changed to radiant energy when such electrons are suddenly slowed down. In diagnostic X-ray equipment most of this energy (approximately 99 per cent) is in the form of heat and a very small part of it is in the form of X rays.

This conversion of energy takes place inside the device known as an X-ray tube which is designed to enable the process to happen as satisfactorily as can be arranged. Because the proportion of heat produced is so very high and the quantity of X radiation is so small in relation to the heat, it cannot be called an efficient process; those who manufacture X-ray tubes must design them so as to make the best of an unhelpful situation.

Since the conversion which is to occur involves the sudden slowing of electrons in rapid motion, the basic features of an X-ray tube in operation must include the following.

1   A source of electrons.
2   A means to put them into rapid motion across a space where there is nothing to impede them so that the rapid motion may be maintained.
3   A means to slow the electrons suddenly.

In the X-ray tube the requirements are met as follows.

1   The source of electrons is a heated filament, which is called the cathode or negative electrode of the X-ray tube. When the filament is hot the agitation of its molecules causes electrons to leave the wire and form a cloud in front of it.
2   The means to put the electrons in motion is a high voltage applied across the X-ray tube, and lack of impediment to their passage is ensured by making the electrons travel across a vacuum.
3   The means to slow the electrons is provided as might be expected by putting something in the way. Basically this is a metal plate, and it is called the anode or positive electrode of the X-ray tube. The area on the anode

which is bombarded by the electrons is called the focal spot. This focal spot becomes the source of the X radiation emitted usefully by the X-ray tube.

4   Since a vacuum must have a wall round it if it is to exist at all, the two electrodes of the X-ray tube (the cathode structure with its heated wire filament and the anode with its focal spot) are sealed into a glass envelope or tube which is evacuated of air.

An evacuated tube with two electrodes is known as a diode. So an X-ray tube is one form of diode which is specialized in its design and operation so that it may be used to produce X rays.

The wire filament of the X-ray tube must be heated and a suitable way is to use electricity and heat the filament by means of a step-down transformer. The high voltage which speeds the electrons across to the anode is conveniently provided by means of a step-up high tension transformer. These arrangements are discussed more fully in Chapter 2, and are depicted here in diagramatic form.

Fig. 7.1 shows the basic features of the X-ray tube and the connections to the transformers. It is important to realize that this simple circuit comprises two separate voltages and two separate currents. One of these is the voltage and current which serve to heat the filament of the X-ray tube and so cause it to be a source of electrons. This voltage (about 10–12 volts) is obtained from the secondary winding of the filament transformer, and the path of the current (about 6–8 amps) is indicated by the dotted arrows in the diagram. The other voltage is the high voltage (upwards from 40 kV to 125 kV in diagnostic equipment) which is applied across the cathode and anode of the X-ray tube to make the electrons travel fast. This voltage is obtained from the secondary winding of the high tension transformer. The electrons travelling across the X-ray tube constitute the current through it.

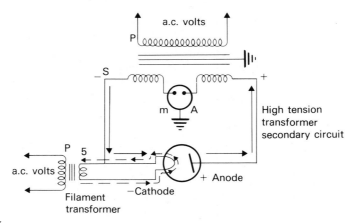

Fig. 7.1

This is the tube milliamperage (up to 5 mA for fluoroscopy and 10–500 mA for radiography, with higher milliamperages still in some cases), and the bold arrows outline the path of the current through the secondary circuit of the high tension transformer. In both cases in Fig. 7.1 the arrows point in the direction the *electrons* flow.

Thermionic emission and the X-ray tube

The process of causing a wire to emit electrons as a result of heat is called thermionic emission, and when this phenomenon takes place in a vacuum diode there are certain features associated with it.

1   The rate at which electrons are emitted by the wire filament depends on the temperature of the wire and its surface area. So raising the temperature of the wire increases the number of electrons which leave and form a cloud round it. This cloud of negative electricity (electric charge) occupying space is called, reasonably enough, a space charge.

2   When an electric potential (a voltage) is applied between the filament and the second electrode which is the anode (essentially a metal plate for receiving the electrons), the electrons will travel across to the metal plate provided that it is positively charged in respect of the filament; it *must* be positively charged in order to hold any attraction for the electrons. In the X-ray tube this metal plate is of very specialized design as will be seen, but this does not alter its essential function which is to attract the electrons from the filament.

3   Since the electrons will flow from the heated filament to the plate only if this is positive and can attract them, when connections are reversed so that the filament is positive, no electrons flow. This why a vacuum diode when it is operating properly passes current in one direction only.

4   When the filament is negative, the higher the positive potential on the anode the more electrons it will collect from the filament. This means that as the voltage across the diode rises, the current through it (number of electrons going across) rises also. A change in the voltage across the diode changes the current through it and the two cannot be changed independently.

5   Eventually *all* the electrons which are being emitted are being collected, and no increase in voltage (positive potential on the anode) can bring any more across. The only way now to get any more electrons across (raise the current through the diode) is to arrange for more to be emitted from the filament by increasing its heat. This state of affairs in which all the electrons which are being emitted are also being collected is known as *saturation*. When the diode is operating in these conditions, alterations in voltage across it do not alter the current through it. Current and voltage can be changed independently of each other; this is the state of affairs that we *want* when using an X-ray tube.

The reader may like to consider a very simple analogy in order to understand clearly these characteristics of conduction through a vacuum diode. Suppose the cloud of electrons in the space around the filament to be a group of children playing in a meadow. The force of attraction coming from the positive potential on the anode is the voice of someone calling them in for tea.

At first the voltage is low and the positive attraction is weak, corresponding to a call in a faint voice; not many of the children will come. As the voltage across the diode increases, the voice may be supposed to be getting louder and more determined; more children will come (the current through the diode rises). Eventually the voice is loud and determined enough (the voltage is high enough) for *all* the children (electrons) to come; now it is no use calling any louder in the expectation of fetching more children in, and at this stage the only way of gathering in more children is to arrange for there to be more there.

This corresponds to the state of affairs when the voltage across the diode is sufficiently high to collect all the electrons. Increasing the voltage does not increase the current through the diode, and the current is altered by changing the number of available electrons; this is done by changing the filament heat. Current and voltage can now be altered independently of each other, and the diode is operating above the saturation point.

It may be emphasized here that very small changes in filament heat result in large changes in current through the diode, so this is a very sensitive control of current. Fig. 7.2 is a graph which shows how the current through the diode increases when the filament-heating current is increased.

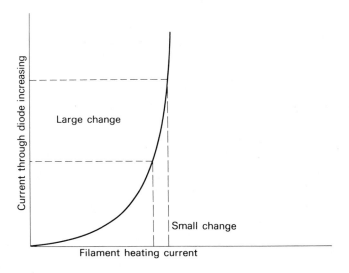

Fig. 7.2

Saturation and the X-ray tube

It was said a little earlier that the state wanted for an X-ray tube is that it should be functioning above the saturation condition. When this is achieved, altering the kilovoltage across the tube does not also change the milliamperage, which is controlled through the filament heat. The radiographer can select kilovoltage and milliamperes independently of each other, and thus finds more convenience and greater control of factors when using the tube.

Let us consider now whether the X-ray tube in fact operates above the saturation condition. The simple answer is that it does not always do so, especially when it operates at high milliamperes. If the tube milliamperage is relatively low (below 100 mA), the filament will not be very hot and the number of electrons which leave it will be relatively limited. Because of this it is easy for even the lowest tube voltage (say 40 kV) to collect all the electrons, and the X-ray tube operates above the saturation point.

High milliamperage, however, requires the emission of electrons from the filament to be much greater. When a heavy electron emission is combined with a relatively low kilovoltage, the electrons will be less inclined to travel towards the anode and will tend to stay in a cloud in front of the filament; this cloud impedes the electrons that do want to go to the anode. This tendency to form a cloud and the consequences of it are known as the space charge effect.

With the anode voltage collecting only some of the electrons from the filament, the tube milliamperage is limited by the number that the anode collects and not the number that the filament emits. Raising the filament temperature does not increase the milliamperage for it results in more electrons being emitted and not in more being collected; more electrons *are* collected when the tube voltage is raised, so milliamperage rises with increase in kilovoltage.

The X-ray tube is now operating below the saturation condition, and the radiographer using it will find that a given milliamperes setting (filament heat) results in different currents through the tube according to the kilovoltage used. For example, with 400 mA selected at 70 kV, a drop to 50 kV might reduce the milliamperage to 350 mA and an increase to 90 kV could increase the tube current to 460 mA, the filament heat remaining unchanged. This is clearly a very unsatisfactory state of affairs for the radiographer. In modern equipment provision is made for this space charge effect, as explained in Chapter 2. Over the range used, kilovoltage and milliamperage can then be selected independently of each other. Even if the X-ray tube is not operating above the saturation condition, the results are the same as if it were, and the space charge effect ceases to be of significance to the radiographer in normal general use of the tube.

Equipment for diagnostic radiography involves two types of X-ray tube which must now be considered in detail. These are (i) the fixed anode X-ray tube, and (ii) the rotating anode X-ray tube.

THE FIXED ANODE X-RAY TUBE

A fixed anode X-ray tube is illustrated in Fig. 7.3.

The cathode

The cathode is the negative electrode of the X-ray tube. It is on the left in Fig. 7.3. Essentially it consists of a metal structure to support the filament which in operation will be heated so that it becomes an electron emitter. The cathode structure not only supports the filament; it is designed to carry out the further function of focusing the electron beam which leaves the filament, as will be described shortly.

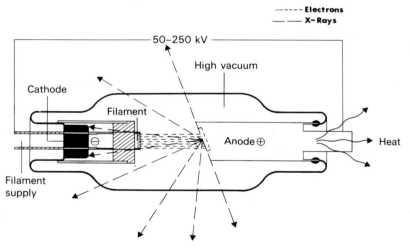

Fig. 7.3 A fixed anode X-ray tube insert. *By courtesy of Machlett X-ray Tubes (Great Britain) Ltd.*

The filament

This is made of tungsten wire. It is tungsten because this metal tolerates being heated to a very high temperature (over 2000°C is required), and it is formed into a close helical winding (i.e. corkscrew or spiral staircase type); this is so that it will have a larger surface from which to emit electrons. As the aim is for the filament to become hot when current passes through it, the wire should have a high resistance so that a given current produces the most heat. It is also necessary for the electron source to be small so that the electron beam may be brought to cover a very small area. For these reasons the wire is very thin.

Since the electrons emitted by the filament are negatively charged particles, their natural tendency will be to spread out away from each other in their passage across the X-ray tube. This must be corrected and the electrons must be brought to impinge upon a small area on the anode. The area covered by their bombardment is the source of the X rays, and this must be as small as possible so that the radiographic images produced may be as sharp in outline as possible. A large area of electron bombardment means a large X-ray source; this would result in certain unsharpness in the radiographic images produced. The simple comparison to be made here is between the sharp shadows produced by a very small light source such as the pencil beam of an electric torch and the diffuse shadows produced by such a light source as a long fluorescent tube.

Focusing the electron beam

The electrons streaming away from the wire filament are brought together by means of the electric field which exists between anode and cathode. The filament sits in a slot in the cathode structure as can be seen in Fig. 7.4 and the electrons leave the filament through the slot. Both the filament and the slot in which it sits are carefully designed in their size and shape, and the filament is carefully positioned within the slot. The shape of the electric field between the cathode and anode which results from the design causes the electrons leaving the filament to come together so that they cover a small area on the anode—i.e. the electron beam may be considered to be focused, the term used of a light beam the rays of which are brought together by means of a lens.

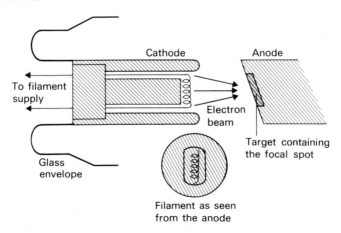

Fig. 7.4

The area on the anode covered by the electron beam is known as the focal spot or the actual focus of the X-ray tube, actual because it is the real size of the X-ray source. The size of this area is determined by just the features that one would expect.

1　By the size and shape of the filament.

2　By the dimensions of the focusing slot and by the depth of the filament in it.

3　By the characteristics of the electric field associated with the focusing slot.

4　By the spacing of the two electrodes—that is, how far apart the cathode and the anode are.

These features are very carefully selected and designed when the X-ray tube is made so that the electron beam covers a very small area on the anode of the tube, this area being of a predetermined size and not a matter of chance. The helical filament in its rectangular slot produces an electron beam which covers a rectangular area, and X-ray tubes having rectangular focal spots are sometimes described as being of the line-focus type. It is of course not a line at all since it is an area, but the term distinguishes this sort of X-ray tube from its predecessors which had circular focal spots. All modern diagnostic X-ray tubes are of the line-focus type.

The rectangular focal spot is about 3 to 4 times longer than it is wide, and its area in square millimetres varies from around 2–3 mm^2 to around 10–15 mm^2. Focal spot sizes are discussed in more detail later in this chapter (page 279).

The anode

We have said that the anode is essentially a metal plate to receive the electrons which bombard it, but it is of very special design. The two most important considerations which govern this design are (i) that the electron bombardment gives rise to a great amount of heat and only a small proportion of X radiation; (ii) that the X-ray tube must be capable of producing images which are sharp in outline and the beam must therefore originate from a small source.

These considerations cause a situation of conflict, for the heat is produced at the area of electron bombardment which is also the X-ray source. Spreading the heat over a large area would help to solve the problem of making an X-ray tube accept it without damage, since a given quantity of heat spread over a larger area results in less temperature rise; but this would mean that the X-ray source was large in size and the images produced by the tube would be unsharp because of this. So the anode of the X-ray tube is constructed with these points in mind and the conflict is resolved as well as possible through its highly specialized design, as explained below.

Heat dissipation and the production of X rays

The area of electron bombardment is the place where both the heat and the X rays are produced. So it is important that this part of the X-ray tube is made of a metal that is able to stand high temperatures without melting, and is able on bombardment to produce X rays as well as possible. The metal used is tungsten and it is chosen for the following reasons.

1   It has a higher melting point than other metals.

2   It has a fairly high atomic number and it is therefore more efficient at producing X rays than are metals of low atomic number. Efficiency of X-ray production increases with the atomic number of the bombarded metal.

3   It is a fairly good conductor of heat. Because of this the heat can be passed reasonably quickly away from the small area where it is being produced, and so the rise in temperature at that area is prevented from being too great.

4   It does not vaporize easily. The presence of metal vapour inside an X-ray tube would spoil the vacuum which is essential for its correct operation.

5   It can be worked and made smooth. These features ensure that it is physically suitable to be used in the manufacture of the anode and that the X rays are produced from a source which is smooth; the significance of a rough-surfaced source is explained on page 269.

Tungsten provides a satisfactory combination of these features. There are other metals which, for example, have higher atomic numbers or are better conductors of heat; but they have lower—in some cases much lower—melting points and would be quite unacceptable because of this.

The piece of tungsten within the X-ray tube which contains the area of electron bombardment is known as the target. It is a small plate about 2 mm thick, rectangular or circular in shape and larger than the focal area upon it which is covered by the electrons. The heat which is produced by the electron bombardment arises (with a small amount of X radiation) at the focal area or focal spot on the target. The X rays are emitted in all directions from the focal spot, and the heat is spread by conduction over the tungsten target.

So long as the tube is producing X rays more heat is being formed at the focal spot. The high melting point of the tungsten target enables it to take this heat, provided that the temperature rise is not so great that the melting point of tungsten (3360°C) is passed. To keep down the rise in temperature at the target, the anode is designed so that the heat can pass by conduction into another metal. The tungsten target is therefore set into a thick copper rod which is massive relative to the small tungsten target. This cylindrical copper block and the tungsten target set into its face together form the anode of the X-ray tube—that is the electrode which will be connected to the positive pole of the supply.

The copper rod prevents excessive rise in temperature because of the following features.

1   It is a good conductor of heat (better than tungsten) and can conduct the heat to the exterior of the tube.

2   Because the anode block is large and because it is made of copper, it is able to accept a great amount of heat without a correspondingly great rise in temperature. The copper block can do this better than a corresponding mass of tungsten because it is a characteristic of copper to be better in this way.

The copper anode with its tungsten target is therefore a more efficient design than a solid tungsten anode which would show a greater rise in temperature for the same heat input. Furthermore, the tungsten anode would not be able to conduct the heat so well to the exterior of the tube.

The anode of the X-ray tube has a sloping face. This slope allows X rays produced at the focal spot to leave the tube sideways, and the radiographer uses a beam which is emitted about an axis at right angles to the long axis of the X-ray tube. In the middle of this beam is (reasonably enough) the central ray which is perpendicular to the long axis of the tube and is surrounded by diverging rays; this is sketched in Fig. 7.5.

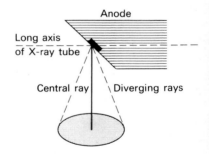

Fig. 7.5

The anode and image sharpness

The slope of the anode face has an importance which must be explained. If it were possible for the eye to see X radiation and an observer (a mythical creature immune to the effects of X rays) could be positioned so that he looked at the anode of the X-ray tube *en face*, viewing it along a line at right angles to its front surface (in Fig. 7.6 the first point of observation), he would see the X-ray source as a rectangle (ABCD in Fig. 7.6).

This rectangle is the area bombarded by the electrons as previously explained, and it is called the actual focus of the X-ray tube. The larger this is, the larger is the area receiving heat from the electron bombardment. On

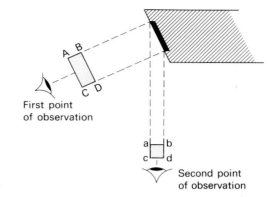

Fig. 7.6

a short exposure a larger area can take more heat than a smaller area can before the temperature rises to the melting point of tungsten. This means that an X-ray tube with a large actual focus can be operated at higher milliamperages without becoming damaged by a melted target. Higher milliamperages allow shorter times of exposure to be used, and there is then less chance of the patient making the image unsharp by movement. So a large actual focus is what a radiographer wants.

At the same time the radiographer has another conflicting demand. This is that the source of the X rays must be small; the X-ray tube can then produce sharper shadows because the geometric unsharpness (that is unsharpness contributed by the size of the source) will be small.

The sloping anode is able to reconcile these two conflicting demands for (i) a large area to take the electron bombardment and (ii) a small X-ray source. The compromise is achieved in the following way.

Suppose that the hypothetical observer looking at the anode of the X-ray tube has now moved his observation point so that he looks up at the anode along the central ray from the position that the film occupies when the exposure is made (in Fig. 7.6 the second point of observation). He will now see the X-ray source not as a rectangle but as a square. This is because the slope of the anode face foreshortens the longer dimension of the rectangle and it now appears as the square abcd in Fig. 7.6.

This square is the projection of the actual focus of the X-ray tube and it is known as the effective or apparent focus. The actual focus is the true size of the X-ray source; the effective focus is the size of the X-ray source as it appears to be when viewed from the film. The actual focus (being the area of electron bombardment as well as the true size of the X-ray source) determines the electrical load which the tube will take (milliamperes which can be used). The effective focus (being the size of the source as it appears to be) determines the amount of geometric unsharpness present in the image; it is *not the only determinant* of this, but it is an important one.

So the sloping anode and the rectangular focal spot provide a focus which *is* large and from the film *looks* small, thus reconciling the conflicting elements in what the radiographer wants in a satisfactory X-ray tube. This method of compromise, which uses the foreshortening of a rectangular focal spot, is called using the line focus principle (a conveniently short way of referring to it provided that you can remember what it means).

The angle of anode slope

The steeper the slope of the anode face, the smaller is the apparent focus for a given size of actual focus. This is shown in Fig. 7.7 which depicts two anodes of different slope, each having the same size actual focus.

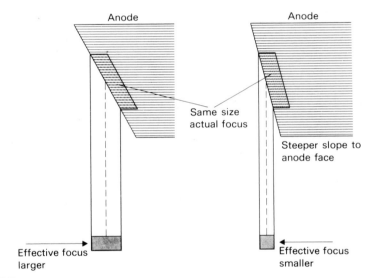

Fig. 7.7

The steeper slope of one of them (the one on the right) projects the focus as a smaller square, and the X-ray tube with this anode will produce sharper images than the other one while taking the same electrical loadings. From this point of view a steep slope is a wanted feature of the anode.

However, a limit is placed by the fact that a steep slope means a narrow useful beam. This is obvious if we again consider the hypothetical observer who can see X rays and can safely move about under the X-ray tube looking up at the source. Last time we thought of him, he was immediately under the central ray. In Fig. 7.8 he would be at C, viewing the X-ray source as a small square, which is the effective focus of the X-ray tube.

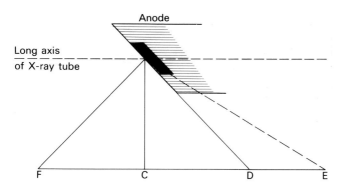

Fig. 7.8

Suppose that he now moves his position along the long axis of the X-ray tube towards the anode end so that in Fig. 7.8 he is at D. He now sees the X-ray source somewhat more foreshortened than it was previously, and he sees it just clear of the lower edge or heel of the anode. Radiation reaching the point D will be nearly enough of the same intensity as radiation reaching point C for the beam to be considered uniform over this extent. (In fact the intensity at D is less than at C, and at C is less than at F. This variation in intensity along the long axis of the X-ray tube is known as the heel effect, and in practice in diagnostic radiography it is generally ignored, the intensity along the line FCD being taken to be uniform. There is also variation in the apparent size of the focal spot as a result of the different foreshortening which occurs at the different viewpoints. It appears smaller at D than it does at C, and smaller at C than it does at F. Theoretically this makes a difference in the sharpness of the image along the line FCD, but this too is usually ignored in practice.)

If the observer moves in Fig. 7.8 to point E he is now in the 'shadow' of the anode and he can see the X-ray source only through the anode block. It would be like seeing the sun through a heavy haze of cloud; the radiation reaching him will be attenuated by the massive copper block, and there is therefore appreciable reduction in intensity of the radiation reaching E as compared with that reaching D. E is beyond the area covered by the useful beam, which is limited by the distance in Fig. 7.8 between D (the last point at which the source was hypothetically viewed from the film clear of the anode heel) and C (the point under the central ray).

Along the axis EDC in the direction of the cathode of the X-ray tube the point F can be taken, which is as far away from C as D is. At F the radiation is still considered to be of acceptably uniform intensity as compared with the intensity at C and the intensity at D. The useful beam covers a circle of diameter FD and radius CD.

Fig. 7.9 shows that as the slope of the anode becomes steeper, D becomes nearer to C and the area covered by the useful beam becomes smaller at a given tube to film distance.

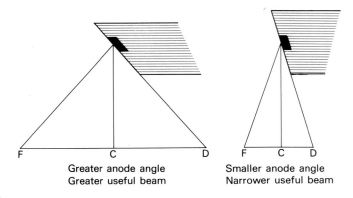

Greater anode angle
Greater useful beam

Smaller anode angle
Narrower useful beam

Fig. 7.9

So something (i.e. steeper slope) that is *wanted* in order to achieve a small effective focus may make the X-ray tube impossible to use satisfactorily with large films and short tube to film distances. Once again a compromise must

Table 7.1

Target angle	Tube/film distance in centimetres	Field size (square) in centimetres
7°	80	20 × 20
	100	25 × 25
	150	37 × 37
	180	44 × 44
10°	80	29 × 29
	100	35 × 35
	150	53 × 53
	180	63 × 63
15°	80	43 × 43
	100	53 × 53
	150	80 × 80
	180	97 × 97
20°	80	59 × 59
	100	73 × 73
	150	110 × 110
	180	130 × 130

be reached, this time between an anode that is (i) too steep for the useful beam to be useful in practice, and (ii) not steep enough to foreshorten the actual focus adequately so that images produced may have small geometric unsharpness. In modern diagnostic tubes this compromise results in an anode angle which, according to the make and type of the X-ray tube, varies from 7 to 20 degrees.

Some examples of the field sizes covered in relation to X-ray tubes with different angles used at various tube to film distances are given in Table 7.1.

Relationship between true source and apparent source

In the absence of our useful mythical observer the apparent source of an X-ray tube can be examined by methods which are explained in Chapter 17.

The devices which are used allow the apparent source to be measured and its size to be known. This apparent source in Fig. 7.10, is the small square ABCD.

The actual focal area covered by the electron beam (true source of the X rays) in Fig. 7.10 is the rectangle EFGH. As explained earlier, the slope of the anode face foreshortens the long dimension of this rectangle and turns it into an apparent square. The degree of foreshortening which takes place depends on the angle of anode slope—that is on the angle between the central ray and the face of the anode, which in Fig. 7.10 is θ. As shown in Fig. 7.7 the smaller this angle, the more is the foreshortening that occurs.

The important features in this foreshortening and the relationship between the size of the true source (in Fig. 7.10 EFGH) and the apparent source (in Fig. 7.10 ABCD) are: (i) the angle θ, (ii) the dimensions of the

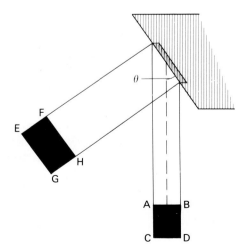

Fig. 7.10

true source, and (iii) the size of apparent source which it is wished to obtain. These features are selected in manufacture so that AB = EG sin θ.

It is therefore possible without breaking up the X-ray tube to determine the size of the true source (actual focus) provided that (i) the angle of anode slope is known, and (ii) there is available an accurately made image of the apparent source so that the length of AB can be measured. Since AB = EF, the size of the rectangle EFGH can then be determined by a mixture of measurement and calculation. For most radiographers this is an academic piece of knowledge, useful sometimes in the examination hall but never in the X-ray department.

On page 223 it was stated that the anode angle varied from 7 to 20 degrees. Anyone mathematically inclined (we will spare the mathematically uninterested by not doing it here) can work out that a 7 degree anode angle results in a true source about 8 times larger than the apparent source, a 10 degree anode angle results in a true source about 6 times larger than the apparent source, a 15 degree angle results in a true source about 4 times larger than the apparent one, and a 20 degree anode angle results in a true source about 3 times larger than the apparent source.

The dual focus X-ray tube

At this stage it is perhaps worth reviewing the problems relating to the size of the focal spot of an X-ray tube which is to be used for diagnostic radiography. The salient facts are as follows.

1   A small amount of X radiation is produced and a great amount of heat which initially is spread over the focal spot—the area covered by the electron beam.

2   The larger this area is, the more heat it will take on a short exposure before the temperature of the focal spot rises to the melting point of tungsten. Larger focal spots therefore permit higher milliamperages to be used without damage to the X-ray tube.

3   Higher milliamperages mean greater intensity of radiation output and this allows the use of shorter exposures. Short exposures are a *necessity* for radiographs of certain patients and of certain organs and systems of the body when movement is probable or certain.

4   *But* a large focal area means a large X-ray source and this results in the geometric unsharpness of the image being large.

5   If the unsharpness from movement is great it does not matter if the geometric unsharpness is very small indeed, for the large movement-blur will invalidate the small geometric unsharpness, and the image will be unacceptable.

6   If the unsharpness from movement can be prevented from being large at

the cost of *some* increase in geometric unsharpness, then this compromise must be accepted as the best means of obtaining the sharpest possible image.

Radiographic examinations present different problems according to the type of subject and the region of the body being examined. In some it is obviously very easy to obtain an image which is satisfactorily recorded and is sharp in outline, even by means of an X-ray tube which is producing a low output of radiation; examples are radiographs of body parts such as the extremities and teeth of co-operative patients. In these cases a radiographer can use with satisfaction an X-ray tube with a small focal area. The geometric unsharpness will be small as a result, and although the tube will not allow the use of high milliamperage and short exposure-times, this will not matter because (i) the body part is not greatly absorptive of X-rays and therefore does not need a large exposure dose and (ii) the risk of movement is not great and very short exposure-times are unnecessary.

In the case of parts of the body which are very radio-absorptive and of regions which contain organs with involuntary movement, a large exposure dose is needed because of the absorption in the subject and short exposure-times become a necessity to reduce movement-unsharpness in the image. The radiographer finds an X-ray tube with a small focal area very unsatisfactory indeed as it does not allow the use of high milliamperage (greater X-ray output) and short exposure times. What is needed in these circumstances is a tube with a larger focal area so that high milliamperages may be put through it on a short exposure without damage. Geometric unsharpness in the image is bound to be somewhat greater than when small focal areas are used; but in these cases which present the risk or certainty of great movement-unsharpness the outlines obtained from large focal spots have less *total* unsharpness than those produced when small focal spots are used. This is because the large movement-unsharpness can be diminished by the use of short exposure-times in combination with high milliamperage.

So clearly a radiographer wants tubes with different sizes of focal spot according to the subject being examined. The willingness of designers and manufacturers to seek a solution to these problems led to the development of the dual focus tube. This is an X-ray tube which has incorporated into it two different focal spots; the larger of the two is known as the broad focus, and the smaller is known as the fine focus. Modern X-ray tubes in general use in hospital X-ray departments are of the dual focus type. Small tubes for use on dental X-ray units and the simplest portable equipment have only one focal spot and are described as single focus tubes.

Dual focus X-ray tubes have two filaments mounted usually side by side on the cathode structure, each filament sitting in its own separate focusing slot. Since the area on the anode covered by the electron beam (focal area) is determined by characteristics of the filament, the broad focus filament is bigger than the fine focus filament—that is, it is a helix of greater length and it is in a longer and wider slot.

On the anode the target accommodates the two different focal areas superimposed upon each other. There is a margin of tungsten allowed round the focal areas so that the heat may spread from the immediate place where it is generated into a surround of tungsten from which it is conducted into the copper rod backing the target of the tube.

Each of the two filaments is heated by a transformer winding. When the radiographer selects the focus that is to be used (which is done by means of selector switches or push-buttons on the control panel), the appropriate transformer winding is energized and the appropriate filament is heated as a result. The circuits are arranged so that it is not possible to heat both filaments at the same time.

The practical arrangement for connecting the two filaments to the transformer windings is by means of *not* four leads (two for each filament) but three (one being common to the two filaments). This arrangement is shown diagrammatically in Fig. 7.11. The high tension switches allow the appropriate filament to be energized according to whether broad or fine focus is being used.

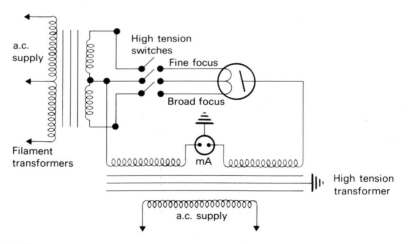

Fig. 7.11

As well as being joined to step-down transformers which heat them the filaments must be connected also to the high tension transformer which provides a voltage to drive the electrons they emit across to the anode. As can be seen in Fig. 7.11 the common lead is used for connection to the secondary winding of the high tension transformer, the X-ray tube in operation forming a complete circuit with this winding. Focal spot sizes and their selection for different radiographic examinations are discussed further in another section of this chapter (page 279).

The glass envelope and the vacuum

The electrodes of the X-ray tube must be sealed into an enclosure since it is necessary for them to operate in a vacuum. The enclosing envelope serves to support the electrodes and maintain the vacuum. The characteristics required in the envelope are:

1 that it should be able to withstand heat and mechanical stress;
2 that it should be an electrical insulator able to withstand high voltage, for if it cannot do this the electric current that is meant to pass in a controllable manner *through* the tube between the two electrodes would simply track along the outside of the envelope very easily indeed and wreck the device;
3 that it should be capable of being sealed to the electrodes with a vacuum-tight, heat-proof seal.

The substance chosen for modern tubes is hard heat-resistant glass. This is not the same thickness throughout, for underneath the anode where the useful X-ray beam emerges the glass is ground away to form a thinner window. This is done because if the X-ray beam emerged through the thick glass envelope, it would be reduced in intensity and changed in quality.

The glass envelope is cylindrical in shape. One of the factors determining its size is the maximum kilovoltage that will be applied across the tube, higher maximum kilovoltages requiring the tube to be larger. The most noticable features of the envelope (in addition to the thinned window) are (i) that the ends are turned in upon themselves, and (ii) that the cylinder is wider in diameter at its middle portion than it is at its ends; that is it is wider over the inner ends of the electrodes and the space between them than it is over their outer ends. In the sections where it is narrow the glass envelope is able to support the electrodes and to form the required seal to the metal parts. In the section where the envelope is wide, the glass walls are kept sufficiently far away from the region of the electrostatic field produced by the high voltage between cathode and anode and from the stream of electrons between the two and from the area where the electrons bombard the target. If the glass walls were too close over the middle of the tube, it might be erratic in operation and the walls might be punctured.

If there is a spoilt vacuum disaster occurs in the X-ray tube. What happens is that the electrons leaving the filament no longer have unimpeded passage to the anode, and they collide with the atoms of whatever gas it is that is in the tube spoiling the vacuum. These collisions deprive the electrons of some or all of their kinetic energy, so that when eventually they do reach the target of the tube the X radiation produced is less intense and less penetrating than it otherwise would be. Furthermore the electrons from the cathode will ionize the gaseous atoms—that is they cause electrons to leave these atoms. This means that there are more electrons travelling to the anode than just those emitted by the cathode, and the tube current increases erratically and becomes much bigger than it should be. The atoms of gas which have lost electrons are positive and are attracted to the cathode of the tube and may damage it. The filament will increase in temperature as a result of being bombarded by the positive ions and this leads to its emitting more electrons. These contribute further to the increase in tube current. The milliamperage thus becomes completely uncontrollable.

It is very important that the tube should be made with a high degree of vacuum, and when it is in operation and its parts become very hot that this vacuum is not spoilt. Unless special attention were paid to this in manufacture of the tube, when the glass and metal become hot they could release gas trapped within them. So during manufacture the components of the tube are very carefully de-gassed. This is done by heating them at various stages to high temperatures while the tube is attached to vacuum pumping equipment.

It becomes hotter than it ever should become when properly used and this process gets rid of most of the lurking gas. When the final vacuum pressure is reached the glass tube is sealed off.

The tube shield

The expression *tube shield* refers to the casing in which the glass X-ray tube is contained. The word shield suggests that this casing has a protective function and so indeed it has. In this context there are two separate risks from which people must be protected. These are (i) the radiation risk and (ii) the electrical risk.

The metal case provides protection against both these dangers. Because it gives radiation protection it is said to be ray-proof, and because it gives electrical protection it is said to be shock-proof. In addition to providing protection, the ray-proof shock-proof case serves also to contain and support the glass tube and so it is often called the tube housing; while the glass X-ray tube itself is often called the insert as acknowledgement of the fact that it is placed within the housing. The housing and the insert together are shown in Fig. 7.12.

The ray-proof housing

The word ray-proof here may be misleading if it is taken at its face value for it suggests that the housing can stop all radiation from coming through. In

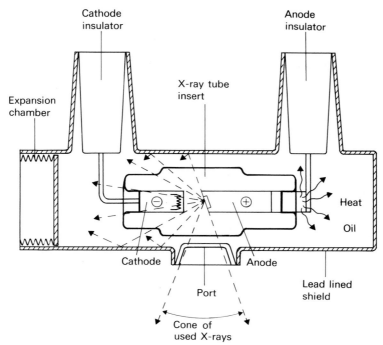

Fig. 7.12   A fixed anode X-ray tube: insert and tube housing. *By courtesy of Machlett X-ray Tubes (Great Britain) Ltd.*

fact it cannot do this. Knowledge of the physics of X-ray absorption informs us that it is impossible to absorb X rays *completely*, but it is possible by absorption to attenuate the X-ray beam so that the amount of radiation coming through the absorber is very small indeed, so small as to be within the limits of safety.

These limits are specified in certain recommendations laid down in approved codes of practice for the use of radiation. Such codes embody statements as to how much radiation may be allowed to come through the tube shield.

The ray-proof housing is necessary because X rays produced at the tube target leave it in all directions. An X-ray tube without any cover is therefore a source emitting radiation all round it. The only *useful* beam is the one used to produce the radiograph; this is a beam of radiation leaving the tube sideways about an axis at right angles to the long axis of the X-ray tube as shown in Fig. 7.5. All other radiation coming from an unprotected tube would simply increase the dose to the patient and to anyone else in the room and do no useful work at all. It is therefore important to provide the X-ray tube with a shield. The useful beam leaves the shield through a plastic-

covered aperture called the tube port or portal, and this arrangement allows
the useful beam to be carefully limited and directed. The rest of the radiation
which comes from the X-ray tube is known as leakage radiation; it is
absorbed in the shield and reduced at least to the low intensity specified in
recommendations for protection.

The shield is made by lining the cylindrical aluminium or aluminium
alloy case with thin sheets of lead which are thick enough and absorb the X
rays sufficiently to reduce the leakage radiation to the required level. The
lead lining does not need to be of the same thickness throughout the shield.
At the anode end of the tube, the heavy copper mass absorbs radiation before
it leaves the glass tube, so in this part of the housing the lead protection is
not required to be so thick.

The cylindrical housing is made with two projections from one side
which are known as cable receptacles; they are called this because the
projections contain insulated sockets or 'pots' into which are inserted the
cables which connect the X-ray tube to the high tension supply. One socket
is at the cathode end of the casing so that the cathode can be connected to
the high tension and the filament can be connected to its supply circuit as
well; the other socket is at the anode end of the casing so that the anode may
be connected to the high tension. More is said of these cables on page 232 of
this chapter.

The insulating medium

It is necessary to surround the X-ray tube inside its housing with some
material which is an electrical insulator and entirely fills up the space
between the tube and the metal shield. The chosen material is a thin purified
insulating oil which is able to serve the double purpose of acting both as an
electrical insulator and as a cooling agent when the tube is in use. More is
said on page 234 in this chapter on the cooling of an X-ray tube. Oil-
immersion of the tube allows the housing to be smaller in size than if the
medium surrounding the tube were air; oil is a better electrical insulator
than air and a bigger volume of air would be needed to insulate the tube
from the metal housing. The oil must fill up *all* the space in the housing so
it is put in very carefully under vacuum conditions. Care is taken to eliminate
air bubbles and the case is hermetically sealed.

When the X-ray tube is in use, the oil receives heat from it and therefore
becomes warmer and expands. Some means must be given for it to expand
safely without its being forced out of the shield or damaging the glass tube.
A diaphragm of synthetic rubber is provided within the housing. (Fig. 7.19.)
As it expands, the warm oil pushes and stretches the diaphragm, and thus
an extra bit of space is made for the oil within the housing. When the oil

becomes cool again and occupies less space the diaphragm relaxes, freed from the pushing action of the oil. Since it is important that the oil does not become so hot as to form a sludge which would alter its insulating properties, the diaphragm is sometimes used as a safety device to prevent the tube from going beyond a certain point of heat. If the oil gets hot enough to expand sufficiently to stretch the diaphragm beyond a certain limit, the movement of the diaphragm operates a microswitch. The operation of this switch prevents another exposure from being made until the oil is cool enough and the diaphragm has relaxed as a consequence.

The shock-proofing

The shock-proofing of the parts of the X-ray set which are at high voltage provides electrical safety (that is security from electrical shock) for staff and patients. An electric shock is the result of current flowing through the body. The danger of high voltage is not in the high voltage itself, but in the fact that high voltages make large currents flow through given resistances. The human body may be considered simply as an electrical resistance in this context.

If the insulation of the equipment breaks down, the high voltage could make current flow through the body of someone in touch with the equipment, and because the voltage is high the current will be high too if the body is presenting as a low electrical resistance. The magnitude of the shock is related to the value of the current which in general terms depends on (i) the value of the voltage and (ii) the resistance of the body. The electrical resistance of the human body is altered by such features as whether the skin is dry or damp, and whether the person is wearing rubber-soled shoes or not, and is standing on a dry or a wet floor. It is important therefore to shock-proof the apparatus—that is to construct it so that if the insulation breaks down current will flow safely to earth, and will not pass through the body of someone touching (or simply being very close to) the equipment.

The parts of the X-ray set which are at high voltage are (i) the X-ray tube itself; (ii) the high tension generator which provides it with voltage; (iii) the conductors which connect the X-ray tube to the high tension generator. Shock-proofing of these parts of the apparatus is achieved by a method which essentially is this: the three elements named above are completely surrounded by an earthed metal screen from which they are separated by insulation.

To earth electrical equipment is simply to connect it to the earth by means of an unbroken conductor which has low resistance. The low resistance ensures that this will be an easy pathway for the current to take, and the vast size of the earth allows it to receive big electric charges without increase in its own electrical potential. So electric charges conducted to earth have been disposed of safely. In practice earthing is achieved by connecting the equipment via a low-resistance copper conductor to a large metal plate buried in the ground.

In simple diagnostic X-ray sets such as small portable and dental sets, the X-ray tube and the high tension transformer can very easily be enclosed in a single shield. The tube-head of such a unit consists of a single oil-filled tank, the outer casing of which is earthed. This tank contains a small X-ray tube and the high tension transformer to which it is connected by wires. The tank also contains the step-down transformer which heats the filament of the X-ray tube. Although this transformer has no high voltage across its primary or its secondary windings, reference to the diagram in Fig. 7.1 shows that its secondary winding is connected to the filament of the X-ray tube and thus directly into the high tension secondary circuit. This is why the filament transformer must be included within the system of protection against high-voltage dangers, and why filament controls used by the radiographer must be in the *primary* filament circuit.

In larger more complex X-ray units it is not possible to enclose the tube and the high tension generator in one tank. So there are three elements in the continuous earthed metal screen which surrounds the high tension circuit: (i) the X-ray tube is oil-immersed within an earthed metal shield, which is also the ray-proof case as previously described; (ii) the high tension generator and the step-down transformer for the filament are oil-immersed within an earthed metal tank; (iii) connection of the tube to the generator and the filament transformer is made by means of a pair of special cables (known as high tension cables) which have a metal sheathing which is earthed. Careful connection of the cables to the tube housing at one end and to the generator tank at the other ensures that the high tension parts are completely enclosed in an earthed metal sheath from which they are separated by an insulating medium; the insulation is oil in the tube housing and in the generator tank and is rubber material in the case of the cables.

High tension cables

The construction of each high tension cable is shown diagrammatically in Fig. 7.13 and is as follows. (The description is somewhat simplified.)

1   Innermost are the electrical conductors which carry the supply to the X-ray tube. These conductors are copper wires. In a cable which is to be used for the anode end of the X-ray tube only one such inner conductor is necessary, but for a cable to be used at the cathode end of a dual-focus tube three are necessary (so that the two filaments as well as being connected to the high tension may be connected to their heating transformers). To save

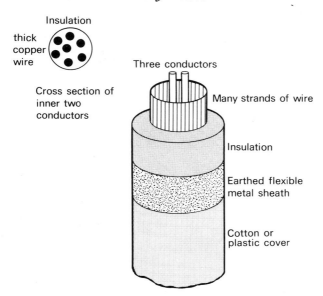

Fig. 7.13

making different cables and to allow interchanging cables, the modern practice is to make both the cathode and anode cables the same—that is with three inner conductors or cores. These are arranged as in Fig. 7.13, the outer one of the three being the common conductor mentioned on page 226.

2   Round the central conductors is the insulating layer of material. This is made of special rubber which has very good insulating properties. It is put round the copper cores in a thick layer. The higher the voltage to which the cable is to be subjected the thicker this layer must be, and the cable will be bulkier, heavier, less flexible and more expensive.

3   Round the rubber is a flexible metallic sheath made of strands of metal plaited or braided together. This metal sheath is connected to earth and constitutes the earthed metal screen which has been mentioned.

4   Over the metal sheath is a further covering which is a plastic sheath. It is designed to protect the flexible metal braiding from damage.

The cables are connected to the tube housing and to the generator tank by means of a plug and socket arrangement. The cable receptacles in the side-arms of the tube housing hold insulator sockets to accommodate the cable ends; they are matched by similar sockets in the tank which holds the high tension generator. The sockets have contacts in their floors which accept the conducting cores of the cables. These cores emerge as 'pins' from the tapered cable ends (see Fig. 7.14) and when the cables are in place the cores are connected via the contacts to the electrodes of the X-ray tube at

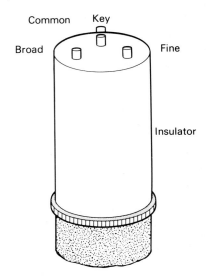

Fig. 7.14

one end, and to the high tension generator and the filament supplies at the other.

Each cable has at each end a metal screw-cap which slides loosely over its outer covering and is screwed into place on the tube housing and on the generator tank when the cable end is pushed home into the appropriate socket. When the screw-cap is in place (i) the metal housing of the tube, (ii) the metal sheathing of the cable and (iii) the metal tank containing the generator are all firmly connected together and are connected to earth. The high tension parts are thus completely enclosed in an earthed metal screen which is continuous.

Cooling the X-ray tube

Almost all the electrical energy put into the X-ray tube is converted into heat as has been explained, while a small proportion of it (about 1 per cent) gives rise to X radiation. This means that throughout the exposure a great amount of heat is developed at the target of the X-ray tube where the conversion of electron energy is taking place. This continues to be developed as long as the exposure lasts.

The amount of heat is related to the product: kilovoltage across the tube × milliamperes through the tube × duration of exposure. The greater these factors are, the more heat will be developed at the target of the tube. During the exposure, the temperature of the tungsten target continues to rise as heat is put in. If a sequence of events for the dissipation of heat were not taking place at the same time, the melting point of tungsten would very soon be reached.

The processes by which heat is dissipated are (i) conduction, which takes place in solids; (ii) convection, which takes place in liquids and gases; and (iii) radiation, which can occur in a vacuum as well as in a space filled by air or other gases. All three processes are utilized in the X-ray tube and its shield.

The first step is for the heat to be removed from the target area. This is done by the tungsten plate passing most of the heat by conduction into the copper block of the anode in which the target is set. Copper is a good conductor of heat, and furthermore this massive piece of copper has the capacity to accept a certain amount of heat without marked rise in temperature; both these features make it a good receptacle for the heat from the tungsten target. The copper anode conducts the heat along its length and thus to the outside of the tube. The target also conveys a small part of its heat by radiation across the vacuum of the X-ray tube to the glass envelope.

Via the anode rod and the glass envelope, the heat thus reaches the oil in which the tube is immersed. Like the copper, the oil is able to accept the heat without great rise in temperature. Convection currents are set up in the oil and the heat is conveyed to the metal casing. It is then conducted through the casing to its outer surface which is in contact with the air in the room. The metal casing then loses heat by convection and by radiation to the air surrounding the X-ray tube.

It can be realized that the quantity of heat which initally is produced over a very small area indeed (the few square millimetres covered by the electron beam in the X-ray tube) is slowly spread through greater and greater volumes (copper, oil, metal of the housing, air in the room). So the temperature is lowered slowly as the heat is passed on its way.

When an X-ray tube is used for fluoroscopy the periods of exposure last several seconds and are sustained in series over a period of time. The tube is then said to be on 'continuous operation'. This can be contrasted with 'intermittent operation' when the tube is being used for general radiography. Most of the exposures are then fractions of seconds or at most a second or two, and they are not repeated at intervals so short that the tube is unable to lose much heat between them (except in certain special examinations).

For continuous operation it is possible to hasten the rate of heat loss beyond that of the natural methods. This can be done by providing an air-circulator—an electric fan—which is contained in a housing that can be mounted on the tube shield. It blows cool air over the shield and speeds up the convection process by which the heat is lost. In practice, however, air-circulators are rarely used at the present time.

Filtration in the X-ray tube

When an X-ray beam passes through materials which are capable of absorbing any part of it and thus altering it, the beam is said to have been filtered. An X-ray beam is produced with many different photon energies in it and a filtering material acts by absorbing preferentially the low energies in the beam. When the beam emerges through the filter without those photons which have lower energy, it has been altered in quality by having a higher average energy. If the low photon energies are left in the beam (that is, there is no filter) they are absorbed by the patient's skin and superficial tissues; they increase the dose to the patient without contributing usefully to the production of the radiograph. So the beam is preferred after it is filtered because it is used then with less dose to the patient and without diminution in its radiographic efficiency.

Coming out of the tube after it leaves the target, the useful beam must pass through (i) the thinned window in the glass envelope, (ii) the oil within the tube shield, (iii) the plastic-covered aperture in the lead-lined shield (called the tube port or portal) which ensures that the oil is kept in and the X-ray beam is allowed out. None of these substances absorbs X rays heavily, but together they add up to a filter which is able to remove the lowest energies from the beam. The filtering action of these three elements in the construction of the tube and its housing is called the inherent filtration of the tube.

The manufacturer of the X-ray tube includes in its specifications a statement of what this inherent filtration is; it is conveniently expressed as the number of millimetres of aluminium which could achieve the same filtering effect as the combined successive layers of glass/oil/plastic which are in the X-ray tube and its housing. The inherent filtration in most modern X-ray tubes is equivalent to about 1 mm of aluminium. (Strictly, 1 mm of aluminium can be *exactly* equivalent to the glass/oil/plastic layers of a particular X-ray tube under only one condition of kilovoltage, milliamperage and voltage waveform.)

It is possible to filter the X-ray beam more heavily than this and remove more of the low energies so that the dose to the patient is further reduced, and the intensity which is radiographically useful is not noticeably diminished. Approved codes of practice may state specifically in terms of aluminium equivalence what the total filtration should be for an X-ray tube used in diagnostic radiology. If the inherent filtration is less than the wanted level, then an additional aluminium filter can be inserted. At the tube port there is a recess external to the plastic-covered aperture in the shield where the filter can be fitted into place. The thickness of the additional filter is chosen so that it and the inherent filtration provide a filtration which is equivalent to the required thickness of aluminium.

Limitations of the fixed anode X-ray tube

The dilemma inherent in the nature and use of the diagnostic X-ray tube has now been discussed in various sections of this chapter. It has been seen that the radiographer wants a large focal area; this allows more electrical energy and more heat to be put in without the temperature of the focal spot rising to the melting point of tungsten, and the tube can therefore be used at greater radiographic output. At the same time the radiographer wants a small X-ray source so that the geometric unsharpness in the image will not be too great.

As already discussed, these conflictions can be partially resolved by the use of a sloping anode face so that the focus when viewed from the film appears smaller than it really is, and by the use of dual-focus X-ray tubes. There is, however, a limit to what can be achieved by the sloping anode face. A very large focus cannot be foreshortened enough to make it appear acceptably small; an anode angle slight enough to achieve the foreshortening required would result in a useful beam which could cover only a small-sized X-ray film, which would not be very practical. As seen on page 223 the focus is projected to seem approximately one-quarter or one-third the size it really is. This is the limit to reduction in apparent size that can be usefully achieved in practice with a fixed anode X-ray tube.

A development in solving these problems has been the rotating anode X-ray tube for diagnostic radiography introduced about forty years ago. It has proved such an advance on the fixed anodes that it has by now entirely superseded these, except for tubes used in dental X-ray sets and in small portable and mobile units of restricted output. The rotating anode X-ray tube is described in the following pages.

THE ROTATING ANODE X-RAY TUBE

A rotating anode X-ray tube is illustrated in Fig. 7.15.

As their names suggest, the essential difference between an X-ray tube with a fixed anode and one with a rotating anode is that in the latter the anode rotates during the exposure.

In a fixed anode X-ray tube the area (a) which is covered by the electron beam and becomes the X-ray source and the area (b) over which the heat from the electron bombardment is spread are the same. In the rotating anode tube, because of the rotation the two areas (a) and (b) are not the same. So it becomes possible to keep the area (a) small while allowing the area (b) to be large. The result is an X-ray tube which permits the use of big electrical loads in combination with a small effective focus and apparent X-ray source. From the radiographer's point of view, this X-ray tube makes

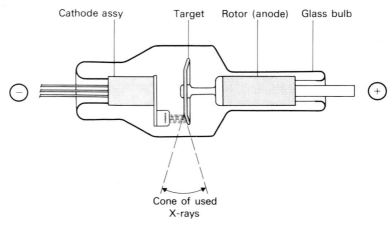

Cathode assy   Target   Rotor (anode)   Glass bulb

Cone of used
X-rays

Fig. 7.15   A rotating anode X-ray tube: the tube insert. *By courtesy of Machlett X-ray Tubes (Great Britain) Ltd.*

it possible to use high milliamperes and short exposure times without any sacrifice in terms of geometric unsharpness.

The cathode and filament

The features of the cathode and its filament are not essentially different from those of the same structures in a fixed anode X-ray tube. The main characteristic to be noted is that the helical tungsten filament has a position in the X-ray tube which is *not* such that the electron stream from it is along the central axis of the X-ray tube. In a rotating anode tube the cathode structure supports the filament in a position which is off-centre to this central axis. The electron stream from the filament travels through the tube along a line parallel to the long central axis and is brought to a focus towards the edge of the anode disc which faces the filament.

A sketch of this arrangment is shown in Fig. 7.16 and it can also be seen in the diagram in Fig. 7.15. The filament is again housed in the supporting structure so that the electron stream is focused, one side of the filament being electrically connected to the cathode structure so that a negative potential is on both. As in the case of the fixed anode X-ray tube, the area covered by the electron stream is determined by the cathode characteristics— size and shape of filament and dimensions of focusing slot or cup—and the spacing of the electrodes in the X-ray tube.

The anode

The anode is a heavy disc mounted on a molybdenum stem which functions as its support. Earlier discs were made entirely of tungsten; modern discs are made of molybdenum faced with tungsten or with tungsten alloyed with rhenium. The diameter of the disc is among the factors which determine the permissible electrical load and larger discs can take higher loads without damage. The range is about 50–100 mm. The disc is not a flat one; its outer rim is bevelled so that the shape suggests a shallow overturned saucer or (considered in conjunction with its support) a rather flat opened umbrella. This can be seen in Fig. 7.15. Viewed from the cathode end of the X-ray tube the anode is a disc with its centre on the longitudinal central axis of the tube; during the exposure the anode rotates about this central axis at a speed of some 3000 revolutions or more per minute.

The electron beam is focused so that it covers a rectangular area towards the periphery of this disc; this is the small dark rectangle in the sketch in Fig. 7.17(a) which shows the anode disc *en face*. Since the cathode structure does not move and the only movement made by the anode is rotation, this

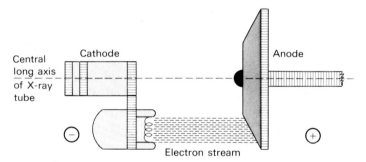

Fig. 7.16

area of electron bombardment does not shift in its placing in the X-ray tube or change its position relative to its location on the anode face—that is below the central axis towards the periphery of the disc.

This rectangular area of bombardment is essentially the same as the line focus of a fixed anode X-ray tube. It is the true size of the X-ray source and it is 3 to 4 times longer than it is wide. As can be seen in Fig. 7.17(b) the bevelled edge of the anode disc functions exactly as the sloped face of a fixed anode and foreshortens this rectangle to a square so that the apparent size of the source is smaller than the actual source. The angle of bevel has usually varied from a target angle of 15 degrees, which gives a true source 4 times larger than the apparent one, to a target angle of 20 degrees, which gives a true source about 3 times larger than the apparent one. However, some modern tubes (see page 273 in this chapter) have a target angle of 10 degrees, which gives a true source between 5 and 6 times greater than the apparent one.

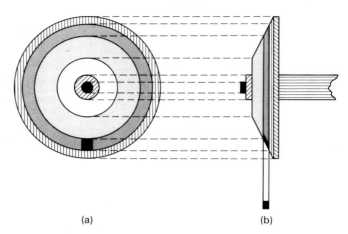

(a)   (b)

Fig. 7.17

The arrangements described take care of the area (a) which is covered by the electron beam and becomes the X-ray source. The area (b) over which the heat is spread is a much bigger one. The rotation of the anode ensures that the portion of the disc which is actually under the electron bombardment is changing all the time. So the area over which the heat is spread is not a small rectangle, but for one complete revolution of the disc is a ring; the outer circumference of this is nearly enough the outer circumference of the anode disc, while its inner circumference depends on the length of the line focus to which the electron stream is focused. This ring is indicated by the dark grey area in Fig. 7.17(a). It is called the focal spot track or target track.

The increased area which receives the heat may be more clearly appreciated if figures are considered. Suppose that the electron beam covers an area (the actual focus) on the anode disc which is 1×3 mm^2: this projects as an apparent focus which is 1 mm^2. For one revolution of the anode disc, the passing ring of the focal track presents an area of which the 3 mm^2 of the actual focus is only from 0.1 up to 1.0 per cent. In these circumstances the area (b) over which the heat is spread is from 1000 down to 100 times greater than the area (a) covered by the electron beam. The tube will allow much more heat to be put into it and will take bigger electrical loads than a tube in which the two areas are the same. It will do this without any increase in size of effective focal spot over a fixed-anode X-ray tube. The great advantage of the rotating anode X-ray tube is that it allows high milliamperage to be used and good radiographic detail to be maintained because there is no increase in geometric unsharpness.

The anode: support and rotation

As can be seen in Fig. 7.15 the support for the anode disc is a stem and this is made of molybdenum. One end of the stem is attached to the disc at its centre and the other end is mounted into a copper cylinder shown in Fig. 7.15. This copper cylinder is known as the rotor because it is the moving part of an electric motor which produces a rotating force. The rotor rotates because electric currents are induced in it, and it rotates on its own support which emerges through the end of the glass envelope.

The emergent end of the rotor support which is the anode shank is used to connect the high voltage supply to the anode of the X-ray tube. The glass envelope is sealed to the rotor support with a vacuum-tight, heat-proof seal. When the tube is fixed into its outer shield, this seal between the glass and the rotor support carries the anode weight—and this is no light matter!

The rotation takes place on ball bearings between the rotor and its support. It is very important to the life of the tube that these ball bearings should always allow free and easy rotation and that everything possible should be done to prevent them from getting too hot. This is why the disc is attached to the rotor by *a narrow* stem of a metal (molybdenum) which is not more than a moderately good conductor of heat. Thus the stem allows only a small amount of heat to pass back from the anode disc to the copper rotor.

The rotor is made of copper because this metal is a good conductor of electricity—an essential feature in the rotor since it is moved by inducing electric currents in it. The outer surface of the copper cylinder is treated to make it radiate heat to a maximum extent so that the heat is radiated out to the glass walls of the tube and away from the ball bearings. This treatment consists of blackening the outer walls of the cylinder.

The ball bearings are made of steel and must be lubricated if they are to continue to let the rotor run freely. The lubrication is specialized because the ball bearings are inside the glass envelope of the tube and therefore are inside a vacuum and are subjected to heat. Ordinary lubricants would spoil the vacuum when they become hot and so they cannot possibly be used. Instead, lubrication is achieved by coating the ball bearings with silver or lead, a thin layer of these soft metals having the required result. The rotor which rides on the ball bearings carries the heavy weight of the anode disc, and to reduce the stress of this the molybdenum stem which connects the disc and the rotor is made as short as possible.

The ball bearings lead a hard life for the rotor rotates fast at every radiographic exposure made. If they fail in service and do not provide free running for the rotor without vibration or do not keep up the required speed of rotation, then such failure in the bearings can terminate the useful life of the tube. The tube cannot be used satisfactorily if the ball bearings are badly worn. Fig. 7.18 sketches a ball race.

The force of rotation for the anode is obtained from an electric motor; this is of a type known as an induction motor. Outside the glass envelope of the tube where the envelope forms a narrow neck around the rotor is placed a collar. This carries the iron core of the motor and its electrical windings.

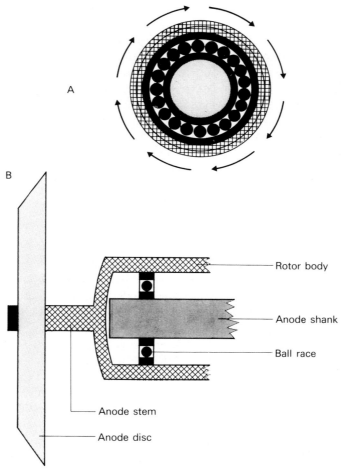

A

B

Rotor body

Anode shank

Ball race

Anode stem

Anode disc

Fig. 7.18 At (a) is a sketch diagram of a ballrace. The grey-shaded inner part represents the anode shank or support which is firmly attached to the inner ring of the ballrace (smaller black ring in the diagram). The ball bearings are in a channel between this inner ring which is fixed and the outer ring (larger black ring in the diagram). The outer ring rotates freely about the inner, carried on the ball bearings. The cross-hatched part in the diagram represents the rotor body firmly attached to the outer ring of the ballrace. At (b) is shown the assembly of the rotor and ball bearings in cross section.

The core and the windings together form the stator; this is the stationary part of the electric motor. The stator can be seen in Fig. 7.19. When the motor is energized, the windings carry alternating current and the rotor is within the magnetic field from this current. The glass neck of the tube which is between the rotor and the windings is made as narrow as possible so that the separation is minimal and the magnetic field most efficiently used.

By the use of special circuits it is possible to obtain a rotating magnetic field from such windings. The rotor then finds itself in a magnetic field which is constantly changing, and since the rotor is itself an electrical conductor the changing field induces electromotive force and current flowing in the rotor. This induction gives to the rotor a magnetic field which is opposite in polarity at any one time to that from the windings, and so there is a force of attraction between the rotor field and the winding field. Since the field from the windings rotates, the rotor field wants to follow it round and as the rotor is free to move it rotates.

When a rotating anode tube is in use for radiography, the anode must be rotating during the exposure, and furthermore it must be rotating at its full speed when the exposure begins. The standard speed is from about 2400 to 3600 revolutions per minute, and it will take the anode about 1 second to reach this speed. In order to make sure before the exposure commences (a) that the anode has begun to rotate and (b) that it is rotating at full speed, the practice is for the manufacturer of the X-ray unit to link the starting of the anode with pressure on the exposure button. The radiographer using the equipment finds that when the button of the exposure switch is lightly pressed the first thing that happens is that the anode begins to rotate. There then follows what is described as the 'prepare' period during which the anode comes up to full speed. At the end of the required interval, a relay operates (it can be heard if the radiographer listens carefully in a quiet room). If the exposure switch is then firmly depressed, the exposure begins. (See page 154 for interlocks in the stator circuit.)

If the radiographer tries to evade the 'prepare' period by depressing the exposure button firmly at once without doing it in two stages, it will be found that the exposure in any case will not begin until the end of the delay imposed to allow the anode to reach its full speed of rotation. When the exposure stops, the electrical supply to the stator windings is automatically cut off and the rotor loses speed and stops. (A braking dc voltage may be applied.)

The careful radiographer using a rotating anode tube listens for these events—the starting of anode rotation and its eventual cessation. If they do not occur properly something is clearly wrong and needs attention. In the event of failure of the anode to rotate, the exposure should not be made.

Initiation of exposure which is linked to anode rotation has a certain nuisance value in some radiographic examinations when it is important to be able to begin the exposure at particular instants in time—for example in an angiographic series or in examining small children when the radiographer wishes to seize an appropriate moment which is all too fleeting with an unco-operative subject of this type. It is possible to arrange to have anode rotation controlled by a key or switch on the control panel if this is wished. When special work is being undertaken, the anode can then be put into rotation independently of the exposure switch and the exposure can begin without previous delay.

When this is done it is imperative that the radiographer should remember to switch the anode off as soon as possible. It is on record that one unfortunate took an angiographic series of films into the darkroom for processing and came back to find the anode not switched off and still rotating. The heat from this continued running of the motor had melted the paint on the outside of the tube housing. This was an impressive sight which caused that radiographer not to forget again and not to need reminding that when the stator windings are energized for long periods, the power consumed must be included in the total heat input to the tube. A modern practice which greatly reduces the risk of overheating is to run the stator at 230 volts at the start for, say, 1 second and then continuously at 40 volts; but even this reduced power input must be taken into account.

The dual focus rotating anode X-ray tube

Unless the rotating anode X-ray tube is for very restricted use, it is of the dual focus type. The cathode structure then supports two filaments side by side or one above the other, one of the two being larger than the other. The area covered by the electron beam from each filament is determined by the size and shape of the filament and the dimensions of the focusing slot in which each sits. The two filaments cover areas on the anode which may be superimposed, may be placed side by side, or may be placed so that one is nearer the centre of the anode disc—i.e. one is above the other when viewed from the film position underneath the portal of the tube.

For the filament connections to their separate heating transformers and to the high voltage supply, reference should be made to the section dealing with this for the fixed anode tube on page 226 in this chapter. Focal spot sizes and their application to various radiographic examinations are discussed in later sections (page 279).

The glass envelope

Fig. 7.3 and Fig. 7.15 show that the glass envelope of a rotating anode X-ray tube is not the same shape as that of a fixed anode X-ray tube. This is hardly surprising in view of that fact that the electrodes within each tube are different in form. The envelope of the rotating anode tube (like that of the fixed anode tube) is narrow at its extremities where it is turned in on itself to form a vacuum-tight seal with the metal parts. At the anode end, the glass envelope forms a long narrow neck to accommodate on its outside the stator core and its windings, and on its inside the rotor rotating freely very close to (but of course not making contact with) the glass (Fig. 7.19).

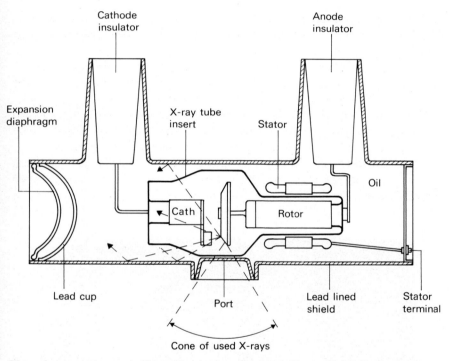

Fig. 7.19 A rotating anode X-ray tube: insert and housing. *By courtesy of Machlett X-ray Tubes (Great Britain) Ltd.*

Just about where the inner end of the rotor narrows to the molybdenum stem which supports the anode disc, the glass envelope widens to become a cylinder of much greater diameter. The central portion of the tube where the anode disc and the filaments are has walls much wider apart to reduce the risk of damage to the glass envelope when high tension is applied between the electrodes. Beneath the anode where the X-ray beam emerges there is a thinner window carefully controlled in thickness so that the beam leaves the tube with less absorption in the glass. The glass used for the envelope is hard and heat-resistant.

As in the case of fixed anode tubes it is very important that the vacuum should be as near perfect as possible. Great care is taken in manufacture to see that this vacuum is created and is maintained as long as possible during the working life of the tube. Pure materials are selected and de-gassing procedures are carried out with the tube and its parts raised to high temperatures.

The tube shield

The tube shield of a rotating anode tube is seen in Fig. 7.19 and Fig. 7.20. The important features of any tube shield have already been described (page 228). The essential points are as follows.

1 That the shield should be lead-lined and ray-proof at least to the extent that the leakage radiation from it is not more than that permitted by codes of practice and recommendations for protection.

2 That the shield should be shock-proof and should constitute an earthed metal enclosure for the tube, this enclosure forming part of that which contains all the high tension elements used for operation of the tube.

3 That the shield should be provided with electrical insulation, this being usually achieved by filling it with an insulating oil which has been dehydrated and degassed.

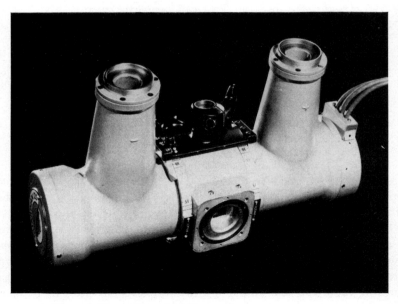

Fig. 7.20 A diagnostic X-ray tube and shield.

4   That the portal through which the X-ray beam leaves the shield should be of such a size and should be provided with lead protection such that the useful beam covers a limited area which is not more than the maximum likely to be required.

5   That the shield should provide sockets or cable receptacles (one for the cathode cable and one for the anode cable) such that the X-ray tube may be safely connected to the high voltage supply via the high tension cables; the shield, the cables and the tank which contains the generator together forming the earthed metal enclosure to which reference has previously been made.

Shields for rotating anode tubes carry in addition to the high tension cables a mains voltage supply to energize the stator windings. This supply is carried by a cable much smaller in size than those for the high tension since this cable carries a small current at a low voltage. This cable enters the shield at the end plate of the casing. The terminal for the stator cable can be seen in Fig. 7.19 which shows a rotating anode X-ray tube in its shield.

The area covered by the useful beam is usually indicated in manufacturers' specifications in terms of degrees from the central beam—for example, X-ray coverage is 17 degrees from the central beam. This coverage is for an area 43 cm² at 1 metre target to film distance.

The exit port of the X-ray tube is lead-lined and often has a little cone shape in lead fitted into it so that the beam leaving the tube is limited. The outside of the shield is fitted to allow beam-limiting devices such as extension cones and light-beam diaphragms to be readily attached to it.

The cable receptacles project to accept the ends of the high tension cables as previously described (page 233) and these are an obvious external feature of any tube shield, whether it be for a rotating anode tube or not. The position of these cable receptacles is described by the manufacturer in terms of the angle between the axis of the X-ray beam and the axis of the cable receptacles. In some modern rotating anode tubes for overtable use, the angle is 90 degrees, as in Fig. 7.21 and other angles such as 180 degrees, 135 degrees and 20 degrees are available.

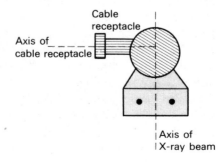

Fig. 7.21

Obviously some angles are more convenient than others according to how the tube is to be mounted and used. What is suitable for an overtable tube may not be convenient for an undertable tube to be used with the table in vertical or horizontal or intermediate positions.

Cooling the rotating anode X-ray tube

Fixed anode and rotating anode X-ray tubes are unable to share the same sequence of events in dissipating heat from their focal areas where it is produced. When the tubes operate, it will be recalled that in the case of the fixed anode tube the first stage in removing the heat from the area of electron bombardment is that it is conducted from the tungsten target into the solid copper rod which backs it. The heavy copper rod passes the heat by conduction so that it is brought externally to the glass envelope into the oil surround. A very small amount of heat (10 per cent) is conveyed to the glass envelope by radiation through the vacuum from the target face.

In the case of the rotating anode tube it is very important that all the heat should *not* be passed back from the focal area. When it reaches the rotor, the heat raises the temperature of the ball bearings on which the rotor rotates on its support. This is something that must be not encouraged but positively prevented by some features of the tube's construction. These are (i) the anode disc is mounted on a narrow stem made of metal which is not a good conductor of heat; (ii) sometimes the target disc is backed with another disc which serves as a baffle, reflecting the heat and preventing it from reaching the rotor and its ball bearings; (iii) heat which does reach the rotor is taken outwards away from the ball bearings by radiation from the blackened outer surface of the rotor to the glass envelope.

The pattern of heating for the rotating anode disc is an alternating heat–cool–heat–cool–heat sequence maintained as the disc revolves. During one revolution of the disc, the focal spot (that is, the area on the focal track which is covered and under bombardment by the electron beam) receives electrons for some microseconds (say 3 to 60 according to the speed of rotation) before the movement of the disc carries it out of the line of the electron stream: the electrons of course then cover an adjacent spot on the focal track which has been moved into position for bombardment.

The bombarded focal spot has its temperature raised by about 2000°C, the heat being intense at the surface of the disc. When the bombarded spot is moved out of the line of fire, it remains outside the electron beam for a period of time which is several hundred times longer than the few microseconds during which it was in place for bombardment: then the rotation of the disc brings it back to the place where it is again bombarded by electrons. So there is a heat–cool–heat sequence repeating itself continuously throughout the exposure at a rate of 140 to 166 sequences per second. The 'cool' periods are much longer than the 'heat' periods and they allow the concentrated heat produced instantaneously at the surface to pass to the deeper layers of the anode disc. The poor conduction of the anode disc results in its becoming red or white hot almost at once when a heavy load is applied, and in this state the anode is able to lose heat by radiation very well indeed. So most of the heat loss is by radiation from the anode disc. Anode cooling is improved if the disc has a black-coated surface on one side and if the disc is larger in area.

Once the heat reaches the glass envelope by radiation and conduction the cooling sequence in a rotating anode tube is the same as in a fixed anode tube. Heat is transferred by conduction through the glass into the surrounding oil, by convection in the oil to the metal casing, by conduction through the casing to its outer surface, and then by convection and radiation to the air of the room. The use of an air-circulating fan to assist cooling when a tube is being run continuously which is described on page 235 is applicable also to rotating anode tubes.

Filtration in rotating anode X-ray tubes

Inherent and added filtration in X-ray tubes have already been discussed in relation to fixed anode tubes (page 236). There is no need to say anything different on this topic when considering tubes with rotating anodes, and the reader who wishes to pursue this matter here should turn back to the appropriate pages.

RATING OF X-RAY TUBES

When a manufacturer provides an X-ray tube he must be able to produce with it certain statements of the conditions in which it may safely be used, and in this context the safety with which we are concerned is that of the X-ray tube itself. The information required is details of the electrical loads which may be applied to the X-ray tube without damaging it and the safe duration of such loads.

The limiting factors are as follows.

1 The temperature to which the focal area is raised by the heat produced when the electrical load is applied. This temperature certainly must not exceed the melting point of tungsten which is 3360°C, the safe level being taken to be 3000°C. Greater electrical loads result in greater heat. The temperature of the focal spot is affected by the rate at which heat is removed from it except at the very shortest exposures.

2   The thermal capacity of the anode. This is the amount of heat which the anode can accept from the target without overheating.

3   The cooling rate of the anode—that is the effectiveness with which it can pass heat on to the oil and the shield.

4   The thermal capacity of the shield. This is the quantity of heat which the shield can accept without overheating.

5   The effectiveness with which the shield can dissipate heat to its surroundings by means of the processes already described—that is its cooling rate.

6   The maximum voltage which the X-ray tube is designed to stand—that is the highest voltage at which it may be used.

At short exposures (less than 1 second) the limitation on the electrical load is based chiefly on how hot the focal area becomes during the instants that the exposure lasts. During longer exposures there is time for the processes to become effective by which heat is transferred from the focal area; on longer exposures the ability of the anode to dissipate heat becomes important. On continuous running (during fluoroscopy) the cooling rate of the anode and the ability of the oil and the housing to dissipate heat to their surroundings are significant.

The limit on the maximum voltage which may be used is set by the design of the X-ray tube, important points being the distance separating cathode and anode, the length of the tube and the thickness of its glass walls. The choice of a given X-ray tube with a particular voltage limitation will be governed by the work for which it is intended to use the tube and the output of the high tension generator which is to supply it.

Thus if you were to equip an X-ray room with a major installation for a great variety of work and you had a high tension generator capable of a maximum output of 120 kV, it would be useless to select an X-ray tube which was suitable for use only to 100 kV. If on the other hand the high tension generator could not provide a voltage greater than 100 kV, it would be unnecessary to go to the expense of purchasing a tube capable of operating safely and satisfactorily at a maximum voltage of 125 kV.

The information which a manufacturer provides concerning loads which may be safely applied is called the rating of the X-ray tube. For any given tube the rating is a complex matter, influenced by many variables, and the manufacturer must accumulate and present to the user of the tube many data concerning it. Information which is given about an X-ray tube may be considered to come under three headings.

1   *Radiographic ratings*   These are statements of the electrical loads which may be safely applied to the X-ray tube for radiographic exposures, and of the exposure times which may be used for given loads without damaging the

tube. These data are often given in the graphical form of a series of curves and such graphs are called rating charts.

2   *Thermal ratings*   These are statements on how much heat can safely be put into the anode of the X-ray tube and into the tube unit as a whole, together with information on the rate at which the anode and the tube unit lose heat. There are also statements on safe repetition rates and numbers of total exposures when an X-ray tube is used for angiography. All this information may be given on charts in graphical form.

3   *Fluoroscopic ratings*   These are statements on how the tube may safely be used for fluoroscopy. This is when the tube is running continuously, being energized for periods which are timed in minutes and not in seconds as with radiographic exposures.

These three different aspects of tube rating will now be considered separately.

Radiographic ratings

The exposure factors manipulated by the radiographer and affecting the radiographic result are (i) milliamperage, which is current through the tube, (ii) kilovoltage, which is voltage across it, and (iii) exposure time, which is the period that the tube is energized by means of this electrical load applied to it. The radiographer needs to use these variables over a wide range in order to achieve the desired radiographic results. These variables of exposure alter not only the radiographic results but also the amount of heat put into the X-ray tube when the exposure is made.

The total heat produced by the exposure is proportional to milliamperage × kilovoltage × time. Since the total heat is proportional to a product of three variables, it is clear that for a given heat input it should be possible to alter individual values of each variable, and that with two of them determined a safe value for the third is fixed.

Fig. 7.22 is a typical radiographic rating chart relating to a particular X-ray tube. It can be seen that the horizontal axis of the graph (abscissa) is marked with values which are maximum permissible exposure times in seconds; people who make graphs like to present time as a long horizontal line perhaps because this is mostly what it feels like! The vertical axis is marked with values which are a range of milliamperes from 10 to 130. Across the graph is a series of curves which represent a range of kilovoltages from 50 to 110 in steps of 10 kV, and two values above 110 kV which are 125 kV and 150 kV.

The radiographer uses such a chart to find out whether a given exposure is within safe limits in this way. When two of the three variables have been

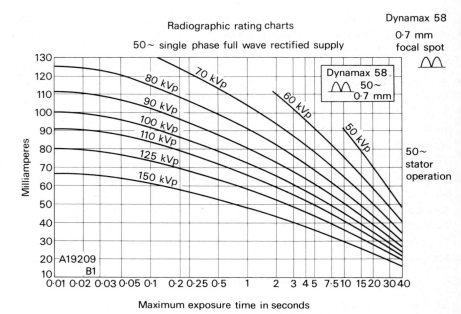

Fig. 7.22 Rating chart. *By courtesy of Machlett X-ray Tubes (Great Britain) Ltd.*

chosen, the maximum permissible value for the third is found by looking on the graphs for the point of intersection of the other two. For a particular kilovoltage curve, safe combinations of milliamperes and time lie underneath the curve (i.e. to the left of the kilovoltage curve on the graph) and maximum safe combinations lie on the curve; unsafe combinations of milliamperes and time lie above the kilovoltage curve (i.e. to the right of the kilovoltage curve on the graph). Thus if the radiographer selects 100 mA at 100 kV, the maximum permissible time of exposure if the focal area is not to overheat is found where the 100 kV curve intersects with the 100 mA ordinate value and is given as 0·02 seconds. If an exposure time of 0·5 seconds and a tube voltage of 70 kV are used, the highest milliamperage which can be selected is just over 100 mA—say 112 mA (560 mAs). If an exposure of 0·05 seconds and 120 mA (6 mAs) are required, the maximum kilovoltage to be used is 80 kV.

Using a rating chart

There are some important points to be kept in mind when using a radiographic rating chart, which should never be casually consulted. These are as follows.

1   The chart consulted must be the one which specifically relates to the X-ray tube in use. If the tube is a dual focus tube, then the chart consulted must specifically relate to the focal spot being used for the exposure.

2   The conditions of operation affect the rating of an X-ray tube. This is explained more fully on page 255 in this chapter and at the moment it is enough to say that for a given X-ray tube and a given focal spot the rating is different according to whether (for example) the tube is operating self-rectified or from a high tension generator equipped with rectifiers. So the radiographer using a rating chart must make sure that the one consulted relates specifically to the conditions of operation which are applicable.

3   A radiographic rating chart expresses limits of load which are safely applied when the X-ray tube is cool and is not already heated by previous exposures. It must be remembered that each exposure puts heat into the tube and a series of exposures individually safe which are repeated rapidly without intervals in which the tube loses heat can build up to an overload on the X-ray tube. An exposure close to the safe limit of load on the chart may be quite safe if it is made, for instance, early in a barium meal session when the tube is cool; but unsafe an hour later at the end of the session when it is made several times in a rapid series of exposures on a duodenal cap. A radiographer using a rating chart of this type must keep in mind its limitations—that it gives information only about single exposures applied to a cool X-ray tube and that it gives no guidance on how often exposures may be safely repeated.

4   If certain milliampereseconds and kilovoltage are safe for a certain exposure time, the same milliampereseconds with another time factor are not necessarily safe calculated on the basis of a simple straight-line relationship—for example, if 50 mAs at 100 kV are safe given as 50 mA for 1 second, it is not necessarily safe to give 100 mA for 0·5 second at 100 kV. This can be checked by reference to the chart in Fig. 7.22. It can be seen that the point of intersection of the 50 mA and 1 second values lies on the safe side of the 125 kV curve, so 50 mA at 100 kV for 1 second (50 mAs) is safe. The point of intersection of the 100 mA and 0·5 second values is well on the safe side of the 70 kV curve but *just* on the unsafe side of the 80 kV curve and far on the unsafe side of the 100 kV curve. So 100 mA at 100 kV for 0·5 second (50 mAs) is decidedly *not* safe. To take another example—reference to the chart at 100 kV curve shows that with an exposure of 0·1 second the highest milliampereseconds which can be used are 92 mA × 0·1 second = 9·2 mAs; with an exposure of 1 second the highest milliampereseconds are 72 mA × 1 second = 72 mAs; with an exposure time of 10 seconds the highest milliampereseconds are 45 mA × 10 seconds = 450 mAs.

Both these examples illustrate the general principles that (i) as longer exposure times are used the milliampereseconds which can safely be applied become greater, or to put it another way the ratings become higher; and (ii) the ratings do not have a linear relation to time, and increasing the time by a factor of 10 does not increase the rating to the same extent.

Why does the rating become higher as exposure times increase? The answer lies in the facts to which reference was made on page 250. On short exposures (less than 1 second) the limitation on the electrical load is based chiefly on how hot the focal area becomes during the instants that the exposure lasts. This keeps the rating low. On longer exposures the ability of the anode as a whole to dissipate heat is an important consideration and becomes advantageous, raising the tube ratings.

Factors affecting radiographic ratings

It has just been shown that one of the factors which alter the rating of an X-ray tube is the duration of the exposure. This might be termed a radiographer-variable since the time of the exposure is altered by the radiographer. The other factors to be considered now are determined by structural features of a given X-ray tube and features of the circuits in which it is to operate. They are as follows:
1   focal spot size;
2   the nature of the circuit which is providing the high voltage for the X-ray tube.

Details of these matters must be included in the rating charts and rating information of any X-ray tube.

Focal spot size

It has already been said that there is limitation of the electrical load because the focal area where the electron bombardment occurs rises in temperature. The larger the area over which the heat is spread, the less is the rise in temperature for a given amount of heat. This means that a greater amount of electric power can be applied to larger focal spots than to smaller ones before the temperature at the area of bombardment rises to the melting point of tungsten. This limitation is the important one during short exposures which are over before the ability of the whole anode to dissipate heat has time to become operative.

To look at rating charts with these facts in mind is to expect them to show (i) that on short exposures larger focal spots have higher ratings than smaller ones, and (ii) that the difference in rating between large and small focal spots is less on long exposures than it is on short.

From a chart relating to a particular X-ray tube, information can be obtained on the maximum milliamperes which can be used at 100 kV for different exposure times, and comparison can be made between the permissible milliamperes on a large and a small focal spot. The information is set out in Table 7.2

Table 7.2 Comparison between 2·0 mm and 1·5 mm focal spots 100 kV

Time in seconds	Highest milliamperes	
	2·0 mm focus	1·5 mm focus
0·1	450	350
5	180	150
10	100	100

To sum up these figures, it can be said that larger focal spots have a higher rating than smaller ones, and the difference between them is greatest on short exposures, when the limit in rating is determined by the temperature rise at the focal area. The difference is least on long exposures when the limit in rating is determined by characteristics of the anode and the tube as a whole. In this particular instance the ratings at 10 seconds are the same for both focal spots.

Nature of the high voltage circuit

Other chapters in this book (Chapters 2 and 3) contain descriptions of the circuits by means of which X-ray tubes are provided with the high voltage which is necessary for their operation. To mention these circuits in general terms here, it can be said that a given X-ray tube may be used in any of the following arrangements.

1 Connected directly across the secondary winding of the high tension transformer. This allows only one half-cycle of the ac sine wave to be used and it is called self-rectified half-wave operation.

2 Connected to the secondary winding of the high tension transformer via a rectification system which allows both halves of the ac sine wave to be used. This is described as single-phase full-wave rectified operation.

3 Connected to a special high tension transformer which is known as a three-phase transformer and feeds the X-ray tube with a supply drawn from all three phases of the mains. The X-ray tube is connected to the secondary windings of such a transformer via a rectification system which allows the use of both half-waves of each of the three phases. This is known as three-phase full-wave rectified operation.

Again information can be sought from a chart relating to a particular X-ray tube in order to find out what difference there is in the rating of the tube when it operates self-rectified and when it operates with full-wave rectification (single phase). The rating chart shows the maximum milliamperes which can be used at 100 kV for various exposure times, and the figures taken from the chart are given in Table 7.3.

Table 7.3 Comparison between self-rectified and full-wave rectified operation 100 kV

Time in seconds	Highest milliamperes			
	Broad focus		Fine focus	
	Self-rect.	F.W. rect.	Self-rect.	F.W. rect.
0·2	150	300	67	125
0·5	140	290	58	110
5	135	275	48	78
10	50	75	35	55
15	45	50	30	48

To sum up: both for large and for small focal spots the X-ray tube has a higher rating when it is given full wave rectified operation then when it is given self-rectified operation. The difference in rating between these two systems of operation is most marked at short exposures and becomes less at long exposures. The explanation of these facts is given in Chapter 3 where the circuits are considered in detail.

The next step is to consider the differences that exist in the rating of a tube which is operated with full-wave rectification on (a) a single-phase supply and (b) a three-phase supply. Again reference can be made to the chart of a particular tube and information can be sought on maximum milliamperes at 100 kVp for various exposure times. Information taken from a chart is set out in Table 7.4.

Table 7.4 Comparison between single-phase and three-phase operation 100 kVp

	Time in seconds	Highest milliamperes 1·5 mm focus	
		Single phase	Three phase
Fine focus	0·03	370	420
	0·05	360	410
	0·5	290	290
	1·0	255	230
	5·0	155	120
	10	100	75
Broad focus	0·03	460	550
	0·05	455	545
	0·5	370	370
	1·0	320	300
	5·0	160	140
	10	100	95

To sum this up: for both focal spots at short exposures the three-phase supply gives a higher rating. At 0·5 seconds the ratings on single-phase and on three-phase supply are the same. At longer exposures the earlier position is reversed and the single-phase supply gives the higher rating. The explanation of these facts is given in Chapter 3 where the circuits are considered in more detail.

Thermal ratings

It has been made clear that a radiographic rating chart as discussed in the previous section gives the limits of loadings which may be applied as single exposures to a cool X-ray tube. It does not provide any information as to how many times and how rapidly a single exposure may be repeated without putting too much heat into the X-ray tube, and how long it takes the X-ray tube to dissipate a given amount of heat. The manufacturer provides further charts in which the answer to these questions may be found. These charts are called heating and cooling curves.

Fig. 7.23 shows two charts, both for the same X-ray tube. The upper one relates to the ability of the whole tube unit (glass insert, oil and casing) to get rid of heat; the lower one relates to the rate of cooling of the anode of the X-ray tube. To plot these charts and subsequently to use them, a special unit is used which is called a heat unit. The heat units (H.U.) produced by an exposure when the X-ray tube is operating are given by this relationship:

For single-phase operation:

$$\text{Heat units} = \text{kV} \times \text{mA} \times \text{seconds}$$

For three-phase operation:

$$\text{Heat units} = \text{kV} \times \text{mA} \times \text{seconds} \times 1\cdot35$$

The factor 1·35 appears because in three-phase operation the wave form of the voltage for the X-ray tube is a rippling and not a pulsating one. The tube produces useful X rays throughout the cycle and given values of kilovoltage, milliamperes and time result in the production of more heat.

It can be seen that both charts have the values marked on the vertical axis as thermal content and the values marked on the horizontal axis as time intervals in minutes. The units for the thermal content are the arbitrary heat units which have just been mentioned. The lower of the two charts has a maximum thermal content of 135,000 H.U. and this means that the anode can accept from the target area 135,000 H.U. without overheating and without reaching the stage of being too hot to take enough heat away from the target area where it forms.

Similarly the cooling chart for the whole tube unit has its highest thermal content given as 1,250,000 H.U. This means that 1,250,000 H.U. is the total heat storage capacity of the tube unit as a whole, and that it can accept this number of heat units without overheating, and without reaching the stage of being unable to pass on the heat quickly enough to the air in the room.

In the chart of anode thermal characteristics the cooling curve is marked. It shows that when 135,000 H.U. have been put into the anode, it will take 6 minutes for the anode to cool to what is considered the zero level of heat units. This is obviously not the same thing as a temperature of zero degrees, and it refers simply to an anode which is at room temperature and has had no heat put into it by the tube's being energized to produce X rays.

The slope of the curve and the figures on the chart show that the anode loses heat most rapidly when it is hottest. Thus when there are 135,000 H.U. on the anode, it cools to 95,000 H.U. at the end of 1 minute of cooling time; this is a loss of 40,000 H.U. At the end of a further period lasting 1 minute, the heat units on the anode have fallen to 68,000 H.U.; this is a loss of 27,000 H.U. in the same period of time. At a later stage when there are only 30,000 H.U. on the anode, the number falls to 15,000 H.U. in 1 minute of cooling time—a loss of 15,000 H.U. So clearly the *rate* of heat loss is highest when the anode is hottest. The cooling chart for the whole tube unit shows the same thing to be true for that as it is true for the anode, the curves being identical in shape.

On the chart showing the anode thermal characteristics there are also four curves which represent four different rates of heat input—255 H.U. per second, 425 H.U. per second, 625 H.U. per second and 850 H.U. per second.

$$\text{Heat units per second} = kV \times mA \text{ (single phase)}$$

Thus any set of tube factors can be converted into a rate of heat input. If the reader thinks about relating these four rates of heat input to tube factors which may be used in practice, it will be realized that they imply low milliamperes. For example, 5 mA at 50 kV means 250 H.U. per second; 4 mA at 100 kV means 400 H.U. per second.

These curves apply strictly to loadings used for fluoroscopy and not to those used for radiographic exposures; and to a maintained heat input rather than an intermittent one.

The curves show that for this particular anode a rate of input of 850 H.U. per second maintained for 6 minutes brings the thermal content of the anode up to its maximum capacity of 135,000 H.U. It must then have a period for cooling before another load is applied. Lower rates of heat input do not bring the number of heat units up to the maximum capacity of the anode at the end of 6 minutes and in fact it looks as if the curves for the lower rates of heat input are then beginning to flatten out. When such curves flatten out, it means that a state of equilibrium has been reached and the anode is successfully passing the heat on to the oil at a rate which is matched to the rate of heat input.

A feature of the cooling chart for the whole tube unit in Fig. 7.23 is that it reveals the influence of an air-circulator on the cooling time which the

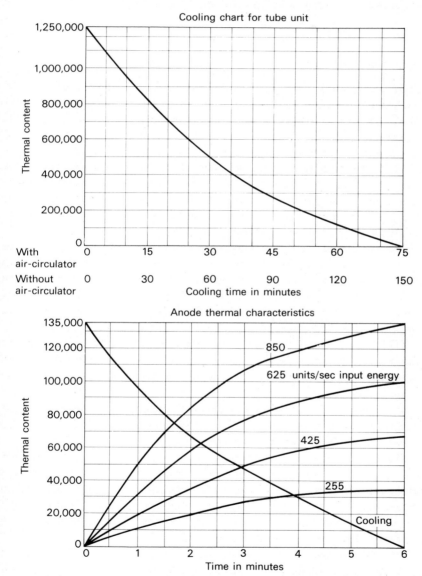

Fig. 7.23 Cooling curves. *By courtesy of Machlett X-ray Tubes (Great Britain) Ltd.*

tube requires to lose a given amount of heat. The air-circulator mentioned is an electric fan contained in a housing mounted on the tube shield; reference was made on page 235 in this chapter to the use of such a device to increase the rate at which the tube unit loses heat. The chart shows that the fan does indeed do this, for the cooling time in minutes required to lose a given amount of heat is doubled when the fan is not there.

Using a cooling curve

The curve showing the anode thermal characteristics may be used to find out whether an exposure which it is intended to repeat in a series will result in the thermal content of the anode rising to or above its maximum capacity. Suppose that it is desired to find out whether an exposure can be repeated 10 times with 0·5 minute of cooling time between each exposure.

The first step is to convert the exposure to the number of heat units which it will place on the anode. If the X-ray tube is operating on single-phase supply, this is done by finding the product $kV \times mA \times seconds$: for three phase equipment this product must be multiplied by the correction factor 1·35. Let us suppose that the answer comes to 20,000 H.U.

The curve of anode thermal characteristics shown in Fig. 7.23 indicates that when the anode has 20,000 H.U. in it, if it is given 0·5 minute cooling time, this value will have fallen to nearly 10,000 H.U. Repeating the same exposure then raises the figure to 30,000 H.U. If again 0·5 cooling time is allowed the anode cools to nearly 20,000 H.U. Repeating the same exposure raises this figure to 40,000 and this falls to almost 30,000 in half a minute.

If this exercise with the chart is repeated until the rise and fall in the heat units with each exposure and its cooling interval are discovered for 10 successive exposures, the results on the next page can be tabled (with some approximations).

It can be seen that at the end of the tenth exposure the thermal content of the tube is well below its maximum capacity of 135,000 H.U. and the 10 exposures can therefore be safely made.

The figure indicates a further piece of information which can be derived from these results. The similarity of the readings on the chart for the ninth and the tenth exposures shows that a state of equilibrium has been achieved between the heat input and the rate at which the anode is passing on the heat, the temperature of the anode rising to about the same level with each repeat exposure after 0·5 minute cooling time.

This will not always be the case. A set of exposure factors which caused a greater number of heat units to be placed on the anode repeated with shorter intervals for cooling could result in an overload of the X-ray tube,

Table 7.5

Exposure	Heat units	0·5 minute cooling	Heat units
1	20,000	fall to	10,000
2	30,000	fall to	20,000
3	40,000	fall to	30,000
4	50,000	fall to	40,000
5	60,000	fall to	50,000
6	70,000	fall to	60,000
7	80,000	fall to	70,000
8	90,000	fall to	80,000
9	100,000	fall to	80,000
10	100,000	fall to	80,000

the thermal content of the anode being above its maximum capacity by the time the series was finished.

An angiographic rating chart

Let us suppose now that the repeated exposure forms a series in an angiographic examination. In such radiographic examinations the repetition rate is high, and the periods of pause which occur in the programme are likely to be very short and to be measured in seconds rather than in minutes. It is best therefore to disregard them as cooling periods.

Fig. 7.24 shows at (a) a radiographic rating chart for an X-ray tube with a 1.5 mm focal spot operating on a full-wave rectified high tension generator on a single phase supply. Let us suppose that we are using this X-ray tube for angiographic radiography and that the exposure factors we plan to use are 300 mA at 100 kVp for an exposure time of 0·05 seconds. We must begin by making sure that this individual exposure in the series is within the limits of safety as given in the radiographic rating chart. The chart at (a) in Fig. 7.24 tells is that this exposure is safe, the maximum permissible time for 300 mA at 100 kV being part of the way between 0·05 and 0·1 second—say 0·07 second.

Fig. 7.24 shows at (b) an angiographic rating chart which the manufacturer provides for the same X-ray tube operating in the same conditions. This chart tells us the total number of exposures which can be made at various exposure rates per second, once we have converted the individual exposure factors into the number of heat units it places on the X-ray tube each time the exposure is made.

In this particular case the heat units are:

$$300 \times 100 \times 0·05 \text{ heat units} = 1500 \text{ heat units}$$

From the angiographic rating chart, the point on the vertical axis which

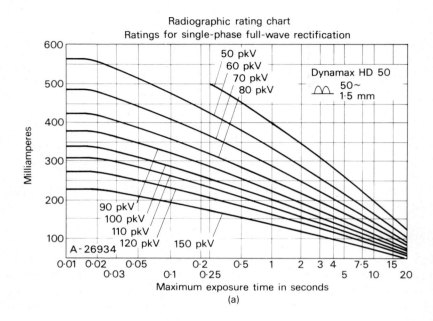

(a)

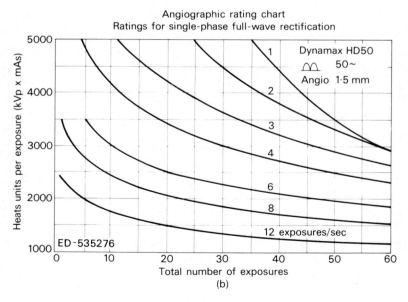

(b)

Fig. 7.24 Rating charts. *By courtesy of Machlett X-ray Tubes (Great Britain) Ltd and Philips Medical Systems Ltd.*

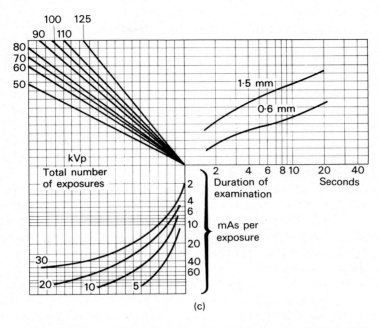

(c)

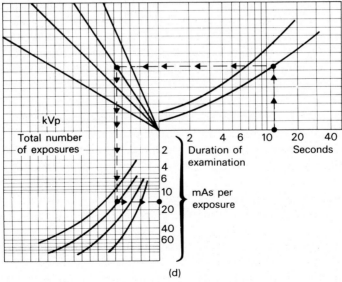

(d)

represents 1500 heat units per exposure can be located. If we look along the horizontal line on the chart from this point, it can be seen that the curve marked 12 exposures per second intersects with the line at the point on the horizontal axis which represents a total number of 20 exposures.

This means that at 12 films per second we could safely make up to 20 exposures and of course any smaller number than 20 would be quite safe. All the other curves of lower exposure rates run off the chart before they intersect with the horizontal line from 1500 heat units; this means that at lower rates of exposure than 12 per second, we could safely take a total of at least 60 radiographs with the exposure factors that we plan to use.

Suppose that we were planning to make a total of 30 exposures in an angiographic series and that the heat units from our set of exposure factors was 2000. What would be the fastest rate we could safely repeat them? The angiographic rating chart can provide the answer to this question. If we look at the chart, we can see that the line from 2000 heat units intersects with the line from 30 total exposures at a point which is on the safe side of the 6 exposures per second curve but on the unsafe side of the 8 exposures per second curve. This means that the fastest rate of repetition which we could use would be 6 exposures per second.

Suppose that we were planning to expose 20 radiographs in the angiographic series and we proposed to make the exposures at a rate of 6 per second. What would be the highest number of heat units per exposure which could safely be placed on the X-ray tube? The answer again is to be found in the chart, which shows that the line from 20 total exposures intersects with the 6 per second exposure rate curve at a point representing 2500 heat units. All we have to do now is to make sure that the exposure factors we select do not put more than 2500 heat units on the tube with each exposure and that the selected exposure factors are safe for an individual exposure as indicated in the radiographic rating chart.

Another type of chart for use in relation to angiography is shown in Fig. 7.24(c) and (d). The method to be used is given below.

1 Determine how long the radiographic programme will take and locate this period of time on the axis marked 'Duration of Examination' in Fig. 7.24(c).

2 Move vertically up from this location to the curve marked for the tube focus to be used. Fig. 7.24(c) shows curves for a 1·5 mm focus and a 0·6 mm focus.

3 From the point located on the curve for the tube focus, move horizontally to the left to meet the line marked for the kilovoltage to be used.

4 From the located point on this line move downwards vertically to meet the curve marked for the total number of exposures to be used in the angiographic examination.

5 From the point located on this curve, move horizontally to the right to read the maximum allowable milliampereseconds recorded on the vertical axis marked in Fig. 7.24(c) 'mAs per Exposure'.

Fig. 7.24(d) shows the same charts as are in Fig. 7.24(c) with the line of progression marked with arrowheads and dashes. The milliampereseconds which are indicated are based on considerations of the heat storage capacity of the X-ray tube. At short exposure times a limiting factor in the rating of the tube is the instantaneous heating of the target; the filament characteristics of the tube also limit the actual milliamperage and the exposure times which may be used. It is therefore essential to make sure that the selected exposure factors are safe for an individual exposure. This is done by using the overload indication of the X-ray set or by consulting a radiographic rating chart for the X-ray tube.

To sum up the uses of rating charts and cooling curves

The figures which have been taken in these exercises with the curves in Figs. 7.22, 7.23 and 7.24 are not in themselves special in any way and other examples could be assumed and used to illustrate the points which are important. These points are as follows.

1 Each exposure puts heat into the anode and the tube unit as a whole. If the intervals between exposures are great enough, the components of the tube unit can lose heat, the rate of heat loss being greatest when the heat is greatest.

2 Charts show the maximum number of heat units than can safely be put into the anode and the tube as a whole.

3 Charts show the rate at which the anode and the tube unit lose heat after a given input.

4 Charts can be used to work out whether it is safe to apply a particular exposure repeated in series during special examinations—for example serial radiography of the gastrointestinal tract and in angiography. Charts are available also which give the radiographic ratings of X-ray tubes for cineradiography; but we decided not to discuss them in this book.

Fluoroscopic ratings

When an X-ray tube is energized for fluoroscopy, the pattern of heat production is different from that of its radiographic use. During fluoroscopy the heat produced is relatively small in amount and it is maintained over a relatively long period of time; during a radiographic exposure the heat produced is great in amount and it is maintained over a very short period of time, in many cases so short as to be classed as instantaneous.

It has already been seen that differences in radiographic rating occur with (i) focal spot size and (ii) characteristics of the circuits in which the X-ray tube is operating. These differences are seen to become less at long exposure times and it is therefore not unexpected that they cease to be significant when the tube is energized for long periods (i.e. minutes, not fractions of seconds) in fluoroscopy. In this type of operation the limit of load is determined by the ability of the whole tube unit to dissipate heat to its surroundings, and the limit is that the rate of heat input should not exceed the rate at which any part of the tube unit can lose heat. The use of an air-circulating fan in raising the rate at which the tube can lose heat has already been seen. When the manufacturer gives the fluoroscopic rating of a tube it is usual for him to say whether it applies with or without the use of a circulator fan.

The fluoroscopic rating may be expressed as the number of heat units per second that can be applied indefinitely with continuous running; or the values of milliamperage and kilovoltage which can be applied indefinitely may be specifically stated. Thus two typical fluoroscopic ratings taken from manufacturers' leaflets are:

1   500 H.U. per second continuous indefinitely with air-circulator fan; without the fan, 500 H.U. per second for 80 minutes continuously. (500 H.U. per second could be 4 mA at 125 kV).

2   2·5 mA at 100 kV continuously with air-circulator fan. (These two ratings apply to different X-ray tubes, and the first one clearly has the higher rating.)

When rotating anode X-ray tubes are used for fluoroscopy it is usual, unless small focal spots are being employed, to energize the tube with the anode stationary as the rate of heat input is low. The life of the ball bearings will be extended if the rotor is not kept running for long periods of time. Fluoroscopic ratings are specifically stated by the manufacturer to apply with the anode stationary.

Rating charts in modern departments

Rating charts and cooling curves are not so familiar to the modern radiographer as they used to be to our predecessors in X-ray departments. The reason for this is that at an earlier stage in the development of X-ray equipment the controls permitted the radiographer very free choice of tube factors. It was possible to select and to apply to the X-ray tube combinations of milliamperes, kilovoltage and time which in fact exceeded the permissible rating and overheated the X-ray tube, so causing damage to it.

A conscientious radiographer who wished to make the fullest use of the equipment therefore required the means to check that a heavy exposure was within safe limits for the X-ray tube. Rating charts for each X-ray tube were kept close at hand and were frequently consulted. Modern equipment has what is called 'overload' protection incorporated in it. This means that the controls are interlocked so that when an unsafe combination of kilovoltage, milliamperes and time is selected an indication (visible by means of a light or audible by means of a buzzer) of the overload state is given and the exposure cannot be made. This allows the radiographer to be independent of a rating chart, saves time, reduces the risk of human error, protects the X-ray tube from one form of mistake and makes a rating chart unfamiliar to the radiographer.

Perhaps this does not matter very much for there is no particular benefit in being familiar with a rating chart unless this familiarity is useful. What is important is that the radiographer should realize:

1   the limitations of the overload protection system which is in use;
2   that not *all* equipment possesses overload protection.

The significant limitation in interlock systems is that most of them (like rating charts) indicate an overload resulting from a given set of exposure factors selected for a single exposure. They do not give warning of overload which occurs through too rapid repetition of a safe exposure, and they do not prevent exposures when the anode has accumulated excessive heat as a result of repeated exposures. Some interlock systems do provide this special protection against overload by the accumulation of too much heat, but most do not and the radiographer using the X-ray set must appreciate the type of overload protection which the set possesses.

All major X-ray sets have some interlock system to prevent overload, but simple equipment of low output (small portable and dental sets) usually has no such protection. The radiographer should keep in mind the possibility of selecting a combination of kilovoltage, milliamperes and time which exceeds the rating of the tube in such equipment. Admittedly this is not a likely occurrence in the use of a dental set with fixed kilovoltage and milliamperes and a limited range of radiographic examinations. It is much more likely when a small portable set is being given the fullest use over a wide range of patients. In doubt, the appropriate rating chart should be consulted—if it can be found.

In a previous section the use of charts was explained for ascertaining the safety of a rapid series of exposures. It is probable that in practice the student may never see such charts consulted for this purpose. When an angiographic programme is being planned, if the combination of kilovoltage, milliamperes and time selected for the exposure is *well below* the overload limit, it is generally assumed that it can safely be repeated according to the required programme. This assumption seems to give a reasonable working rule; the radiographer should nevertheless keep in mind the possibility of overloading the X-ray tube in this way.

FAULTS IN X-RAY TUBES

With use, X-ray tubes are bound to undergo changes which can be likened to a process of ageing, and they may also develop faults as a result of misuse which is mechanical or electrical. The deteriorating processes and the faults can develop in any part of the tube, and wherever their origins they will affect the operation of the tube as a whole. The locations can be as follows.

1   The glass envelope.
2   The anode, the rotor, the stator windings.
3   The filament.
4   The vacuum. This is not a *part* but it is certainly a feature of the tube which has been shown to be most important.

Some of the processes which can occur in X-ray tubes are considered below under these separate headings.

Faults in the glass envelope

A noticeable feature of an X-ray tube which has been used for a long time is change in the colour of the glass. This is the result of constant exposure to radiation and to the expert the degree of staining indicates how much work the tube has done. It is mainly the expert who will observe it for of course the radiographer who is daily using the tube will not be able to see the colour of the glass insert.

A feature which appears with misuse is the formation of a mirror surface on the inside of the glass envelope. Heavy exposures result in some vaporization of the metal parts of the tube because of the high temperatures to which they are raised. The vaporized tungsten is deposited as a thin layer on the inside of the glass envelope, producing a mirror-like reflecting surface. The tungsten deposits come from the filaments and from the anode; their source can be identified by their distribution within the glass.

It might be supposed that the tungsten deposits would act as a filter, reducing the X-ray output of the tube, but in fact it seems that the filtration effect of the thin tungsten layers is negligible. More important is the fact that the presence of the metal film reduces the insulating properties of the glass and thus makes it more liable to puncture when it is under electrical stress with high kilovoltages applied to it. A puncture in a glass envelope, even if it is a minute hole, spoils the vacuum and leads to the destruction of the tube in the manner described on page 228 in this chapter.

The glass envelope, of course, can be more than merely punctured. Stress fractures can occur in glass as in human bones, and where the glass is sealed to the anode it is under mechanical stress from the weight of the anode. To the expert who examines a failed tube these stress fractures are identifiable by their appearance and their smooth edges.

The glass of the X-ray tube is susceptible in the way of most glass to careless handling. This means in practice carelessness with the whole tube unit, which is accessible to casual manhandling whereas the glass insert by itself is not, once it has left the factory. So radiographers should pay attention to the safe passage of the tube unit when X-ray equipment is being moved—whether it is simply a matter of running a tube column along its floor track, adjusting the position of a ceiling-mounted X-ray tube, or the greater adventure of moving mobile equipment about from place to place. There is a true story of a mobile X-ray set that proved so mobile as to run itself down a flight of stairs, unseen by anyone but heard by the whole hospital. Oddly enough, the glass insert survived the experience. This should not lead radiographers to think that every such accident will bring little damage and it should encourage thought on the subject of unsafe places in which to leave mobile equipment unattended.

Faults in the anode, rotor, stator windings

The anode

Every exposure heats the target area to a high temperature and on a short exposure there is a great difference between the temperature on the surface of the tungsten where the electron bombardment occurs and at a depth in the tungsten. This leads to an effect which is that the originally smooth surface of the target track takes on an appearance not unlike the type of paved pathway known as 'crazy paving'; the process is called crazing of the target track or erosion of the target track.

Roughening of the surface of the target is worse in a tube that is maltreated (i) by being loaded above the safe rating value and (ii) by being used without attention to the possibility of overheating the anode by repeated exposures which individually are within safe rating limits. The roughening will affect sharpness of outline in the radiographic image. It will also reduce the radiation output as indicated in Fig. 7.25 for the hillocks of the roughness in the tungsten act as filters and reduce the intensity of radiation leaving the tube, especially towards the anode side of the central ray. This means that as the X-ray tube becomes older it produces a beam less uniform in intensity over the area it covers. This reduction of output due to a rough target is a reason why it may become necessary to increase the exposure values above those which are used when the tube is new.

Heavy radiographic exposures made on a cold target can cause the anode disc to split radially. This damage does not necessarily preclude further use of the X-ray tube so long as the radial crack which results is very narrow. The presence of such a crack may make little difference to the operation of

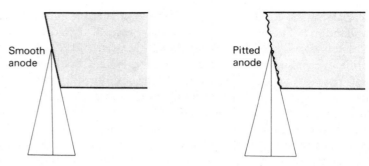

Smooth anode

Pitted anode

Fig. 7.25

an X-ray tube. A wide crack is more damaging since it results in imbalance of the anode and the bearings become noisy: this is always a sign of trouble! Furthermore, the electrons from the filament may travel through the crack to bombard the glass envelope and a melted spot and a puncture can result.

The tendency to crack arises from the circular stresses to which the anode disc is inevitably subjected. Modern anodes have been developed with very narrow radial cuts made in the disc (for example, six spaced at 60° intervals round the circle). These cuts interrupt the circular stresses and the anodes (called stress-relieved anodes) are protected against cracking even when cold.

If an X-ray tube with a stress-relieved anode of this type is used for fluoroscopy, then the anode must rotate to avoid the situation of the focal spot being stationary over a slit while the tube is energized. For X-ray tubes which are for radiographic application only, without fluoroscopy, in situations where heavy loadings are to be made, stress-relieved anodes are the best type to use.

For X-ray tubes which do not have stress-relieved anodes, a warming-up technique may be applied if the tube has been unused for more than 30 minutes. The procedure is as follows:

1 select broad focus;
2 make an exposure with these settings: 70 kV, 200 mA, 1·0 second;
3 at intervals of one minute, make three more such exposures (that is, a total of four exposures with the above factors).

An overheated anode disc is liable to distortion which may result in changes in the anode angle so that it becomes smaller. This leads to a narrowing of the useful beam and the X-ray tube no longer provides full coverage of large-sized films.

Uneven distortion of the anode disc causes enlargement in one direction of the effective focal spot of the X-ray tube. The result of this is greater geometric blur in parts of the radiographic image.

An anode which is severely distorted leads to increased noise from the ball bearings.

The rotor and its bearings

The rotor is constructed from more than one metal, for the anode has a molybdenum stem and the body of the rotor is copper. Since the rotor and the stem become hot, the thermal expansion coefficients of the several metals are important and differences between them can lead to mechanical changes after much use. When the rotor becomes imbalanced there is increased bearing noise.

Wear in the bearings is a deteriorating process that occurs in X-ray tubes. The factors which affect this deterioration are:
1   the speed of rotation;
2   the effects of loading the tube when the anode is cold;
3   the dry lubrication which must be used and is not as effective as lubricating oils and greases;
4   the heat to which the ball bearings are subjected; even with good design of the anode and careful use of the X-ray tube, the bearings can reach a state of being almost red hot.

Once the bearings have begun to deteriorate, the situation may become steadily worse and defects in the bearings are very common causes of tube failure. The smooth rotation of the anode at its proper speed is vital to the continued life of the X-ray tube and is important in the formation of the radiographic image.

The stator windings

If a fault develops in the stator windings there is no power supply to make the anode rotate. Unless a safety device is incorporated in the circuit to prevent an exposure taking place, when the exposure button is pressed home from the 'prepare' position by someone who has failed to notice the absence of the sound of the anode rotating (it is not loud in a tube with good bearings) the load that should have been applied to a rotating anode will inadvertently be applied to a stationary one. This is very likely to overload and overheat the anode, and can result in an anode disc which is cracked right through.

In practice manufacturers usually try to protect the tube against this type of accident by arranging circuits which prevent the exposure from taking place when the stator is without its power supply. (See page 154.)

Faults in the filament

Failure of the filament to heat when its circuit is energized may be due (i) to a break in the filament itself, or (ii) to a fault in the circuit which supplies it with power. Since the filament is heated for every exposure and the heat vaporizes tungsten from it, the filament as it becomes older becomes thinner. Even if the X-ray tube is tenderly handled to protect it from mechanical damage and carefully loaded always within safe limits, it is clear that after long use the filament may become so thin as to break. It is then not possible to use the X-ray tube.

Excessive evaporation from the filament makes an X-ray tube unstable so that it becomes unsatisfactory long before there is a fracture of the filament.

This wearing of the filament takes place more rapidly if the tube is always loaded at high milliamperages which require greater filament heat and shorten its life. Filament life can be extended during use of the tube if the filament is energized only for the shortest possible periods; in practice this means switching on the filament supply only when necessary and keeping the exposure button on 'prepare' for no longer than the shortest possible time. Energization of the filament to the value required for the selected milliamperes is usually linked with the 'prepare' position of the switch so that it is at the last moment before exposure that the full filament heat is achieved. This considerably extends filament life. The extra power applied to the filament to bring it up to the needed value just before exposure is called the filament boost.

Failure (whatever its cause) of the filament to heat means that the tube will not pass current and will not produce X rays; there will be no reading on the milliampere meter when the exposure is made and the developed film is predictably unexposed and blank.

Sometimes a break in the filament or a fault in the circuit supplying it produces an intermittent failure in milliamperes through the tube. One instantaneous exposure may be made successfully, another cannot be made at all, and another made with the milliamperes 'coming and going', the meter needle being erratic in movement to and fro across the scale between zero and the expected value.

Faults in the vacuum

The ways in which failure in the vacuum destroys an X-ray tube have already been described on page 227 of this chapter. With long use an X-ray tube may become 'gassy' so that the vacuum is spoilt. When this happens the milliamperage (as has been shown) becomes erratic and 'runs away' so that it reaches high values. This state of affairs is revealed by the milliampere meter, the needle of which swings over sometimes as far as it can on the scale. A gassy tube will go from bad to worse if it continues to be used, and the best course of action is to stop using the unit until a tube replacement can be obtained.

CHARACTERISTICS OF X-RAY TUBES

Modern tubes have developed from their predecessors. Specifications which today's manufacturers state relate to important characteristics of X-ray tubes which have shown development in the last 40 years. The specifications of an X-ray tube today mention the following:

1   the target angle;
2   the target material;
3   the focal spot sizes;
4   the maximum voltage;
5   the heat storage capacity and maximum cooling rate of the anode and of the tube as a whole;
6   the fluoroscopic maximum continuous ratings;
7   the maximum radiographic ratings, having regard to certain variables which are:

(a) the frequency of the stator supply (which affects the speed of rotation of the anode);

(b) the focal spot sizes;

(c) the nature of the generator (single phase or three phase) which supplies the X-ray tube;

(d) the time of exposure, typically quoted ratings being for 0·01 s, 0·1 s, 1·0 s, 10 s and 100 s.

This range of information is needed today because of the developments which have occurred and have led to the use of:

1   target angles which are less than 15 degrees;
2   anode discs which are not made of solid tungsten but of combinations of metals;
3   faster speeds of rotation for the anode than 3000 revolutions per minute;
4   the grid controlled filament so that the X-ray tube can itself act as a switching device to initiate and end the exposure.

Reduced target angle

Earlier in this chapter (page 220) the importance of the target angle was discussed. It was shown that as the face of the anode becomes more steeply sloped (smaller angle) more foreshortening occurs and the area of electron bombardment is bigger in relation to the effective focus. This can be put another way and we can say that the smaller the target angle, the greater is the electrical load which can be put on the X-ray tube for the same size of effective focus.

The important disadvantage in using a small target angle is that the useful X-ray beam covers a smaller area at a given tube to film distance. The useful X-ray beam (as seen on page 221) is a beam which is of acceptably uniform intensity over the film surface. In any X-ray tube there is loss of intensity towards the anode end of the tube because of the cutting-off effect of the anode mass, and this lack of uniformity becomes worse as the X-ray tube becomes older and the anode loses its smooth surface over the focal track. An eroded anode results in an increased reduction of intensity as compared with a smooth one.

In the past target angles of 15–20 degrees have been used as being the best compromise between too little foreshortening and too much anode cut off. Today the use of special anode materials results in a target track which maintains its smoothness much better than does a pure tungsten track. This means that the rate of loss of uniformity in the beam which is due to the rough target track as the tube ages is much diminished. It has been found that smaller target angles can be employed in practice, and X-ray tubes are now available with target angles of 10 degrees and 7 degrees.

The beams from such X-ray tubes cover fields of the sizes given on page 222.

The figures do mean that there are some restrictions in the use of such tubes.

The reduced target angle foreshortens a relatively large area of electron bombardment so that it projects as a very small focus. These modern tubes can therefore have a very small effective focus (0·3 mm) and yet can still take a relatively heavy electrical load—for example, 110 kVp and 100 mA for 0·1 second on a tube with a reduced target angle (this tube also had the advantage of increased speed of anode rotation which is described on page 276 in this chapter).

A development in the use of smaller target angles is an X-ray tube which has two different target angles incorporated in it; such an X-ray tube is described as a double angle or bi-angular tube. The anode of a double angle tube has two focal tracks arranged on the anode as two concentric rings. In one design the inner track is for the fine focus and the outer track is for the broad focus; the cathode has two filaments arranged one above the other, and each covers with its electron beam a rectangular area on one of the focal tracks. The surface of the anode disc is bevelled at two angles (see Fig. 7.26) so that the inner target ring (fine focus filament) is on a part of the anode face which is at a steep angle which is approximately 10 degrees. The outer target ring (broad focus filament) is on a part of the anode face which has a different slope, the anode angle being 18–20 degrees.

In this way the steeper angle is used to make the fine focus of the X-ray tube effectively very small. Yet it will take electrical loads comparable with those of the broad focus on a target of conventional angle. This allows the use of a fine focus for radiographic examinations such as angiography and gastroenterology in which it could not previously be employed.

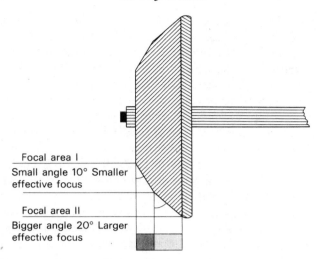

Focal area I
Small angle 10° Smaller
effective focus

Focal area II
Bigger angle 20° Larger
effective focus

Fig. 7.26

In another design it is the broad focus filament which is focused on the inner ring with its steeper slope. The inner ring is of smaller circumference which means lower rating because there is a smaller area receiving the heat for one revolution of the disc. The area to receive the heat can be increased by making the shorter inner focal track wider; the steeper target angle ensures that this wider track is sufficiently foreshortened to make the broad focus not so large in projection as to be unacceptable.

New target materials

In the previous section it was said that a target material is being used which retains its smoothness better than tungsten does as the tube ages. The material concerned is an alloy of rhenium and tungsten (10 per cent rhenium) which is used to face the anode disc. This resists the roughening process much better than a pure tungsten target does, and because the target surface does not deteriorate so quickly higher electrical loads can be applied to it during its working life. Rhenium and tungsten targets therefore increase the permissible ratings of X-ray tubes.

Another material now being used for anode discs is a combination of tungsten and molybdenum. Molybdenum has the advantages of being not so dense as tungsten and of ability to accept a given amount of heat with less rise in temperature. So in comparison with a tungsten disc of the same weight, a molybdenum disc could safely take more heat and therefore bigger electrical loads would be permissible. In comparison with a tungsten disc able to take the same heat input, the molybdenum disc would be lighter— an important consideration from the point of view of the ball bearings which must carry the weight of the anode disc as it rotates.

It is, however, not possible to use a disc with a pure molybdenum face to receive the electron bombardment because molybdenum has a lower melting point and a lower atomic number than tungsten. So what is used in practice is a molybdenum disc with a coating of tungsten over the target track; or a coating of 10 per cent rhenium–90 per cent tungsten over the target track. The molybdenum disc may be alloyed with titanium and zirconium.

Another material which has been used as a base for anode discs is graphite applied as a thick layer behind molybdenum. Graphite (carbon) has a higher melting point than tungsten ($3510°C$ compared with $3380°C$) and has a specific heat which is 10 times that of tungsten. This last fact gives graphite a heat storage capacity which is much greater than that of an equal volume of tungsten (the heat storage capacity of an anode disc is always proportional to its volume). Improved heat storage capacity is thus gained through the use of graphite without paying the price of an increase in anode volume and hence in the weight of the disc. Graphite (carbon) has a low atomic number in relation to tungsten (6 compared with 74) and this makes it entirely unsuitable as an area for the production of X rays. Graphite is therefore used as a heat sink behind a rhenium-tungsten-molybdenum disc. The main problems that have arisen with graphite and these combinations relate to differences in thermal expansion and to the lower thermal conductivity of graphite.

Fig. 7.27 is a diagram to illustrate these compound anodes that we have been discussing.

Speed of anode rotation

The rating of a rotating anode X-ray tube is influenced by the speed of rotation of the disc, being increased for short exposures at faster speeds of rotation. For example, an anode disc with diameter 100 mm rotating at 12,000 r.p.m. has double the rating in comparison with the same size of disc rotating at 3000 r.p.m. The size of the disc is mentioned because larger discs have higher rating, but it is not a practical proposition to attempt to make a tube with a very large disc. The added weight would give the ball bearings a difficult time, and the size and weight of the whole tube unit might give the radiographer using it a difficult time. To increase tube rating by increasing the anode's rotational speed is a much more attractive idea. A special supply to the stator windings is required but this is not difficult to arrange.

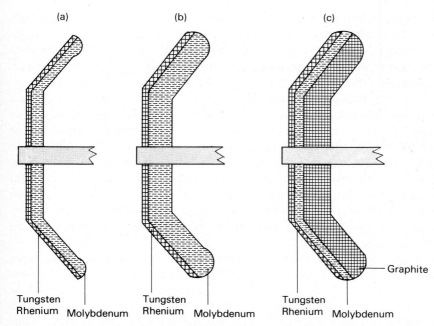

Fig. 7.27 At (a) and (b) are anode discs with tungsten rhenium alloy on a molybdenum base. (b) has a greater heat storage capacity than (a) because it has greater volume but (b) also has greater weight than (a).

At (c) is a rhenium tungsten alloy on a molybdenum-graphite base. The disc at (c) has greater heat storage capacity than the one at (b), since its volume is greater, with a saving in weight. At equal heat storage capacities, molybdenum has half the weight of tungsten: graphite has one fifth the weight of molybdenum.

The stator supply

For high speed anodes the stator supply must be increased in frequency from the 50 cycles per second usual in the United Kingdom to, for example, 150 cycles per second if the anode is to rotate at 9000 instead of 3000 r.p.m. The most modern way of doing this is an electronic device for converting frequency to a new value.

It is always difficult when one aspect of an X-ray tube is improved to avoid worsening some other feature. Here the rating is improved by increased anode speed—the disadvantage is that it then takes longer for the anode to reach full speed, and the users may object to the length of the delay that is imposed before the exposure can begin. The high speed anode can be accelerated in a shorter time if more power is used in the motor, but the high voltages then needed on the stator windings and the high power input may be inadvisable.

At the end of the exposure the anode must stop rotating and with high speed anodes it is usual to incorporate a braking device. This is to avoid some hazards from vibration if such an anode is allowed simply to slow itself down and stop from a high speed of rotation. The braking device continues to work even if the unit is switched off as soon as the exposure ends.

It is only at short exposures that the high speed anode shows the greatest improvement in rating over its fellows with conventional anode speed. For example, at 0·01 second a high speed anode with 0·3 mm focus may take at 100 kV nearly twice the milliamperage that can be taken by another tube with the same size of focus but with its anode rotating at conventional speed—120 mA as compared with 70 mA. At 1 second the relative maximum milliamperages at 100 kV of these two tubes may be 95 mA and 60 mA, so the difference between them is decreasing. At 10 seconds the relative milliamperages are 50 mA compared with 40 mA, and at 100 seconds the difference has disappeared.

In the foregoing paragraphs, features of modern rotating anode tubes have been described. By way of summary it can be said that these features are (i) lesser target angle, (ii) superior target material and constructions to relieve stress, (iii) high speed rotation of the anode. They all contribute to increased rating for small effective focal spots at short exposure times. They have resulted in the production of X-ray tubes with 0·3 mm focal spots which allow the use of such factors as these: 0·1 second, 100 mA at 110 kV. This is about four times the maximum milliamperage allowed on a 0·3 mm focus in an earlier type of tube and makes the 0·3 mm focus much more useful. The range of use covers enlargement techniques, cine-radiography, angiography, gastroenterology, and fluoroscopy with image intensifiers.

Grid-controlled X-ray tube

Chapter 5 considered in detail the important matter of control of the duration of the X-ray exposure. Here it can be said that control of the length of time that the exposure lasts involves two separate elements. These are:

1 the *timing* of the period of exposure,

2 *switching* the circuit which supplies the X-ray tube—i.e. the circuit which supplies the X-ray tube must be closed at the beginning of the exposure so that current can flow and must be opened at the end of the exposure so that current stops flowing.

Timing and switching involve quite separate elements in the equipment. Here we look briefly at a special form of switching which is achieved by alteration in characteristics of the X-ray tube itself.

The object of switching is to make current flow through the X-ray tube at the beginning of the exposure so that it produces X rays and stop at the end of the exposure so that it ceases to produce X rays. The switching will be done truly at the heart of the matter if the X-ray tube can be made to do its own switching by becoming conductive (a closed switch) at the beginning of the exposure and non-conductive (an open switch) at the end of the exposure.

However, there are problems connected with switching a high tension circuit such as that of which the X-ray tube is a part, and for many years it was not possible to achieve the switching by altering characteristics within the X-ray tube itself. It is only comparatively recently that techniques have been developed which incorporate switching within the X-ray tube itself.

One way in which this is done is to put a wire-mesh grid across the opening of the cathode slot where the filament sits. When there is a negative voltage on this grid it is said to be negatively biased. This negative voltage can be made sufficient for the grid to act as a complete barrier to electrons which want to leave the filament, and the X-ray tube is then non-conducting and acts like an open switch. By applying positive voltage to the grid the negative bias can be reduced so that the grid ceases to be a barrier to the electrons. The X-ray tube then becomes conductive and acts like a closed switch, producing X rays as a result of the electron flow through it. In this state of affairs the X-ray tube conducts just for the period of time that the positive voltage (1–3 kilovolts) is applied to the grid.

Another way of using the effect of grid control is to do without the wiremesh grid across the cathode slot; the filament is insulated from the cathode head and the bias voltage is applied to the head. This is sufficient to produce cut-off—that is it forms a barrier to the electron flow. Some modern X-ray tubes have grid control for the fine focus only and some have it for both focal spots.

Grid control of the X-ray tube is a method of switching which allows extremely short exposures (a few milliseconds) to be used since the positive voltage can be applied as a 'pulse' of brief duration. These short exposures can be repeated rapidly since the switching is without inertia. There is no mechanical movement associated with it and it works by changes in the electrical characteristics of the wire-mesh grid.

Focal spot sizes in X-ray tubes

When a manufacturer sells an X-ray tube he specifies the size of its focal spot, or rather of its focal spots since most X-ray tubes for general use are of the dual focus variety and have both a broad and a fine focus. This statement of size is given in millimetres and it describes the effective or apparent focus—that is the small square which the actual focus appears to be when it is viewed from the film (see page 219 of this chapter) and which is the apparent size of the X-ray source. Thus when a certain X-ray tube is said to have a 2 mm focus, what is meant is that the actual focus projects as a square of sides 2 mm in length.

The range of sizes encountered in diagnostic equipment is indicated below.

1   0·3 mm. This is a very small focus which in the past has been able to take only very limited loads but in certain modern tubes can take higher loads than before.

2   0·5–1·0 mm. Focal spots in this range are considered as fine foci.

3   Above 1·0–2·0 mm. Focal spots in this range are considered to be broad foci.

In dual focus tubes the different sizes are combined in various ways. Thus manufacturers produce a range of tubes with such focal spot combinations as these:

(i)	0·3 and 1·0 mm	(ii)	0·3 and 1·5 mm
(iii)	0·3 and 2·0 mm	(iv)	0·5 and 1·5 mm
(v)	0·5 and 2·0 mm	(vi)	0·6 and 1·0 mm
(vii)	0·6 and 2·0 mm	(viii)	0·7 and 2·0 mm
(ix)	0·8 and 1·8 mm	(x)	1·0 and 2·0 mm

The radiographer should understand the principles which underlie selection of focal spot size for any particular radiographic examination, and why the fine (or small) focus is used for one examination and the broad (or large) focus for another. The reader is referred back to page 224 of this chapter and the section on the dual focus X-ray tube. Here perhaps it may be helpful to make three general statements on focal spot sizes and their use in radiography.

1   Focal spots in the range from above 1·0 mm to 2·0 mm are used for all radiographic examinations which require a large exposure dose (because the body part is absorptive) and a short exposure time (because movement in the subject or part of the subject is probable or certain). The use of these focal spots results in greater geometric unsharpness but greatly reduces motional unsharpness, and the end result is therefore a sharper image than would be obtained from using a small focus.

2   Focal spots in the range 0·5–1·0 mm are used for those radiographic examinations in which the risk of movement is not very great. In general they are used for the examination of bony parts of the body.

3   The 0·3 mm focus which takes a very limited load has a special application in radiography for it is used in enlargement techniques. In these a long distance between the subject and the film is deliberately employed in order to obtain an image which is 2 or 3 times larger than the true size of the part under examination. The long subject-film distances result in great blurring

of detail unless they are used with a very small X-ray source in order to reduce the geometric unsharpness to which they give rise.

Typical for an 0·3 mm focus is an X-ray tube with a 70 mm diameter disc, a compound anode with a 10 degrees target angle and grid control available for this focal spot. With the anode rotating at a standard speed, the rating at 0·1 second and 100 kV is limited to 48 mA (that is, 4·8 mAs); with the anode given high-speed rotation, the rating rises to 89 mA (that is, 8·9 mAs).

An 0·3 mm focus can be used for fluoroscopy with the anode rotating. As we have already noted, at long exposure times and on continuous running the size of the focal area ceases to be the limiting factor in the load which may be applied and the limit then rests on the characteristics of the anode and the whole tube in dissipating heat. The resultant increased rating at long exposure times is clearly shown in the ratings of an 0·3 mm focus at 100 kV for different times of exposure and for fluoroscopy as given below:

Table 7.6

Seconds	Maximum mAs
0·01	0·49
0·1	4·8
1	43
10	340

Fluoroscopy: 500 H.U. per second, which can be continued indefinitely if there is an air-circulator fan, irrespective of the size of the focus.

Since an 0·3 mm focus used for fluoroscopy must have the anode rotating, the heat of the stator input must be reckoned among the total heat input. The heat of the stator input will be about 80 H.U. per second.

A METAL X-RAY TUBE

An X-ray tube has been designed in which the envelope of the tube insert is not made entirely of heat-resistant glass as for the tubes which we have previously discussed in this chapter. Instead the tube envelope is made of metal bonded closely and securely to end-pieces which are of glass. Fig. 7.28 is a sketch of such a tube insert to show the metal envelope. As can be seen in Fig. 7.28 the metal cylinder is placed so that it is around that part of the insert where the electron beam is focused between the cathode and the anode. The X-ray beam comes out through a beryllium window in the tube envelope and there is a further aluminium window built into the tube-shield. These window arrangements are designed to improve the inherent filtration for the X-ray beam.

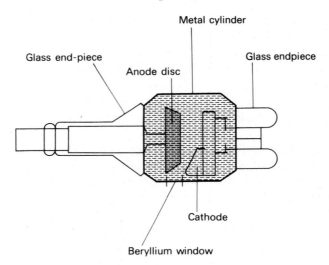

Fig. 7.28

The use of the metal cylinder is said to permit the tube to operate safely with a higher filament emission than can be allowed for X-ray tubes with inserts made entirely of glass: this greater filament emission implies the use of higher tube currents. To compare kilowatt ratings, see Table 7.7.

Table 7.7

Focal spot size mm²	Metal tube kW	Conventional tube kW
0·3	15	12
0·6	35	25
0·7	50	—
1·0	—	50
1·2	100	—
1·5	—	100

This X-ray tube is described as being suitable for exposure techniques which use high milliamperages at low kilovoltage settings with very short exposure times. An anode disc with large volume ensures that the tube has a high heat storage capacity and the tube shield is matched to these thermal characteristics of the anode.

So the tube is suitable for operation at high output with short exposure times repeated as a sustained series with no cooling intervals. These abilities suggest the use of this metal X-ray tube for angiography.

X-ray tubes for mammography

In radiographic techniques for mammography, the quality of the radiation used is extremely important. This is because the normal and the pathological structures to be delineated in a radiograph of the breast have very similar abilities to absorb X rays. Hence there are very small differences in intensity of the X rays transmitted through these various structures. If the X rays used to make the record are very penetrating, these small differences are smaller still. The penetrating power of the X rays used must be such as to maintain these small differences and certainly not such as to reduce or annihilate them. Thus an X-ray beam of soft radiation (long wavelengths) is required.

The importance of using X rays of certain long wavelengths produced at low kilovoltages has led to the development of special X-ray tubes for mammography. In the design and construction of such tubes there are features which make them suitable for the task. The special features which may be incorporated are as follows.

Closer spacing of cathode and anode

An X-ray tube which is to be operated at low kilovoltages (not more than 50 kVp) may safely have its cathode and anode closer together than is permitted for tubes with higher voltage ratings. With the two electrodes closer, a higher milliamperage may be obtained for the same filament heat; or the tube may be operated at a lower filament heat for a given milliamperage. Lower filament heat results in less build-up of evaporated tungsten on the glass wall of the tube and there is longer filament life.

The closer anode-cathode spacing reduces the maximum kilovoltage for which the tube is rated, the upper limit being about 50 kVp. This hardly matters in a tube to be used for mammography because higher kilovoltages do not produce suitable radiation.

Molybdenum anode

The wavelength of the radiation used for mammography being so important, a requirement in the X-ray tube is that it should produce intense radiation within a narrow band of certain long wavelengths. One way of obtaining high intensity within a narrow band of wavelengths is to use strong characteristic radiation produced at the anode of the tube. Molybdenum anodes have some characteristic radiation with wavelengths considered to be suitable for mammography. So special X-ray tubes for this technique have been made with molybdenum anodes; both fixed anodes and rotating anodes are used.

Beryllium window: thinned glass window

If the X-ray tube has a beryllium window through which the beam of radiation is emitted, then the filtering effect is less than that provided by the conventional glass window. The lowered inherent filtration in a tube with a beryllium window aids the intensity of X-ray output, particularly of soft radiation which is absorbed by heavier filtration. The radiographer wants to use soft radiation for mammography so it is an advantage to reduce any filtration which removes it from the beam. Another useful way of reducing the inherent filtration is to make the ordinary borosilicate glass window thinner than in a conventional X-ray tube; the glass contributes the heaviest filtering effect. Making the glass window thinner lowers the maximum kilovoltage rating of the X-ray tube because there is more risk of puncturing with the high tension a thinner window. Again, this does not matter because a mammographic tube does not need a high kilovoltage rating.

Molybdenum filter

X-ray tubes with molybdenum anodes to be used for mammography are fitted with a very thin molybdenum filter. By its selective absorption this filter removes from the beam, as it emerges from the X-ray tube, certain wavelengths which are not in the narrow band of intense wavelengths which it is wished to use.

Focal spots

Opinions vary as to the best size of focal spot to use for mammography. If we were dealing with inanimate subjects we could reach the conclusion that small focal spots must be used if fine patterns of calcification are to be detected because with a small X-ray source the geometric blurring is less. In practice, with a living subject movement can produce so much blurring that it totally invalidates the reduction in geometric unsharpness given by the use of a small focal spot. It may well be much better to use a larger focus if it permits shorter exposure times because of its higher milliamperes rating. Thus we can reduce what might otherwise be an intolerable unsharpness due to motion, paying the price of some increase in the unsharpness due to geometry of shadow-formation. Focal spots of about 0·8 mm to 2·0 mm may be encountered in mammographic tubes.

The features mentioned which make an X-ray tube suitable for mammography make it unsuitable for other work and such a tube is therefore designed not to be used for anything else. It is a justifiable part of the X-ray department's equipment if much mammography is to be done.

Choice of an X-ray tube

Much attention is being paid now to the many elements which constitute the total process that leads to a radiographic image. We have to consider a progression in which the first step is an X-ray tube producing X rays which are directed towards the patient. Emerging from the patient is a pattern of varying X-ray intensity produced by the varying absorptive powers of the different tissues of his body.

This X-ray pattern is received by whatever imaging system is used; it may be radiographic film or a fluorescent screen with image intensifier or (in newer techniques) a xerographic plate or an imaging (ionization) chamber. Every step in this progression plays a part in the resolution in the final visible image. Resolution means here the making of the separate parts of a subject distinguishable by the eye.

As we have seen, as a source of X rays the X-ray tube contributes an unsharpness in the image; lack of sharpness of course impairs resolution. It is now being seen that to pay a great deal of attention to improving the resolving power of all the other steps in the progress while neglecting the X-ray tube is to waste some endeavour. From this emerges the concept of the best X-ray tube for the job you want it to do, rather than one willing carthorse of an X-ray tube doing all the jobs you have for it to do.

Thus a new range of X-ray tubes from one manufacturer includes those with the following applications and characteristics.

1 For neuroradiology, heat storage capacity 300,000 H.U., 7 degrees target angle, focal spots 0·3 and 0·6 mm.

2 For angiography, heat storage capacity 400,000 H.U., 12 degrees target angle, focal spots 0·6 and 1·2 mm.

3 For mammography, heat storage capacity 300,000 H.U., 10 degrees target angle, focal spot 0·6 mm.

4 For general radiography, heat storage capacity 300,000 H.U., 12 degrees target angle, focal spots 0·3, 0·6 and 1·2 mm.

5 For general radiography, heat storage capacity 300,000 H.U., 15 degrees target angle, focal spots 0·6, 1·0 and 2·0 mm.

Students may wish to test their powers of recall by comparing 4 and 5 and answering this question: why does the tube with the smaller minimum focal spot size also have a smaller target angle? If you do not know the answer, please turn to pages 220 and 223.

TUBESTANDS, CEILING TUBE SUPPORTS (TUBE HANGERS, CEILING CRANES)

The function of a tubestand or similar equipment is to support the X-ray tube so that it can be applied by the radiographer to the examination of patients. The purchasers of X-ray apparatus probably give more thought to the choice of the generator or table than to the details of design in the tubestand or ceiling crane which is to go with it. Nevertheless, it is an important item of X-ray equipment and has to fulfill certain requirements if it is to make the X-ray tube fully and easily usable.

1   The support should be adequately rigid so that vibration of the X-ray tube is avoided.

2   All movements of the support and of the X-ray tube about it should be smooth, as unrestricted as possible and easy to perform.

3   It must be possible to make certain precise angulations of the X-ray beam.

4   It must be possible to direct the X-ray beam parallel to the floor as well as in a perpendicular direction.

5   The controls providing for the tube movements should be readily accessible.

Tube supports are found in a variety of designs and two main categories; (a) tubestands and (b) apparatus which suspends the tube from the ceiling.

Tubestands

A typical tubestand consists of a column of heavy gauge steel tubing which is mounted on a carriage and by this means can move between tracks on the floor and ceiling (in some cases the overhead mounting may be along one wall); the floor track is often recessed.

On this vertical column a cross-arm supports the X-ray tube. This cross-arm is on ball races and can be moved (a) up and down the column, (b) at right angles to the column, (c) in a rotational motion about the vertical axis of the column. The X-ray tube can be (a) rotated upon the cross-arm and (b) tilted about an axis parallel to itself.

By these means provision is made for the following excursions of the X-ray tube.

1   *Longitudinal travel* (parallel to the X-ray table) for at least 3·5 m (12 feet), or for greater distances if required, within the limits of the length of the room.

2   *Horizontal travel at right angles to* (*i*). The extent of this transverse movement is usually of the order of 90 cm (36 inches). It is restricted in one direction by the length of the cross-arm itself and in the other direction by the configuration of the bracket holding the X-ray tube—it is not usually

possible to move the X-ray tube nearer to the vertical column than about 75 cm (30 inches). However, a movement of this extent is adequate to allow the X-ray tube to cover the width of a bucky table, or stretcher or litter, on which a patient may be lying; or to be centred upon other apparatus in the room, such as a chest stand or vertical bucky. The cross-arm carries a scale which is calibrated in centimetres or inches. The centre of the excursion is marked zero and the scale gives the distance of the tube from the centre at any point on either side of it within the limits of the available movement. Very often there is audible indication—a little 'click'—when the tube is central on the cross arm or the tube may locate itself in the central position by means of suitable keying.

3 *Vertical travel up and down the column.* The extent of this depends upon the height and detailed design of the column. It usually affords a maximum focus-bucky or focus-table distance of at least 1·25 m (50 inches) and in some cases of 2 m (6 feet). At the other limit of its travel it is possible to lower the tube to within about 75 cm (30 inches) from the floor. Scales on the vertical column refer to each of these distances.

4 *Rotational travel about the vertical column.* Some manufacturers permit the rotation about the column to be 360 degrees. In the interests of the high tension cables it is perhaps better if the movement is limited to something less than a complete revolution. For example, 300 degrees or even 270 degrees allow plenty of scope for manœuvring the X-ray tube and may prevent a succession of heedless users from damaging the cables by winding them ever more tightly round the column; the inevitable result of persistent rotation of the X-ray tube in one direction only. Often automatic locations of the tube are provided at 90 degree intervals and a manual control is used to lock the tube at any intermediate angle.

5 *Rotation on an axis parallel to the cross-arm of 180 degrees to 180 degrees.* Automatic locations of the tube may be effective at 90 degree intervals and a manual lock fixes the tube at any other required angle. Freedom of rotation and precise movements on this axis are important to the radiographer, since many radiographic techniques require accurate angulations of the tube towards the feet or the head of a patient who may be lying on the table or sitting erect at a vertical bucky. Manufacturers usually provide angulation scales which are easy to read, marked at intervals of 1 degree and prominently situated on the tube mount.

6 *Rotation round the tube's own long axis.* Rotation round the tube's axis is necessarily restricted by the nature of the bracket holding the tube and will vary in extent with the details of the tube mount's design. In one example the tube can be rotated up to 30 degrees on either side of the vertical. In another the total angulation is 125 degrees; this is divided unequally on either side of the vertical, being in one direction restricted to 20 degrees.

The lock and scale for axial rotation of the tube should be prominently placed—like their companions—on the front of the tube mount, where the radiographer can easily manipulate the one and read the other. However, this is not always the case, no doubt because these angulations are less often required and for this reason are perhaps thought to be less important. Radiographers sometimes cannot read the scale from their normal working position and may find the lock inaccessibly placed for easy manual operation.

The brakes

Electromagnetic brakes operated by push-buttons or switches on the tube mount are usually provided for the three directions of travel; longitudinal (floor), transverse (cross) and vertical. When the main power is 'off', these brakes and all related tube movements are usually free. Independent manual controls are included, and when a unit is left overnight it is good practice to see that the tube is run down the column to a safe position on the table—for example over the pillow—and that the manual locks are tightened.

In some instances a circuit may be so arranged that brakes become operative when the circuit is incomplete and are released when the circuit is 'made'. This means that when the mains supply is switched off in the room the brake in question is locked; it seems a sensible provision in respect—for example—of rotational movements when the weight of high tension cables might pull a tube from the position in which it had been left and cause damage to it.

Tube suspension and counterweighting

The cross-arm carrying the X-ray tube is suspended by a variety of means: a single-wire cable may be employed; sometimes twin-wire cables are used; and in another example a dual system consists of a cable and a chain. The tube is counterweighted in its vertical motion, the counterweights being usually—although not necessarily—placed within the tube column. In some cases the tube is instead counterpoised by means of springs within the column.

When the suspension is by means of a single cable, a 'fail safe' mechanism is essential; otherwise, fracture of the cable could result in the rapid descent of the cross-arm and tube, to the detriment equally of the tube itself and of any patient so unfortunate as to be on the X-ray table at the time. A simple, effective device of this kind is depicted in Fig. 7.29.

The tube column is grooved on one aspect to provide a channel in which a brake block within the carriage casting of the cross-arm can move. A

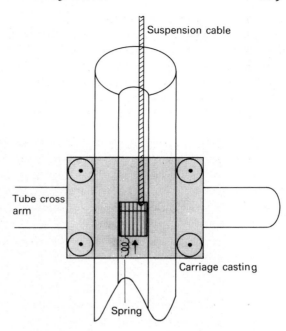

Fig. 7.29 A fail-safe device for a suspension cable.

spring fixed at one lower corner of the brake block provides a force which would push it out of alignment in its groove, were it not for the upward counter-pull of the suspension cable. If the cable snaps, this counter-pull is at once removed: the brake block is thrust askew by the spring and becomes stuck in its channel thus arresting the downward rush of the carriage, cross-arm and X-ray tube.

Ceiling tube supports (tube hangers)

Arrangements which support the X-ray tube by a suspension from the ceiling are available in a variety of designs from different manufacturers and are known by a number of names. In the United Kingdom, *ceiling tube support* (Fig. 7.30) and in the U.S.A. *tube hanger* are perhaps the best known descriptions; the terms *ceiling crane* and *ceiling suspension* are also used.

Typical apparatus of this kind is sketched in Fig. 7.31. It will be seen that it consists of three principal parts.

1 The main supporting unit or carriage from which the X-ray tube is suspended by a telescopic system.

2 A pair of rails on which the tube carriage travels in a direction designated as transverse since it is often at right angles to the X-ray table. These rails

are really a second carriage (sometimes called the transverse carriage or bridge) since they are themselves mounted on—

3 longitudinal tracks which are fixed usually to the ceiling as illustrated but sometimes to a wall or to a combination of the ceiling and a wall.

Depending upon the dimensions of the transverse carriage and the length of the ceiling track, the X-ray tube can be moved about the room over a considerable floor area. The standard length of the ceiling track varies

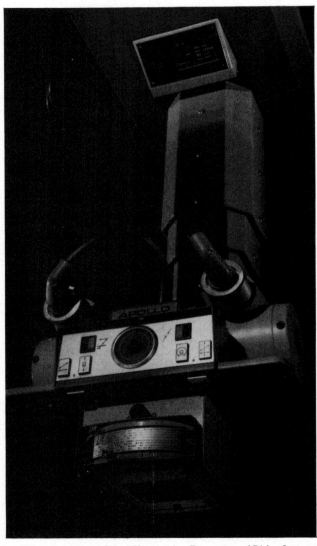

Fig. 7.30 A ceiling tube support for an X-ray tube. *By courtesy of Picker International Ltd.*

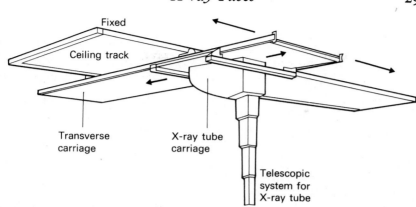

Fixed

Ceiling track

Transverse
carriage

X-ray tube
carriage

Telescopic
system for
X-ray tube

Fig. 7.31

between different examples—for instance 3·6 m (12 feet) and 4 m (13 feet 9 inches)—but in most instances the run can be extended if the length of the room and the nature of the work make this appropriate. The transverse travel of the tube is limited by the length of the bridge: 2·6 m (8 feet 6 inches) and 3·5 m (11 feet 6 inches) are typical examples.

Tube movements and their control

The movements of the X-ray tube which can be obtained from a ceiling suspension are similar in nature to those already described for a tubestand but differ, of course, in degree. They are listed below with some additional comment.

Horizontal travel

The term horizontal travel includes movements of the X-ray tube in directions which are both longitudinal (parallel to the long axis of the X-ray table) and transverse (at right angles to the table). The area covered may be most of the X-ray room.

The tube movements are controlled by electromagnetic brakes operated by push-buttons; these are sometimes on the tube mount, sometimes on a separate control handle. Various examples of the equipment have (a) both horizontal movements motorized, (b) only the longitudinal movement motorized, (c) neither movement motorized.

Usually some indication is available when the X-ray tube is over the midline of the table. This may take the form of a pilot lamp on the tube mount or an automatic location of the tube carriage at the central position on the bridge.

Vertical travel

A ceiling height of not less than 2·9 m (9 feet 6 inches) is required for satisfactory ceiling suspension of the X-ray tube. If the ceiling is too low, the maximum focus-table top distance obtainable is inevitably decreased. If the ceiling is too high—more than 3 m (10 feet)—there are minor complications of installation, since the joists which carry the ceiling tracks must be fitted from suitably lower points: this is no matter of difficulty as a rule. A much more important aspect of installation is that the ceiling track is required to be level within critical limits.

Assuming a ceiling height—or its equivalent—of 2·9 m (9 feet 6 inches), the maximum focus-table top distance which is available varies between different examples: 1·2 m (48 inches) and 1·5 m (60 inches) are typical examples.

A helpful feature of ceiling tube suspensions is that the X-ray tube can be lowered without difficulty, often closer to the floor than is the case with some tubestands. Minimum focus-floor distances vary between 50 cm (20 inches) and 87 cm (35 inches) depending on the type considered. There should be on the overhead carriage clear, preferably illuminated scales indicating both the focus-table top and focus-floor distances. Like the horizontal movements of the tube, the vertical movement may or may not be motorized. Electromagnetic brakes operated by push-buttons or switches on the tube mount are used to control it in either event. Counterweighting suspension is usually by dual cables for safety. These cables may be arranged so that as long as they are taut a microswitch in the brake circuit remains 'closed'. Should the cables slacken or fracture, the switch becomes 'open circuit' and the brakes operative, thus preventing the descent of the tube.

Rotation

Rotation of the X-ray tube is usual in two planes:
1 about the axis of the telescopic hanger;
2 about the transverse axis of the tube.

In some cases 360 degree rotation is allowed in each plane. In other examples the movement may be restricted to 270 degrees to prevent tangling of the high tension cables as the result of indiscriminate revolutions. Automatic location of the tube by keying at 90 degree intervals is a frequent feature.

As (2) is the plane of tube tilts required in many radiographic techniques, it is usual to show these angles on a prominent scale on the control panel on the tube mount.

The advantages of ceiling suspension of the X-ray tube in certain situations are obvious.

1 The floor of the X-ray room in the vicinity of the X-ray table is free of obstruction and access to the table is easy from all sides.

2 One X-ray tube can readily serve two or more tables in the same room or can easily examine a patient brought into the room in a bed or on a stretcher or litter.

3 Exposures using a horizontal beam—for example the lateral radiograph of the femoral neck—can be made with equal facility from either side of the table.

4 Teleradiography—that is, the use of an anode-film distance of at least 1·8 m (6 feet)—is easily achieved in the case of a patient standing in front of a floor- or wall-mounted cassette holder.

5 The tube can be easily aligned with additional equipment such as a vertical bucky.

6 The X-ray tube is always out of the way when not in use.

7 In a small room, maximum use is made of the available space.

8 When the X-ray tube has to be moved mechanically for the purpose of tomography, the drive is more direct in the case of the ceiling suspension than when it must be made from the floor, via a tubestand and cross-arm: the motion is consequently better controlled and shake of the X-ray tube less likely to be present during exposure.

While there are a number of advantages associated with ceiling suspension, it would be wrong to suppose that this is invariably the best method of support. In Chapter 12 reference is made to some special features required in a table which is used for myelography. One of these features is a second image receptor fitted to the side of the table and energized by the overtable tube in order to permit examination of a prone patient from the lateral aspect. In these circumstances, a ceiling-supported tube may limit the adverse table tilt to something like 25 degrees if the suspension is not to be dragged from the ceiling: a floor to ceiling tubestand does not have this disability.

Chapter 8
The Control of Scattered Radiation

In diagnostic radiography secondary radiation is useless radiation. It makes no favourable contribution to the formation of the X-ray image and it seriously deteriorates contrast in the radiograph.

It is not the role of this book either to explain the production of secondary radiation when an X-ray beam traverses a patient or to demonstrate how radiographic contrast is reduced. However, we *are* concerned with the practical use of diagnostic X-ray equipment. This equipment inevitably is affected in its construction and function by the need to employ the X-ray beam as usefully as possible and to save radiographs from the deleterious influences of secondary radiation. We will therefore consider very briefly some of the physical problems involved.

THE SIGNIFICANCE OF SCATTER

It may be helpful at this stage to make a summary statement of the kinds of X radiation reaching the film during a radiographic exposure. These are:

1 primary radiation which is variously attenuated by the patient's tissues and thus produces a pattern of response from the film that we recognize as the radiographic image;

2 secondary radiation which is largely Compton scattering of the primary beam within the patient and of which an unspecifiable proportion is moving towards the film and will necessarily result in a density on the film.

It is this forward-moving scatter with which the diagnostic radiographer is concerned. Some significant aspects of it should be considered.

1 The amount of scatter produced increases rapidly with the volume of material irradiated. This means that it is greater (a) when the patient is obese; (b) when a thick body part is X-rayed, for example the pelvis as opposed to the ankle; (c) when a large exposure field is used, for example a full radiograph of the abdomen as distinct from a localized view of the gall bladder in the right hypochondrium.

2 The energy of the scattered X-ray photon is less than the energy of the primary one. Even so, in the case of most diagnostic X-ray beams, some scatter will certainly be energetic enough to reach the film. When high

kilovoltages are employed for radiography, less of the primary beam is scattered but the scattered photons have greater energy and more of the scatter is in a forward direction. Consequently a much larger proportion of these photons reach the film.

So far as the radiograph is concerned there is more scatter at high kilovoltages: in fact there may be more scattered than primary radiation incident on the film.

3   The diagnostic radiographer recognizes the presence of scattered radiation as an overall density on the film which is not productive of image detail to any extent. It is therefore fog. The effects of such overall density are (a) a decrease in the light-transmitting ability of the film and (b) a lessening of contrast, which is the ratio between adjacent optical opacities.

There are two avenues of approach to the project of protecting radiographs from the effects of scatter when thick body parts are X-rayed. These are:

1   limiting its formation by devices which reduce the volume of irradiated material;

2   preventing whatever scattered radiation is produced either from arriving at all upon the film or from affecting it so much.

Mechanisms which limit the formation of scatter are *cones, diaphragms* and *compression bands*. Mechanisms which diminish its action on the film are *secondary radiation grids* and—in a very small way—*intensifying screens*. These will now be considered separately in greater detail.

BEAM LIMITING DEVICES

Cones and diaphragms

Cones and diaphragms are usually associated together as they operate in the same way. Both are metal devices which restrict the size—or rather area—of the beam which is employed. It is evident that the smaller the area of the patient which is exposed to radiation the smaller also must be the volume of irradiated tissue and the less the resultant amount of scatter.

Radiographic cones

As a rule, cones are tapered metal structures which may be fitted to the X-ray tube at the beam's exit port. They are usually manufactured either of brass or steel and are open at both ends; the end nearer the tube is often the apex of the cone, while the wide part is directed towards the film. There is little difficulty in understanding the use of the cone shape in view of the divergent character of the primary X-ray beam. Sometimes a radiographic cone is a steel cylinder which may be extensible in length; or the cone may be tapered towards the film, as in the case of those supplied with dental X-ray units (however, this is a misleading appearance as the 'cone' here is merely a radioparent attachment to make beam centring easier and is not a true radiographic cone).

Radiographic cones come in a variety of sizes which result in different areas of radiation field. They cannot be employed properly unless the radiographer is aware of the size of field produced by any given cone used at the chosen anode-film distance.

Factors which influence the field area are:

1   the anode-film distance (A);
2   the length of the cone (L);
3   the distance between the narrow end of the cone and the focal spot of the X-ray tube (F);
4   the large diameter of the cone (D). The associated small diameter is implicit in the geometry of the cone.

From the knowledge of these measurements it is possible to compute the size of field on the film by employing the following expression:

$$\text{Diameter of the film field} = \frac{A}{L+F} \times D$$

However, it is probable that very few radiographers make use of this equation, or even need to do so. In many instances the manufacturers of the equipment print a numerical factor on the side of each cone. This number divided into the anode-film distance provides the diameter of the radiation field. For example, a cone might have a factor of 4. Used at an anode-film distance of 100 cm (40 inches), this cone would give a circle of radiation 25 cm (10 inches) in diameter; if the anode-film distance were 90 cm (36 inches) the circle on the film would have a diameter of 23 cm (9 inches).

In the absence of such a cone factor, radiographers tend to employ cones on an empirical basis. They know from experience that a particular cone used with particular X-ray equipment at a certain anode-film distance results in a field area large enough to come within the boundaries of a specific size of film, or that it will completely cover some smaller film.

If a film is to be completely covered, the diameter of the coned area must be at least equal to the diagonal of the film concerned. To have it much greater than the film diagonal is obviously to waste the purpose of the cone, since an unnecessarily large area—and therefore volume—of the patient is irradiated. On the other hand, to be over-ambitious and employ too small a cone may result in the necessity to repeat an exposure if the resultant radiograph does not include the full area of clinical interest. It is certain that the early efforts of all student radiographers include at least some 'coned off' disasters.

Fig. 8.1(a) shows that when a circular cone is used to cover a film completely the cone is not employed to the best advantage. There is irradiated a considerable area (volume) of the body which, though beyond the boundaries of the film, nevertheless provides a potential contribution of scattered radiation to the radiograph. (This is not true if the part X-rayed is a limb, as the 'surround' is then air which does not appreciably scatter X-ray photons.) Fig. 8.1(b) illustrates the greater efficiency of beam limitation produced when the radiation field 'fits inside' the edges of the film.

Expertly used, cones are highly effective and must be reckoned as one of the two best methods of controlling scatter in diagnostic radiography. However, it is not always possible to 'cone down' even to the extent indicated in Fig. 8.1(b); this could, for example, result in the omission of the peripheral parts of the diaphragm from a radiograph of the abdomen.

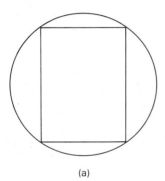

(a)

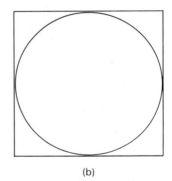

(b)

Fig. 8.1

Radiographic diaphragms

The problems of fitting circular fields of radiation to non-circular patients and films can be skirted by making the field rectangular. Such a rectangular field is provided by radiographic diaphragms, which exist in either of the following forms.

1 A simple tablet of heavy metal has a central rectangular aperture for the X-ray beam and can be slotted into a fitting on the tube port in a similar manner to a cone. It is usual to have available a number of diaphragms which will have each a different sized aperture in order to suit the differing dimensions of X-ray films and the varying needs of radiographic subjects; for instance, a narrow 'slit' diaphragm is appropriate for the examination of the petrous temporal bone in the skull.

2 An adjustable diaphragm system. For general radiography the adjustable diaphragm system is now almost universally used. It is convenient, as it does not require the radiographer continually to change attachments to the X-ray tube nor does it preclude the additional use of a cone when a circular localized field is appropriate and desirable.

The adjustable diaphragm system

Adjustable diaphragms on the X-ray tube are an arrangement of two pairs of movable leaves of metal—usually lead—situated in the X-ray beam; each pair moves in a line at right angles to the other. Fig. 8.2 is a sketch of such a

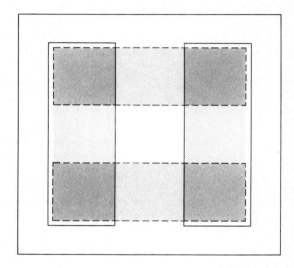

Fig. 8.2

system from the direction of the focus of the X-ray tube. Fig. 8.3 is the 'elevation', showing how the pairs are arranged in a near relationship, above and below each other, and also the chamfered design which enables the leaves to close completely at the midline. Each pair of leaves is operated independently of the other by means of a control knob on the casing. The area of the field produced is thus continuously variable in either direction, from zero up to a certain maximum.

As in the case of the cone, the geometry of projection determines the size of field produced by any given aperture, whether we consider a fixed diaphragm or moveable diaphragms. The field in each direction is determined by the same factors:

1 the anode-film distance (A);
2 the distance between the diaphragm and the focal spot of the X-ray tube (F);

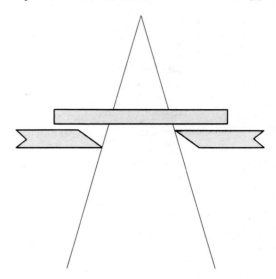

Fig. 8.3

3   the size of the aperture (*D*).

Just as in the case of the cone, we can say of each pair of diaphragms that they result in a field edge on the film in accordance with the following relationship:

$$\text{Extent of field on film} = \frac{A}{F} \times D$$

However, it is unlikely that working radiographers make use of this expression to compute their practices with diaphragms, particularly diaphragms of the variable type just described. It is customary for manufacturers to calibrate the control knobs of these so that the operator knows that a certain position of each knob results in a certain dimension of the field at a given anode-film distance. Such control knobs and scales can be seen on the light-beam diaphragm which is fitted to the X-ray tube shown in Fig. 7.30 on page 290.

Perhaps even this information is scarcely used since variable diaphragms of the kind discussed are usually associated with an illuminated mirror which provides visual evidence of the field area. It is probable that the majority of radiographers select the diaphragm positions by sight, to include on the radiograph only the requisite area of the patient. Radiographers who work in this way should remember that the area indicated on the presenting skin surface is projected on the film as a somewhat larger field of radiation; the visible boundaries selected on the patient should be a little less than the dimensions of all the structures which the radiograph is required to display.

A light beam indicator built into a variable beam collimator is one of several beam centering devices and will be separately discussed in a later section of the chapter (see page 304).

Before leaving variable collimators we may note that these are an equally suitable beam limiting device for an X-ray tube in the undertable position used for fluoroscopy. In this case they are remotely operated from the image receptor's carriage. Formerly control was usually by means of a Bowden cable but at the present time the diaphragms are likely to be motor driven. No calibration of their position is necessary since the operator will adjust them visually during fluoroscopy. In the U.K. and elsewhere approved codes of practice refer to the collimating system of an undertable X-ray tube.

Demarcation of the radiation field

The use of a diaphragm—whether fixed or in the form of adjustable leaves— may not necessarily produce a sharp demarcation of the boundaries of the radiation field. A penumbra is often noticeable on the radiograph; if the diaphragm is adjustable this occurs particularly along the edges which are at right angles to the tube's axis and are usually delineated by the pair of leaves further from the focus. This penumbra is due to the following factors.

1   As the diaphragm is relatively near to the tube target its situation results in a large amount of geometric unsharpness. This may not be very significant except to the 'artistic' appearance of the radiograph.

2   The presence of extra-focal radiation. This is radiation arising from other internal parts of the tube than the focal area itself. It is due partly to the scatter which occurs as the primary beam traverses the glass wall of the tube and the surrounding oil and so on, but more significantly to X rays produced from parts of the target beyond the focus. Such X rays are generated by electrons which bounce from the area of original impact and then fall on the target at points other than the focal area. Unfortunately radiation produced in this way—unlike scattered radiation—is almost as penetrating as that from the focus itself and consequently the situation cannot be improved by increased filtration in the tube shield. The effect is worse in a rotating anode tube because there is much more tungsten in this type of anode; in the case of the fixed anode the bouncing electrons fall on copper and less extra-focal radiation is generated.

Extra-focal radiation cannot be completely removed from a rotating anode tube but the effects of its presence—which are degrading to radiographic detail—can be minimized by the following methods.

1   A lead collimator built into the window of the tube shield and serving as a fixed diaphragm at the tube port. It should have as small an aperture as

possible, consistent with adequate coverage of films in general use. This fitting should be standard on modern rotating anode tubes.

2   A double-leaved diaphragm. This apparatus operates similarly to the single adjustable diaphragm already described, being merely a reduplication of this system; there are four pairs of moveable leaves instead of two. Each two pairs work in association in the manner indicated in Figs. 8.2 and 8.3 and the groups are mounted one above the other. The increased efficacy of the double leaved diaphragm depends on the ability of the second set of leaves to absorb extra-focal radiation which passes the proximal pairs. This is undoubtedly an improved system. However, there are entailed at the same time increases in mechanical complexity, in size and weight of the equipment and also, inevitably, in its cost.

While it is general practice to use a cone or diaphragm for medical radiography, even if none were employed the size of the beam would still be limited to a certain degree; though it would be unnecessarily large in most cases. In Chapter 7 the main attributes of an X-ray tube shield are described and the student will find here reference to two self-contained features which result in limitation of the size of the primary beam:

1   the dimensions of the aperture in the tube shield by which the useful X-ray beam leaves;

2   the angle of anode inclination—the steeper the anode angle the stricter is the 'cut off' of radiation towards the anode end of the X-ray tube.

Radiation protection

In this chapter we are concerned with the unpleasant radiographic results of scattered radiation and particularly with equipment which is intended to ameliorate these. However, beam limiting devices—whether cones or diaphragms—are a means also of restricting radiation dose to a patient and others. In this respect they may be subject to certain recommendations in an approved code of practice which should advise that a beam collimator always should be in place and should offer the same degree of protection as the tube housing (see Chapter 7, page 288).

Compression bands

A compression band is not a beam limiting device, as this term is appropriate only to equipment which restricts the area of the primary beam. However, it is fitting enough to include it in the present discussion since—like beam limiting devices—a compression band can be said to reduce the amount of scatter present, even although in rather a devious way. This is because for any given area of the patient irradiated a compression band can be used to diminish the volume of tissue through which the X-ray beam must pass.

Essentially its function is to 'flatten' the patient—or rather that part which is X-rayed—and by displacing adipose tissue to either side of the primary beam it precludes such tissue from the emission of secondary radiation. Furthermore, by reducing body thickness a compression band may enable a lower kilovoltage to be used than would otherwise be needed for adequate penetration. This effect is outstandingly demonstrated in the Manchester techniques for obstetric radiography.

A radiographic compression band is simply a long strip of linen or nylon about 20–35 cm wide. It is attached at the ends to either side of the X-ray table by means of two fitments which can occupy any opposite positions on the length of the table. One of the fitments may be merely a pair of hooks which will engage with the side rails of the table when cross tension is put on the band. Their partner is a roller into which the band can be slotted and which can be rotated by means of a ratchet and handle. The roller winds the band tightly across the table and thus across the body of the table's occupant. The usual application is to the abdomen. The ratchet mechanism includes provision for the easy release of compression.

Compression bands are simple and effective devices of which perhaps too few radiographers make routine use. They cause appreciable improvement in radiographic contrast and they carry bonus advantages as a comfortable means of immobilizing a recumbent or erect patient during any of a number of examinations.

BEAM CENTRING DEVICES

Beam centring devices are very common radiographic accessories. The term refers to any piece of apparatus which provides the radiographer with a pre-indication of the direction of the central ray. In themselves beam centring devices have no effect whatever upon the formation or limitation of scattered radiation but it is convenient to consider them at this time since one at least is directly associated with an adjustable diaphragm system. Furthermore, when the position of the central ray is visibly and precisely pre-indicated, the radiographer should be encouraged to make accurate limitation of the primary beam.

In the following paragraphs four kinds of beam centring device will be considered:
1 simple centre finder;
2 Varay lamps;
3 light beam delineator;
4 optical delineator.

Centre finder

Fig. 8.4 is an illustration of a simple centre finder consisting of a telescopic steel pointer which is fitted to the tube port and can occupy the position of the central X-ray beam. This particular one extends from about 36 cm (14 inches) to about 59 cm (23 inches). It is hinged so that it can be displaced 90 degrees to either side while the X-ray exposure is made. No doubt the main disadvantage of the device is that sooner or later every radiographer forgets to do this and obtains a radiograph in which the image is devastatingly obscured by the metal parts of the centre finder. The centre finder shown can be removed from the tube port and replaced by a cone. In some portable X-ray units, however, it is permanently attached.

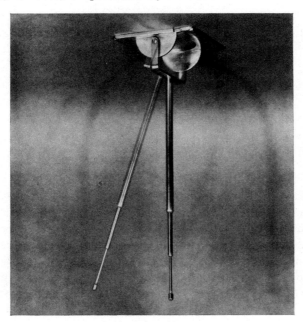

Fig. 8.4   A centre finder. *By courtesy of Picker International Ltd.*

Varay lamps

Varay lamps have the advantage that they do not need to be moved, either during the X-ray exposure or to permit the use of a cone; they are attached to the tube outside the radiation field.

Fig. 8.5 illustrates the principle on which two Varay lamps can be mounted at right angles to produce intersecting cross-lines of light. Each lamp is a little metal cylinder from which light emerges only through a small slit occupying part of the circumference near one end. This results in a

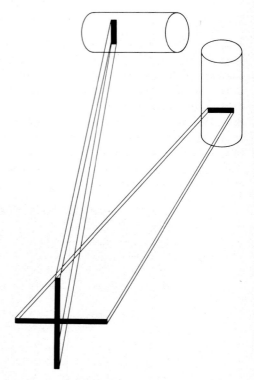

Fig. 8.5 A pair of Varay lamps
mounted on the X-ray tube shield at
right angles to each other produce
intersecting lines of light.

narrow beam of light appearing as an illuminated line on any surface upon
which the lamp is directed.

To form a centring device on an X-ray tube two lamps are fixed at 90
degrees to each other, close to the tube port. One of these has its slit aperture
parallel to the long axis of the tube and will produce a line of light
longitudinal to the table and the patient. The beam from its partner is at
right angles to the tube axis and will make a line crosswise to the table and
the patient. The point of intersection of these indicates the axial line of the
primary X-ray beam.

It is to be emphasized that Varay lamps do not 'frame' the radiation field
in the manner of other delineators described. They simply produce two
lighted cross-lines which intersect at the centre of the field. They are
accurate and always in place and do not add significantly to the weight of
the X-ray tube.

Light beam diaphragm

A light beam diaphragm or delineator is an adjustable collimator of one of
the kinds described in the previous section of this chapter, with which is

combined a method of illuminating the field such that the lighted area corresponds to the area of the X-ray beam. Altering the area of the beam by means of the diaphragm controls similarly changes the area of light falling on the subject.

The light is produced by a small lamp bulb—sometimes similar to that used in certain car head lamps—and a mirror is used to display the light in the same direction as the X-ray beam. A small central area, marked on the Perspex front window, is opaque to light. This results in a dark spot at the centre of the light field which corresponds to the projection of the central primary X-ray beam.

The scheme is depicted diagrammatically in Fig. 8.6. The mirror is (a) approximately at 45 degrees both to the beam of light and to the primary X-ray beam; (b) equidistant from the filament of the lamp and the focus of the X-ray tube. The mirror is of thin silvered glass, or alternatively metal foil, and does not appreciably attenuate the X-ray beam at the kilovoltages normally employed for diagnostic radiography. However, it will have a significant filtering effect if an unusually low kilovoltage is used, for example 25–35 kVp during mammography. Unless the collimator has a plastic mirror, provision must be made for the removal of the light beam diaphragm from the tube during such examinations.

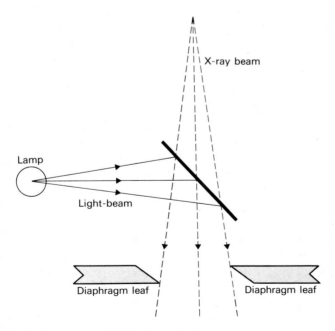

Fig. 8.6 Principal components of a light beam diaphragm.

If the beam delineator is to be easily visible in daylight the lamp must be high powered and consequently its life is relatively short. To prolong this as much as possible the lamp is operated by means of an automatic time-switch which will break the circuit after about 30 seconds. This period is adjustable to some extent but radiographers who do not find the allotted time sufficient for their centring manœuvres should beware of overlengthening it if they are to avoid the tiresome frequent necessity to replace lamp bulbs.

The majority of light beam diaphragms possess the following additional accessory features:

1   control knobs which face the operator and are calibrated with scales of area and distance as explained previously (see page 299);

2   a slide at the distal aspect which will accept a supplementary cone when required;

3   a rotational movement which permits the delineator to be turned from its normal alignment with the axis of the X-ray tube, in order to cover a cassette placed at an angle with the table edge—for example during radiography of an extremity.

Occasionally the mirror in a light beam diaphragm goes out of adjustment so that the light field and the X-ray field are no longer coincident. This is to be suspected whenever radiographers confronting radiographs which are off-centre are heard regularly to protest, 'But I *did* centre it.' The presence of the condition can be proved by means of one of the simple tests described in Chapter 17.

Optical delineator

Generally speaking, the worst disadvantage of the beam delineator just described is that in bright daylight or strong artificial light it may be impossible to discern either the boundaries of the field or the position of the central spot—especially on dark subjects: an instance is a brunette who is having her nasal sinuses X-rayed. It is estimated that the radiographer will scarcely distinguish the demarcated area when the brightness of the room is ten times or more greater than the brightness of the light field. Such a situation can easily occur whenever clear sunlight enters an X-ray room or films have to be taken of a patient in an operating theatre.

In theory the problem could be overcome by putting into the light beam diaphragm a lamp of higher power. However, this brings other difficulties associated with the greater heat which would be produced and the dispersal of such heat from an enclosed radiation-proof system.

The disadvantages of a lamp and mirror system are avoided by an optical delineator of the kind illustrated in Fig. 8.7. This has the familiar box of paired diaphragms and employs a similar radiolucent mirror to the light

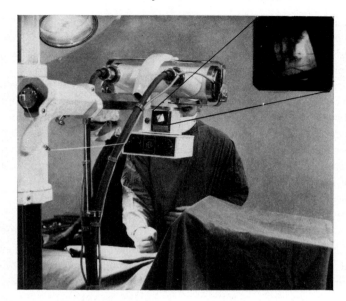

Fig. 8.7 An optical beam delineator. *By courtesy of Picker International Ltd.*

beam delineator. However, instead of a lamp this apparatus is provided with a reflex optical system through which the patient is viewed. The visual impression obtained is that the observer is looking at the patient from the same point of view as the focus of the X-ray tube. The image in the lens is smaller than is the reality and consequently more brilliant; it will always appear brighter than its background whether the ambient lighting is strong or weak.

Inherent in the optical system is a left-to-right reversal of the image as it is apparent to the observer. This does not result in anatomical reversal of the patient but merely turns him head-to-tail. This peculiarity is one to which most radiographers should be able to adjust with practice, but difficulties of recognition often occur in the operating theatre when the subject is draped with towels.

Cross-lines engraved on the viewing lens should intersect at an opaque spot in the centre of the diaphragm's exit window. When this is so the observer's eye is 'looking' along the path of the central X-ray beam.

In addition to the above essential characteristics the optical delineator possesses three refinements described below.

1   A means of varying the angle of the viewing device from the horizontal to about 14 degrees below. This is necessary if the viewer is to be equally accessible (a) to radiographers of differing heights; (b) at elevated positions

of the X-ray tube. In Fig. 9.15 the little 'tunnel' of the viewer can be seen just above the radiographer's right hand.

2   A lead-lined housing for the mirror and optical system and lead glass in the viewer. These are to prevent the leakage of scattered radiation.

3   The facility of replacing the optical system with a light source in situations when it is hardly possible to use the viewer; for example when the tube is brought to table level and the beam directed horizontally for the lateral projection of the femoral neck. This replacement converts the optical delineator to a conventional light beam diaphragm but as the lamp housing is attached outside the diaphragm box its ventilation is easier than usual and a lamp of higher wattage becomes appropriate.

THE SECONDARY RADIATION GRID

We have now to consider necessary equipment which can limit the effects of scattered radiation on the film, as distinct from reducing the amount of scatter formed. In this role intensifying screens play a very small part.

As much scattered radiation is of longer wavelength than primary radiation it excites the screens less strongly. Consequently there is a lower density upon the film from the scattered component than from the primary rays and contrast is improved. However, this is only a minor consequence. Much more efficacious protection of the film is given by a secondary radiation grid, of which radiographers usually speak more simply as a *grid*.

Principles of the grid

A secondary radiation grid is composed of a large number of thin strips of lead separated from each other by some interspacing material which is penetrable by X rays. The grid is placed between the patient and the film in the manner depicted in Fig. 8.8. The diagram illustrates how the primary beam is able to pass through translucent spaces in the grid, while scattered radiation which deviates in direction from primary tends to strike the lead elements and is absorbed before it reaches the film. This is the bare, simple principle on which all secondary radiation grids operate. In practice there are a number of complicating factors which influence the relative efficiency of grids and may make one grid preferable to another in a particular situation. These are further discussed below.

The grid ratio

In effect a secondary radiation grid presents to the X-ray beam a number of

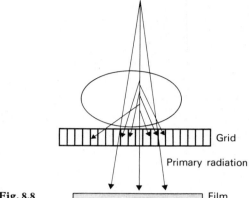

Grid

Primary radiation

Fig. 8.8   Film

radiolucent channels through which radiation can reach the film. Fig. 8.9 indicates two such channels in different grids.

In Fig. 8.9(a) we see a short, wide channel through which the primary beam can easily pass. However, at the same time some scattered radiation is admitted if its deviation from the primary ray is not sufficient for it to strike the lead 'walls' alongside.

In Fig. 8.9(b) the radiolucent channel is both longer and narrower. Radiation which deviates even slightly from the primary beam will be absorbed; but equally any primary beam not in alignment with a channel also will be absorbed and will fail to arrive at the film. When the radiolucent interspaces in a grid are long and narrow, as opposed to being short and wide, there is a greater likelihood of primary radiation being lost in this way. Thus all grids:

1   absorb scattered radiation;
2   absorb a smaller proportion of useful primary radiation.

A grid which possesses a high degree of efficiency in (1) is associated with greater losses in respect of (2). The fact that some primary radiation inevitably *is* absorbed is part of the reason why the use of a secondary radiation grid always necessitates an increase in radiographic exposure by a factor of approximately 3 or 4 depending on the grid.

The difference between Figs. 8.9(a) and 8.9(b) is in a factor known as the *grid ratio*. The grid ratio makes a statement about the width of the radiolucent channel through which primary radiation must pass in order to reach the film and form an image upon it. Formally stated, the grid ratio is an expression of the height of the lead strips (in effect the grid thickness) relative to the width of the interspaces; 8 to 1 and 10 to 1 are examples of the ratios commonly possessed by secondary radiation grids in general use.

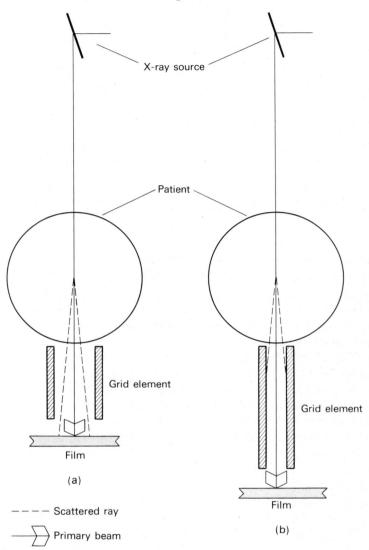

X-ray source

Patient

Grid element

Film

(a)

Grid element

Film

(b)

– – – – Scattered ray

──▷ Primary beam

Fig. 8.9

The grid ratio is not a complete statement of the efficiency of a grid (this will be considered more fully on page 312) but it is a generally accepted statement since it measures the two important—but mutually hostile—effects just considered. A grid of high ratio, relative to another of lower ratio—

1   blocks a greater proportion of scattered radiation;

2 restricts the passage of primary radiation to a greater degree and consequently requires the use of increased exposures.

The grid lattice (lines/cm)

In considering whether a particular grid is acceptable or not, a factor known as the grid lattice is as important as its ratio. The grid lattice is the number of lead strips to each centimetre or inch of the grid's width.

This number has a significant radiographic effect since whenever a secondary radiation grid rests upon a cassette, so that it is interposed between a patient and the film, inevitably the images of the lead strips are recorded on the film as a regular sharp pattern of clear lines. If these lines are uniform, fine and sufficiently close together the eye is unable easily to resolve them and they disappear—or very nearly disappear—for most observers. Conversely, if the linear pattern is composed of coarse, well separated stripes its image is dominant. It can severely detract from and even destroy the appreciation of detail in the radiographic image proper. Consequently, a grid with a large number of lines to the centimetre or inch is much preferred to one of a coarse lattice.

In the construction of a grid to a given lattice, the number of lines to the centimetre or inch is dependent on (a) the thickness of each strip; (b) the distance between individual strips. Not surprisingly thick lead strips are more prominent on radiographs than thin ones. However, a thin strip has the disadvantage that it may incompletely absorb a scattered ray which strikes it. One of the benefits of a high grid ratio is that scattered photons have a greater chance of encountering more than one strip and thus of being eliminated even if the strips are thin. Manufacturers have to strike a balance between strips so thick that the grid wholly destroys recognition of radiographic detail and strips so thin that very little absorption of scatter is obtained from using the grid.

Grids of the 'fine line' type are troublesome to produce and consequently expensive. The lead strips have to be arranged uniformly over the whole grid and the individual surfaces of the strips placed to face each other without misalignment. None of this is easy to achieve and the thinner the strips and the closer they are together the more difficult the grid becomes to manufacture. The magnitude of the maker's problem is reflected in the cost to the purchaser: anyone who has seen a secondary radiation grid being made can understand why even the simplest of them is expensive.

The grid lattice or number of lead strips to the centimetre or inch is now commonly stated simply as the number of lines. In general use are focused grids having 30 lines/centimetre (75 lines/inch) and parallel grids having

32 lines/centimetre (85 lines/inch). Those with 40 lines/centimetre (100 lines/inch) or more have special applications for high detail work.

Geometrical cut-off

Geometrical cut-off is properly defined as the proportion of the primary beam which the lead strips of a grid absorb. It is expressed as a percentage; for example in a certain grid it is 12·5 per cent, this being the amount of primary radiation lost as a result of the geometry of the strips. The thickness of the strips, their spacing and their height each has an influence upon geometrical cut-off. The amount of cut-off can be calculated, but the actual numerical value obtained is not of much practical significance to radiographers; few of us know what it is in respect of any of the grids we use. However, we are well aware of the effects of geometrical cut-off which can result in underexposure of the radiograph in certain circumstances. These will be discussed further when grid structure is considered (see page 314).

The spacing material

The purpose of a spacing material in a grid is exactly as the name implies: it holds the lead strips apart. It must be rigid in order to maintain thin strips precisely in position but it should not absorb the primary beam. Ideally it would absorb no primary and all stray radiation but in practice it can do neither. Any interspacing material may absorb some part of the primary beam as well as being a filter for residual scattered rays; the relationship of the one function to the other necessarily figures in the assessment of a grid's efficiency.

At the present time the spacing material used in grids is likely to be either a radiolucent metal, such as aluminium, or an organic material (plastic). Wood is also used. Metal more effectively filters secondary radiation—though this occurs only to a small extent at best—but at the same time it takes more of the primary beam. Further absorption occurs in the aluminium envelope in which many grids are sealed in order to increase mechanical robustness. This means from the user's point of view that, for the same ratio, a grid which has aluminium spacing requires the use of a higher kilovoltage to produce comparable film blackening.

The assessment of a grid's quality

Helpful assessments of relative efficiency between different grids are complicated to make. A grid is efficient if it absorbs the highest amount of scattered radiation and the least amount of primary radiation. Since the grid ratio is an important determinant of the fraction of scattered radiation removed by a grid it is often employed as a statement of efficiency or quality. However, the grid ratio pays no regard to several other significant factors. These are:

1   the thickness of the lead strips;
2   the composition of the lead—that is the amount of lead (in grammes) which is actually present in each square centimetre of a strip;
3   the nature of the spacing material.

A further source of complexity in attempting to make statements about the usefulness of a grid is that in the course of its work no grid has to handle radiation of only one wavelength. Obviously it will be employed over a range of kilovoltages, with associated implications of change in the penetrating characteristics of both primary and scattered radiation.

When secondary radiation is large in quantity and of short wavelength—that is when kilovoltage is high—a grid of high ratio is necessary for the efficient absorption of scatter. On the other hand there are radiographic situations in which the increased exposure required by such a grid would be unacceptable. In regard to the grid lattice, while a fine-line grid is needed for good cranial radiography, another of fewer lines to the inch might be appropriate for subjects of bold contrast, such as barium studies, or for employment in a bucky diaphragm which moves the grid during the exposure (see page 318). When a mobile X-ray unit is to be used, the handiness of a light grid might make it preferable to one containing more lead per unit area, even although the latter would be a more efficient absorber of scatter for the same transmission of the primary beam.

Considerations such as these make it impossible to give a single, simple opinion on what makes a grid 'good' or 'bad'. Radiologists and radiographers often have very fixed ideas about grids—and manufacturers provide both a wide selection from which to choose and the means easily to change grids in their equipment—but concepts of quality are so inextricably associated with the work which a particular grid is required to do that any real criterion is difficult to establish.

The structure of grids

The parallel grid

In Figs. 8.8 and 8.9 the lead strips of the grid were shown in a parallel arrangement. A grid constructed in this manner is described as a parallel grid. It has a number of disadvantages and one asset, this being that it does not matter which aspect of the grid faces the X-ray tube. Parallel grids are still made and used, although it is questionable whether they need really continue to be so.

Geometrical cut-off

The disadvantages of a parallel grid are referable to the geometrical cut-off which it produces. This can be understood when we consider the direction of radiation at the edges of an X-ray beam as opposed to its central part. Fig. 8.10 illustrates how the centre of a beam is parallel to the lead strips and will mainly pass through the interspaces of the grid; while peripheral rays travel radially from the X-ray tube and are oblique to the lead strips.

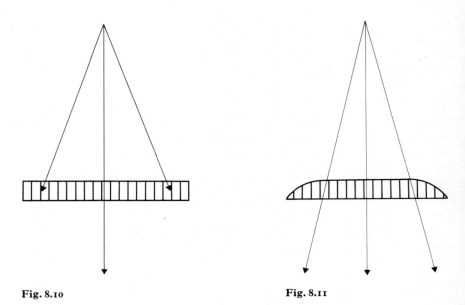

Fig. 8.10   Fig. 8.11

This has two effects on the radiograph:
1   loss of density along two edges of the film owing to heavy absorption of the primary beam;
2   projection of the lead strips as wider than they really are and thus potentially greater interference from 'grid lines'.

The unfavourable effects of geometric cut-off in this type of grid can be minimized in the following ways, none of which is ideal.
1   Increase in the anode-film distance (this implies the availability of heavier tube loadings).
2   Keeping the grid ratio low which deteriorates efficiency.
3   Constructing the grid so that it is thinner at the edges than at the centre. This is illustrated in Fig. 8.11; it further lowers the grid ratio.
4   Using only the centre of the field. This might be feasible in respect of the skull, for example, but it is certainly inapplicable to most abdominal subjects.

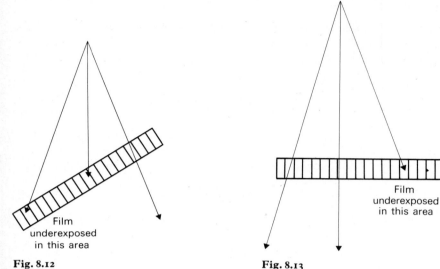

Fig. 8.12   **Fig. 8.13**

Malpositions of the grid

If a parallel grid is misaligned with the central X-ray beam the radiograph again suffers from the effects of geometrical cut-off. The two ways in which this is likely to happen are described below.

1   Tilting the grid so that the lead elements are no longer parallel to the beam (Fig. 8.12); as can be seen this results in loss of density along a central band and at one side of the film.

2   Incorrect centring of the X-ray beam which produces underexposure of the radiograph at the edge *away* from the tube's displacement (Fig. 8.13).

The higher the grid ratio the worse these effects are. Grids of high ratio consequently need very careful use, especially in situations when tilting of the grid and incorrect centring are likely to occur; those which spring to mind are ones involving patients on stretchers, in bed, or in the operating theatre.

The malpositions (1) and (2) are essentially the same in principle as any angulation of the X-ray beam made *across* the elements of a grid. This is to be remembered when radiographers use techniques which depend upon beam angulation. A single angulation can usually be made by tilting the X-ray tube in a direction *along* the grid elements, as this produces no cut-off. Techniques requiring two angulations of the tube (for example, one applicable to the anterior part of the mandible) prohibit the use of a secondary radiation grid altogether.

The focused grid

In the construction of the focused grid the lead strips are arranged to form the radii of a circle of which the X-ray tube is the centre. The principle of this is illustrated in Fig. 8.14.

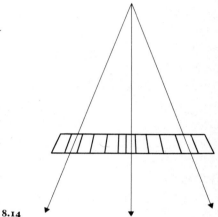

Fig. 8.14

Malpositions of the grid

Focusing the grid in the way described reduces geometric cut-off in areas away from the beam's centre. Furthermore, unlike the parallel grid, geometric cut-off remains about the same whatever the grid's ratio. However, there are limitations to the use of the focused grid and the following points should be kept in mind.

1   As the grid structure postulates one position of the X-ray tube (at the centre of a circle), in theory the anode-film distance cannot be varied. In practice some latitude exists: a grid which has a ratio of 8·5 to 1 and is focused at 90 cm (36 inches) can be used at distances between 75 cm (30 inches) and 130 cm (51 inches) without an intolerable increase in geometric cut-off. This latitude becomes less with increasing grid ratio and decreasing focal distance of the grid.

2   When a focused grid is employed at an anode-film distance which is either too short or too long for it the radiograph is underexposed in areas away from the centre.

3   When the X-ray tube is centred incorrectly across the elements of a focused grid, the radiograph is more seriously underexposed along the edge *towards* which the X-ray tube is displaced.

4   A focused grid necessarily has only one aspect which may face the X-ray tube. This aspect is always indicated on the grid, as also is the length of the

focus. If the grid is inadvertently used in the reversed position there is severe geometric cut-off along both edges of the film.

The principle of the focused grid is well suited to the development of grids of high ratio. A grid having a ratio of 16 to 1 may be chosen for radiography at kilovoltages of 110 or more. Grids of this kind are invariably focused grids. As indicated in the previous pages, grids of high ratio—whatever their kind—require accurate positioning and accurate centring of the X-ray tube. Furthermore, focused grids demand relatively discriminating selection of the anode-film distance.

No doubt parallel grids continue to have adherents, particularly for ward work at moderate kilovoltages, because:

1 parallel grids are generally of lower ratio;
2 anode-film distances are less critical;
3 it is immaterial which aspect of a parallel grid is placed to face the X-ray tube.

The converse of these points makes the use of the focused, high ratio grid technically more demanding for the radiographer.

Cross-grids

So far in our discussion we have depicted grids two-dimensionally in diagrams and have considered the absorption of scatter which is moving *across* the grid. No account has been taken of what happens to radiation scattered in a direction parallel to the grid elements, for the good reason that very little happens: such scatter may be absorbed to some extent by the interspacing material and by the grid envelope but scarcely at all by the lead strips.

In most instances the absorption of only the cross-scatter is sufficient and such absorption accounts for the greater part of all scatter produced. Sometimes, however—for example perhaps in simultaneous bi-plane angiography—it may be desirable to eliminate scattered rays travelling in each direction. This can be done by means of a cross-grid.

A cross-grid in fact is a combination of two grids arranged one on top of the other so that their elements intersect at 90 degrees or at some other selected angle. Cross-grids of different types are available and each component grid may be of parallel or focused construction.

The problems associated with a cross-grid are:

1 it is difficult to prevent grid lines from showing on the radiograph at the points where the lead strips cross each other, even if the grids are moved during the exposure (see page 318 and following pages);
2 the X-ray tube requires particularly careful positioning so that the beam

is perpendicular and central to both grids. Virtually no angulation of it is permitted.

The cross-grid is an efficient absorber of scatter. However it is to be noticed that each component grid has only half the ratio of the total grid and is therefore absorbing less of the scatter travelling across it than would a simple linear grid of the same ratio as the combination. Furthermore, the geometrical cut-off becomes twice as great.

We cannot say that a cross-grid absorbs much more scattered radiation than a linear grid of the same ratio; their absorbing powers in fact are comparable. We *can* say that, whereas the linear grid absorbs rays scattered mainly in one direction, the cross-grid accounts for it in two directions. Its use is appropriate to situations where a high ratio grid is considered necessary and it is desirable to protect the radiograph from scattered rays travelling transversely and lengthwise to the film.

GRID MOVEMENTS

A secondary radiation grid, as we have seen, is composed of a large number of strips of lead. Its use is bound to result in a pattern of parallel radio-opaque lines over the whole radiograph. If these lines are thin, close together and uniformly arranged their presence does not strike the eye obtrusively. However, a fine line grid is difficult to manufacture and costs rise with increasing slenderness of structure. Such a grid is likely to be of high ratio and needs precise use by the radiographer as we have seen.

There is an alternative and long-established method of causing grid lines to 'disappear' and that is to move the grid sideways during the exposure. This results in such blurring of the images of the strips that a definable impression is no longer received by the eye. A grid which is arranged to move in this way is called a Potter–Bucky diaphragm, or more commonly a bucky, for the reason that these were the names of two people who were among pioneers in the construction of secondary radiation grids.

To be successful any bucky mechanism has to meet the following list of requirements.

1 It must set the grid in motion fractionally before the radiographic exposure begins and not permit the motion to cease before the exposure finishes.

2 The motion must be smooth to avoid vibration of patient or cassette and its rate effectively uniform throughout the exposure.

3 The grid must move at an appropriate speed and over a sufficient distance to blur the images of the lead strips to an adequate extent. It must not be significantly off-centre in respect of the X-ray tube at any moment during

the exposure and in theory should be centred on the midline of the table when half the exposure has occurred.

4 The mechanism of the grid movement should be simple. An elaborate movement is more likely to fail. It requires space which will prevent the patient from being close to the film and may make the equipment—if it is a serial changer, for example—cumbersome to use.

The bucky assembly

Whatever kind of grid movement is employed it is presented ·to the radiographer as an integral part of the X-ray table or of any specialized unit to which it is essential. The total bucky assembly incorporates:

1 a frame which holds the grid and allows grids to be readily interchanged;
2 the grid itself—usually 46 × 43 cm (18 × 17 inches) in the case of a table;
3 the grid mechanism;
4 situated underneath all the other items, a robust steel tray in which can be placed any size of cassette and which includes a locking device for the cassette (this often automatically centres the cassette in the tray). The tray can usually be removed quite easily: it may be necessary, for example, to replace it with a special fitting designed for a multisection cassette (see Chapter 13, page 449) or to use it externally as a support for a cassette in the case of a vertical bucky.

In the classic bucky table the whole arrangement is mounted on bearings which allow it to move along a pair of rails for most of the length of the table-top. The grid and film can thus be positioned together in any appropriate place beneath a patient recumbent on the table. A lock is provided to hold the bucky at the selected site: this lock usually is an electromagnetic mechanism and is switch-controlled. The grid and its movement are not visible to the operator without removal of the table-top.

A bucky diaphragm is normally found in the following classes of X-ray equipment.

1 A standard bucky table. In this case, if the overtable X-ray tube is ceiling hung, the switchblock on the tubehead should include an indicator—usually a green or yellow lamp—to establish when the tube is centred crosswise to the bucky: an associated switch for control of the X-ray tube's position is necessary.
2 A tilting table for fluoroscopy and general radiography.
3 The serial changer of such a fluoroscopic table (see Chapter 12).
4 Tomographic units (see Chapter 13).
5 Skull tables (see Chapter 15).
6 A vertical bucky.
7 A universal bucky.

Numbers (6) and (7) are variations of the same idea and enable a moving grid to be employed for radiography of an erect patient. The bucky assembly is mounted on a steel column or pair of columns, very much in the manner of an X-ray tube on a tubestand (see Chapter 7, page 286). It is counterweighted or counterpoised on its support and can be moved upwards and downwards to suit different heights of patient. Accessories such as a compression band or a head-clamp or a cassette-holder can be attached to it.

The universal bucky is the more useful apparatus of the two since it can be employed horizontally as well as vertically and at any intermediate angle. In one example the bucky can be rotated on its support so that the tray is accessible to the radiographer from more than one direction in relation to the column.

When the universal bucky is in the horizontal plane a stretcher trolley, of which the top is made from a radioparent material, can be positioned above it and the combination employed as a standard bucky table. This alliance commends itself for accident and emergency radiography since a seriously injured or ill patient can be put on the trolley in the casualty receiving room and does not need to be subsequently lifted to a table in the X-ray department.

There is more than one way of making a grid move during a radiographic exposure. Below are described two typical mechanisms, one being described commonly as a reciprocating grid and the other as a vibrating grid.

The reciprocating movement

When operated by a reciprocating movement, the grid is driven continuously to and fro from one side of the table to the other during the X-ray exposure, without attention.

One type of reciprocating mechanism is simply depicted in Fig. 8.15. The grid is propelled in one direction by the combination of two springs and a speed control kept constant with an oil dashpot. These features are seen in the upper part of Fig. 8.15.

The oil dashpot

The oil dashpot consists of a barrel and plunger device, resistance to the movement of the plunger through the cylinder being offered by the presence of the oil. The diagram depicts the working arrangements of this principle: the plunger is fixed and the cylinder—being linked to the grid—moves along the plunger as the grid moves, from side to side of the diagram.

The speed of the grid's travel can be altered by rotation of the small knob at the end of the plunger. Turning this revolves one of two opposed discs

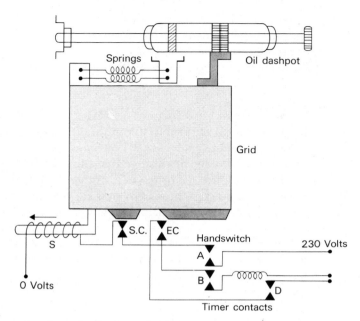

Fig. 8.15. A reciprocating bucky mechanism.

upon the other, so that a number of perforations in each are either in register with each other or more or less out of register. These circumstances permit the oil to flow relatively freely in the cylinder if the discs are at their widest aperture and limit velocity when the perforations are partly or wholly closed.

Adjustments of the dashpot's speed is normally made not by the radiographer but by the maintenance engineer who checks the operation of the equipment. The mechanism cannot—and need not—provide a precise control of speed. High precision would be superfluous refinement but, nevertheless, it is necessary to obtain some degree of accuracy as the grid's excursion has radiographic significance.

The traverse across the film is no more than a few centimetres in extent; it must be at least equal in length to several interspaces of the grid or the image of the lead elements will be insufficiently blurred. A grid—particularly one having few lines to the inch—which moves slowly during a very rapid exposure will cause the appearance of lines on the radiograph because of an inadequate extent of travel. On the other hand, a very brisk, quick movement of the grid may result in such vibration of the whole bucky assembly as to introduce movement unsharpness in the radiographs. (The radiographer, who must watch helplessly while the equipment shakes during exposure, can become very irritable!) For these reasons the contribution of the oil dashpot is important to the movement. Its functions are:

1   to control and smooth the speed of the grid;
2   to enable adjustments of this speed to be made from time to time.

The solenoid and its circuitry

The power which drives the grid across the table in the direction opposite to the pull of the springs comes from a solenoid S. Fig. 8.15 depicts the grid in its resting position and the student should note that the solenoid contacts (SC) are closed and the exposure contacts (EC) are open. The diagram shows two other pairs of contacts—those at A and B—which are closed through a relay which operates when the handswitch is put at 'expose'.

Closing the contacts at A applies a voltage (230 volts) to the solenoid S though the solenoid contacts (SC): the energized solenoid pulls the grid smartly across the table—in about 0·1 second—in the direction of the adjacent arrow. Owing to the projections constructed on the grid carriage where shown in the diagram, this motion has the following electrical effects.

1   The exposure contacts (EC) close and remain closed until the grid returns finally to its resting position.

2   There is a complete circuit through the exposure contacts, the contacts in the handswitch and the timer contacts at D, which are closed when the timer is set. This circuit supplies a voltage to the exposure switching circuit and the radiographic exposure begins.

3   When the solenoid has driven the grid to the limit of its excursion in one direction the solenoid contacts are permitted to open, thus de-energizing the solenoid.

However, though the solenoid has lost power, the springs are now under tension and supply the energy which results in the grid returning more slowly in the opposite direction across the table. When it does this, the solenoid contacts are closed once more and the solenoid is re-energized, resulting in a repetition of the original movement. The two springs and the solenoid continue to alternate as the source of power and keep the grid perpetually in a side-to-side motion until release of the handswitch breaks the circuit at A and permits the grid to be drawn by the springs to its resting position.

The student should note that the grid's movement begins before the radiographic exposure begins, and will continue after completion of the exposure—which is normally terminated by the timer contacts D—so long as the radiographer maintains pressure on the handswitch. Indeed in these circumstances the prolonged reciprocations of the grid become characteristically audible.

The solenoid imparts a more rapid motion to the grid than does the combination of the springs and oil dashpot. This is an important feature of the reciprocating movement. By utilizing the solenoid for the initial travel and the springs and oil dashpot for a subsequent phase the bucky becomes equally suitable for short and long exposures.

The reciprocating movement described is only one of several which have been devised and of which any may be encountered by student radiographers on different varieties of apparatus. They nearly all share the feature that the speed of the two strokes is not the same in each direction: in most mechanisms the first, or forward stroke, is faster than the second or return stroke, with an obvious advantage in respect of short exposures. Generally speaking, from a practical point of view the simpler the mechanism the better.

In the oscillating movement which we shall consider next we meet twin virtues of spatial economy and extreme simplicity of function and construction.

The oscillating (vibrating) movement

With the oscillating movement, just as with the reciprocating one, the grid moves to and fro across the film throughout the exposure and without attention from the radiographer. However, it has not so much an impelled motion as a free swing from side to side. This can be obtained merely by mounting the grid on a spring at each corner and giving it a push from time to time, causing it to vibrate upon the springs. There are other means of oscillating a grid and this one is sometimes described as a vibrating grid to distinguish it among them.

An oscillating grid movement of this kind is shown in Fig. 8.16. In this particular case the springs are of the variety known as leaf springs: they are strong, flexible steel strips and one is mounted in relation to each of the four corners of the grid in a frame in the manner indicated. At S a movable bar is operated by a solenoid. When this solenoid is energized—through the X-ray exposure switch—it flicks in the direction of the arrow and strikes a projection on the grid. An alternative arrangement would be to employ a solenoid to pull the grid towards itself and then release it.

In either instance the effect is the same: the grid sways to and fro on its springs, at first with relative freedom but gradually lessening in extent until eventually the movement ceases altogether. However, about a minute will have elapsed before the grid is finally stationary and this is an ample exposure interval for all usual radiographic needs.

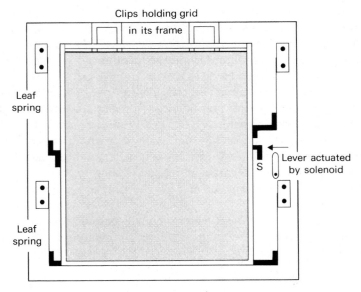

Fig. 8.16. An oscillating or vibrating bucky mechanism.

The stroboscopic effect

The stroboscopic effect which may be produced by a moving grid can be responsible for the appearance of grid lines on a radiograph. The word 'stroboscopic' merely implies the characteristic of occurring in successive phases or a motion of a periodic nature and is therefore appropriate in the context of the electrical functioning of an X-ray unit.

Unless the equipment is of the constant potential type (see Chapter 3, page 121), it is producing effective X rays in a succession of pulses which are directly related in frequency to the cycles of the power supply. A grid movement which is driven by an electric motor is subject to a corresponding succession of impulses. If these synchronize with the X-ray waveform the radiographic effect may be that the grid has not moved.

This will happen if, between one peak of the X-ray waveform and the next, the grid should move a distance which exactly equals or is a multiple of one grid interspace. The effect is perhaps more readily understood if the reader imagines what it would be like to be in a moving vehicle from which it is possible to see only one in a row of similar vehicles moving in a line parallel to the first. If the observed vehicle is moving at exactly the same rate as one's own the effect is that no movement has occurred. The same result would obtain if a stationary observer were to take regular glances through his window at the moving row of vehicles: if the glances and the motion were synchronized he would always see a vehicle in the same space and would believe that no motion was present.

In the same way a synchronized grid appears not to move in respect of the film and the radiograph is spoiled by the appearance on it of the grid strips. It is to avoid the possibility of such synchronism that grid movements often employ spring tension in the methods we have described in preference to a drive from an electric motor. If an electric motor is used—and in some cases it is—then precautions are needed against the possibility of grid synchronization.

THE ASSESSMENT OF GRID FUNCTIONS

Bucky mechanisms

The grid movements which have been described both differ from each other electromechanically and result in dissimilar patterns of the grid's speed during the exposure. In the case of a vibrating movement, the pattern is more or less sinusoidal, with a decreasing amplitude of the wave forms as time passes (see Fig. 8.17a).

The reciprocating movement with which we are concerned takes the grid faster in one direction than the other, but there is no alteration in the amplitude of the pulse with time, nor in the period of each completed cycle. Fig. 8.17b depicts the speed pattern of such a reciprocating grid. It may be noted that the forward speed of this grid is relatively higher than the vibrating grid is likely to achieve even on the first stroke.

If 'grid lines' are not to be apparent on radiographs, the inter-relationship of the grid's speed and the duration of the exposure interval is important: during a short exposure a grid, of a given lattice and excursion, must move faster than if the interval is long.

To a degree, the type of movement which may be preferred is a matter of opinion and is rarely a determinant in the selection of a particular equipment: radiographic tables and stands usually are chosen from a consideration of other features than the nature of the device which the designer has deemed appropriate for driving the bucky grid. However, for the interest of readers who may wish to make some comparison of reciprocating and vibrating movements, some salient points are tabled below.

Reciprocating	*Vibrating*
Relatively elaborate mechanism which needs space.	Simple, effective mechanism.
Subject-film distance is generally greater.	Subject-film distance is reduced.

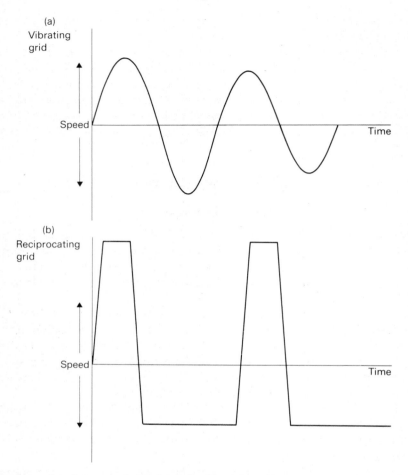

(a)
Vibrating grid

Speed

Time

(b)
Reciprocating grid

Speed

Time

Fig. 8.17. Speed patterns of vibrating and reciprocating grid movements.

The oil dashpot can be unreliable in operation if:

(a) leaking glands permit the entry of air;

(b) the viscosity of the oil alters because of ambient temperature changes. The result is an uneven motion and vibration which in turn may lead to the recording of grid lines, or to movement un-sharpness of the image, or both.

Smooth movement which should not give rise to image-degradation.

Relatively longer traverse of the grid and therefore increased geometrical cut-off in respect of any particular grid (the grid is further off-centre during more of the exposure).

Small traverse of the grid, therefore less cut-off and a decreased grid factor compared with the same type of grid employed in a reciprocating movement.

BUT

Reciprocation may be thought potentially more efficient during very short intervals of exposure.

BUT

Oscillation possibly might not be sufficiently fast during a very short exposure interval.

Fixed grids

In many X-ray departments the student will find examples of X-ray equipment in which the use of a moving bucky mechanism is not feasible: for instance, tables for rapid serial angiography and some tomographic systems. In these circumstances the apparatus employs a fine-line stationary grid.

If such a grid is acceptable during exacting procedures where the production of high detail is difficult for several reasons, it is logical to ask whether much simpler radiographic situations really need a moving grid at all. Would not a plain bucky table be just as satisfactory if the cassette tray were fitted with a good fine-line grid of adequate ratio which did not move during the exposure?

When a grid is moved by either of the means described certain theoretical disadvantages are implied.

1 Unless the exposure is very short, the grid is necessarily stationary during the instants of the exposure in which it reverses its direction of travel, no matter whether the drive is of the reciprocating (see page 320) or the oscillating (see page 323) variety.

2 The grid may suffer from the stroboscopic effect (see page 324).

Either of these features may—but in practice very rarely does—result in the appearance of grid lines on the radiograph. Moving grids generally have a lower ratio and a coarser lattice than those intended for stationary use. In the circumstances described, the linear pattern produced would no doubt be intrusive and the theorist, if he wishes, may advance this possible risk as a feature favouring the fixed grid in all X-ray apparatus where the use of a grid is appropriate.

Much more relevant, however, are the practical arguments of simplicity in place of elaboration, reduced space between the patient and the film and increased lightness of the apparatus in handling. Radiologists and radiographers for so long have been using moving bucky mechanisms that attitudes—if not grids—have become fixed. Some 're-education' may be required before everyone recognizes that an efficient fixed grid is all that is needed.

Chapter 9
Portable and Mobile X-Ray Equipments

It is very often necessary to produce radiographs of people who for one reason or another are unable to come to the X-ray department; perhaps the patient is too ill to be moved about the hospital, or is immobilized in bed in traction apparatus or is undergoing surgery in the operating theatre. When it is impossible to bring the patient to the equipment it clearly becomes necessary to take the equipment to the patient. For this purpose we use portable and mobile equipment.

The two terms are not interchangeable. The word portable means what it says—that is that the X-ray unit is capable of being carried, with the implication that it does not need (in theory anyway) more than one able-bodied person to do the carrying at any given time. This carrying may be simply about the hospital, or it may be a longer excursion to take X-ray equipment to a patient's home or to some place distant from the hospital. Portable equipment is very simple to use and can be packed into carrying cases and so transported—how easily must depend on the portable unit, the porter and the passage to be made. Even at its worst it should not be very difficult—if you have enough hands or a car!

The term mobile also means what it says—that the X-ray equipment is capable of being moved. It is mounted on wheels and can be pushed by human (or in some cases mechanical) power so that it can be moved about the hospital with reasonable ease. Mobile equipment is larger and heavier than the simple portable sets. It cannot be separated into smaller components and it does not lend itself to use outside the hospital. So even to someone who does not know very much about X-ray equipment there will be differences apparent between the two. To the initiated there are further differences which must be fully explained in this chapter.

Since both portable and mobile X-ray sets are commonly operated by being connected to the electrical supply through a plug fitting into a wall socket, the differences in the mains requirements of these two types of unit are a good point at which to begin.

329

MAINS REQUIREMENTS

How much electricity is needed to operate an X-ray set? This was explained in Chapter 1 when it was made clear that the current drawn from the mains supply at a given voltage will vary in amount according to the rate at which electrical work is to be done—that is how much power is to be consumed.

The voltage can be considered as the electrical pressure with which the electricity is delivered; the current is the rate of flow of electricity when any electrical equipment is in operation. A high current could be likened to the flow of water from a tap which is fully opened; a low current to the flow from one which is partially closed.

So far as X-ray equipment is concerned the current drawn is related to the X-ray output. X-ray sets which function at high maximum kilovoltage and milliamperage draw large currents (although for very short periods of time). Any X-ray set which must not draw a large current must be limited in its radiographic output. The small portable set which can be taken away from the hospital to be used in a patient's house *must* be capable of being operated from a low current supply. This limits the X-ray output which it can be expected to give.

The large mobile unit which is used in a hospital setting is likely to be connected to a power supply which can provide a bigger current. This power supply may be part of a specially wired installation, in which case the currents drawn can be compared with those used by major generators in the department. Where the power supplies allow of higher currents the permitted X-ray output can be correspondingly greater, as will be seen in the following sections where details of the radiographic loadings of the sets are considered.

In the United Kingdom, wall sockets for domestic use give a power from which the maximum permissible currents are usually up to 13 amperes and in hospital 30 amperes and even 50 and 60 amperes wall sockets are encountered when special arrangements are made for the use of high-powered mobile X-ray sets. Electric plugs which fit into the wall sockets providing these different supplies can be distinguished from each other because as the maximum current load for which it is designed becomes greater, the plug must be larger and the cable to which it is joined must be thicker. The plug has the 'pins' which emerge from it of rectangular cross-section ('square'-pinned plug) and these fit into rectangular slots in the wall socket. The important point is that the current values assigned to these wall sockets and plugs are maximum continuous values.

If an attempt is made to operate any X-ray set at a greater output than can be supplied from the wall socket in use (that is, to draw much more current than the stated maximum) the result may be a blown fuse, especially if it is an ordinary copper wire fuse. (In practice it *is* possible to draw currents which are above the stated maximum, provided that it is for short instantaneous exposures.) Fuses are discussed in more detail in Chapter 4. Here it can be said simply that a fuse is an electrical safety device which protects a circuit from being overloaded—that is from having too large a current flowing in it which would overheat the circuit and cause damage. The simplest form of fuse is a wire which after a given time melts and breaks when it becomes heated by excessive currents. The broken wire means discontinuity in the circuit and this stops any further flow of current. X-ray sets must be used within the limits of the power supply available and these limits are important primary considerations.

Cable connections to wall plugs

Any portable electrical equipment is connected by a length of cable to the plugs which fit wall sockets from which the supply is taken. Cable connections to the three-pin plugs described in the foregoing section must be made by means of a three-cored cable—that is, a cable which has three conductors in it.

Fig. 9.1 is a sketch of the arrangement. An outer cover of insulation (rubber or plastic) contains three separately insulated conductors within it. Each conductor consists of several strands of copper wire surrounded by its own sleeve of insulating material. The insulation is a different colour for each conductor as explained below.

The wall sockets provide connection to one of the supply lines and to the neutral line in the system of distribution (see Chapter 1). Of the three

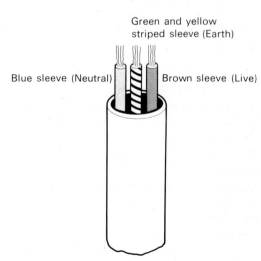

Fig. 9.1

conductors in the cable, one is intended for connection to the 'live' line, one is intended for connection to the neutral line and the third provides connection to earth for electrical safety if the insulation breaks down. Modern cables have a colouring in accordance with international practice. The system is BROWN (a 'warm' colour) for the LIVE line, BLUE (a 'cold' colour) for the NEUTRAL line and spring-like yellow and green stripes for the earth connection. When a cable is attached to its plug, the person doing the job must make sure that the connections are correct.

Fig. 9.2 shows a sketch of a typical three-pin plug. When the screw seen below the centre-pin in the front of the plug is loosened, the back can be

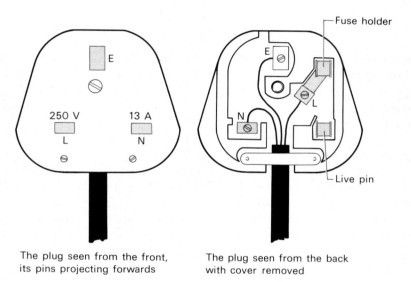

The plug seen from the front, its pins projecting forwards

The plug seen from the back with cover removed

Fig. 9.2

lifted off. The three conductors are then seen placed in the plug with the striped earth conductor lying up the middle joined to the long central pin at the top of the plug. The blue neutral conductor is on the left and the brown live conductor is on the right as the plug is viewed with its back uppermost; they are each joined to one of the two shorter pins of the plug. The insulation is stripped from the end of the conductors and the bare wires are held under the screw which keeps each of them in place at the back of its appropriate pin. N and L are marked on the plug as a reminder to the person wiring it as to which pin is which. The live conductor has a fuse holder alongside it. Its connection to the pin is through a fuse which will be placed in the holder when the plug is assembled and connected for use.

PORTABLE X-RAY EQUIPMENT

The features of an X-ray set can be considered under five simple basic headings. These are:

1   the X-ray tube;
2   the tubestand;
3   the high tension generator;
4   the control unit;
5   the radiographic output and the mains requirements.

The X-ray tube and the high tension generator

In order to make the equipment simpler, lighter, less expensive and easier to move, it is usual for a portable set to be constructed with the X-ray tube and its high tension generator enclosed in one earthed metal tank which is filled with oil. This is sometimes described as a tank construction, and the whole enclosure is called the tubehead. Chapter 7 has included a description of the electrical safety achieved by the total enclosure of the high tension system of an X-ray set in one continuous earthed metal sheath. With larger mobile sets the X-ray tube and the high tension transformer may be in separate oil-filled housings, with connection between the two made by means of metal-sheathed high tension cables. In a portable X-ray set the essence of this system is maintained by enclosing the X-ray tube and filament transformer and high tension transformer all together in the one housing.

When this is done, no high tension cables are necessary and the only leads which go to the tubehead are low tension ones which carry the supply from the controls. These are usually embodied in a sheathed insulated cable containing more than one conductor. This is known as a multi-cored low tension cable. Fig. 9.3 is a block diagram of the essential features.

The tube is a small stationary anode X-ray tube operating self-rectified and connected directly across the secondary winding of the high tension transformer. The tank construction is a practical arrangement and results in a piece of equipment which is easy to handle and does not take up much space.

A small stationary anode X-ray tube with an effective focus of 1·0 mm is a tube with a relatively low radiographic rating; but in any case the limit on the current which this generator is permitted to draw from the mains when it operates means that high radiographic output cannot be expected from it. The characteristics of the tube and its high tension circuit which limit rating are therefore of less importance. What has been achieved is a piece of equipment which is portable, easy to manoeuvre and capable of being used

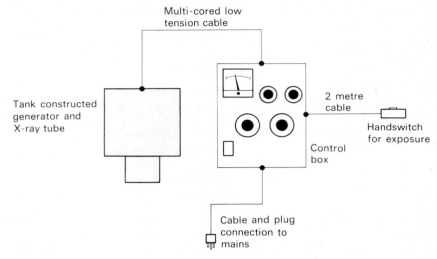

Multi-cored low
tension cable

Tank constructed
generator and
X-ray tube

2 metre
cable

Handswitch
for exposure

Control
box

Cable and plug
connection to
mains

Fig. 9.3

in many different locations even from supply points which yield a low current (and/or provide a relatively low voltage). These advantageous features must be paid for by the acceptance of a reduced radiographic output.

The oil-filled tubehead is exactly comparable with the housing for an X-ray tube itself as described in Chapter 7. The tank is filled with oil to insulate and cool the components contained in it, and it is vacuum-sealed. There are similar arrangements to allow for expansion of the oil when it is hot by providing an expansion bellows or an expansion chamber. Lead protection is included in the housing so that the leakage radiation is reduced to the desired level. There are facilities for attaching to the tube-head beam-limiting devices such as cones and diaphragms and beam-centring devices such as a light beam or a telescopic metal centring rod.

The tubestand

Fig. 9.4 shows a typical portable set with the tank-constructed tubehead mounted on a movable stand and a separate control unit. The tubehead detaches from the stand and the separate items (tubehead, stand and control desk) are suitable for being carried out for use in a patient's house. In Fig. 9.4 the tubehead is shown attached to a support which is on a carriage mounted on the vertical column of the movable stand. Also shown in the illustration is a handle which can be rotated. Turning the handle moves the carriage up and down the vertical column so that it ascends or descends

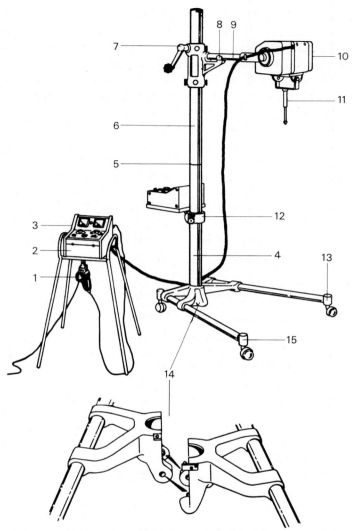

Fig. 9.4 A demountable portable set. The key to the numbered items is given below.

1 Hand-timer
2 Stand for control box.
3 Control box.
4 Lower part of vertical column.
5 Indicates where the vertical column divides into two parts for easy transport.
6 Upper part of vertical column.
7 Handle for raising and lowering carriage of the cross-arm.

8 Bracket on carriage which supports the cross-arm.
9 Cross-arm.
10 Tubehead.
11 Centre-finder.
12 Support for the control box (as alternative to the tubular stand).
13 Castor.
14 Base support for vertical column.
15 Castor.

By courtesy of Picker International Ltd.

relative to the ground. Thus the tubehead can be raised further above the ground (if the carriage is ascending relative to the vertical) or lowered nearer to the ground (if the carriage is descending relative to the vertical). In equipment available today the range for the tube-focus to floor distances may be from 690 mm at its lowest to 950 mm at its highest when the X-ray beam is projected downwards. With the tubehead turned through 90 degrees to give a horizontal-beam projection, the range for the focus to floor distances may be from 775 mm to 1035 mm.

The type of movement is known as a rack and pinion. Its essential parts are a toothed or grooved wheel (the pinion) arranged in relation to other sets of teeth or grooves (the rack) in such a way that they mesh together. When a rotary movement is given to the pinion by means of a handle, the pinion (here constituted by the carriage carrying the tubehead) moves either up or down: clockwise rotation of the pinion moves the carriage up and anticlockwise rotation makes the carriage descend. An outline of the arrangement is sketched in Fig. 9.5.

The control unit

For the X-ray set illustrated in Fig. 9.4 it can be seen that the control unit is housed in a small box or control desk. In all equipment which is portable, the controls are not elevated beyond the essential needs for useful operation of the X-ray tube. The low tension cable coming from the tubestand as indicated in the block diagram in Fig. 9.3 plugs into a socket on the control unit. Another socket on the control unit takes the plug of a thinner cable

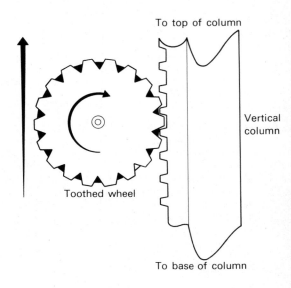

To top of column

Vertical column

Toothed wheel

Fig. 9.5   To base of column

which has the handswitch at its further end: the handswitch carries the pushbutton to initiate the exposure. The cable connecting it to the control unit should be at least 2000 mm in length to meet the requirements of current codes of practice. A third lead from the control unit is the mains lead which is fitted at its further end with a plug that goes into the wall-socket at the outlet point of the supply. All these connections are indicated in the block diagram in Fig. 9.3.

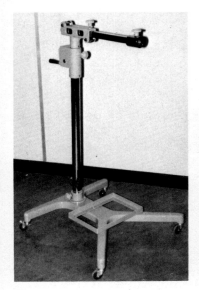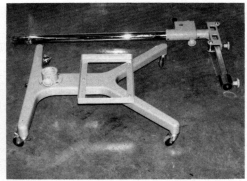

Fig. 9.6 A modern demountable stand for a portable X-ray set. It can be seen that the vertical column which bears the carriage and the cross-arm for the tube unit can be taken apart from the base for easy portability. The tank constructed tubehead to go on the stand is not shown: it attaches to the free end of the cross-arm. *By courtesy of Medical X-ray Supplies Ltd and Shimadzu Medical X-ray.*

Fig. 9.7 is a sketch to show the basic controls of a simple portable X-ray set. The features shown in the diagram are:

1 a mains ON/OFF switch;

2 an indicator lamp which shows when selected factors for the X-ray tube represent an overload beyond its radiographic rating;

3 a line voltage compensator;

4 a kilovolt selector;

5 a pre-reading kilovolt meter (this meter may serve also for use with the line voltage compensator);

6 a milliamperes selector;

7 a timer;

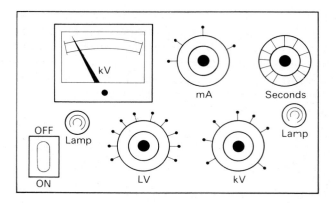

Fig. 9.7

8   an indicator lamp which shows when the X-ray tube is energized during the exposure.

For a typical modern unit, the following specifications are given.

Line voltage compensator

The line voltage compensator is a manual control with seven settings. There is a 4 V difference between each setting.

Kilovoltage selector

The kilovoltage selector is a manual control with 9 settings. It gives a range of kilovoltages from 40 kV to 100 kV for radiographic exposures.

Milliamperes selector

The milliamperes selector is a manual control which allows pre-selection of the tube current chosen for the exposure. There is a choice among three settings for radiography. These are: 10 mA, 20 mA and 30 mA.

The timer

The radiographic timer is electronic. It provides a range of times from 0·1 seconds to 10 seconds in thirteen steps.

Radiographic output. Mains requirements

The relationship between the radiographic output of an X-ray set and current taken from the mains has already been indicated (Chapter 1, page

16, and Chapter 9, page 330). For portable sets which are taken and used at many different points of supply, it is of fundamental importance for the radiographer to realize that the mains current which is drawn at a given voltage becomes bigger as the radiographic output (expressed as the tube load in milliamperes and kilovolts) becomes greater; and that a given tube load draws greater mains current at lower supply voltage than it does at higher supply voltages.

Radiographic exposures constitute intermittent use of power, the current being drawn for a few seconds or fractions of seconds only. Because the current taken from the mains for a radiographic exposure flows for such a short period of time, it is often possible to draw current which is in excess of that for which the circuit is fused without a blown fuse being the result, particularly if lead alloy (and not copper) wire fuses are used. It is to be noted that X-ray equipment which is very simple may not provide protection against overload of the X-ray tube.

Whether any safety devices are or are not incorporated, portable equipment should always be used very carefully, and radiographic factors should be selected which are within the rating of the X-ray tube.

A portable set may in fact be provided with an overload protection circuit. The following ratings might be given for its operation:

Tube kilovoltage	Tube milliamperage	Time (seconds)
100	10	10
80	20	5
60	30	2

The power required here is 3 kVA and the set is operable from standard wall-sockets with the connecting plug fused at 13 A.

MOBILE-X-RAY EQUIPMENT

The term mobile X-ray equipment covers a range of apparatus with considerable differences between its two extremes. At the one end is equipment which in its radiographic output and its mains requirements differs little from the type of portable unit which has just been described. At the other end is equipment giving radiographic output comparable with that obtainable from major X-ray sets which are fixtures in the X-ray department. Such mobile units have mains requirements which may demand special installations and wiring, for if used at their full output they draw such current from the mains that they need at least a 30 amperes supply.

Typical of low-powered mobile equipment is one which operates at 10 mA to 30 mA with a range of tube voltages from 40 kVp to 90 kVp.

Typical of high-powered mobile equipment is one which operates at up to 300 mA with a maximum tube voltage of 125 kVp. In between the two extremes are mobile sets operating with maximum tube factors of the order of 50–60 mA at 90 kVp, 100–150 mA at 95 kVp, 40–50 mA at 110–120 kVp.

Some of the high-powered mobile sets do not seem so readily mobile when the energy used to move them comes from one person pushing and in some cases a motor drive is provided. This is very useful while the motor works, but in the event of its failure all the motor can do is to add to the weight that must be pushed!

Simple portable equipment has just been described in terms of five headings which cover essential features of the equipment. It may be useful to do the same for a high-powered mobile set so that differences between the two types of equipment may be shown. A typical high-powered mobile set is illustrated in Figs. 9.8, 9.9 and 9.10.

The X-ray tube

The X-ray tube for a high-powered mobile set such as the one illustrated is

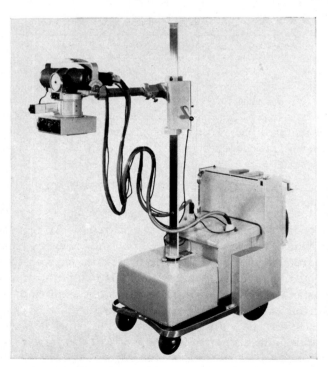

Fig. 9.8   A high-powered mobile equipment set. *By courtesy of Picker International Ltd.*

a dual focus rotating anode X-ray tube. It has focal spot combinations of about 1·0 mm for the fine focus and 2·0 mm for the broad focus.

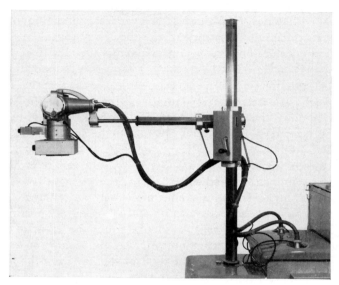

Fig. 9.9 The telescopic cross-arm on a mobile X-ray set. *By courtesy of Picker International Ltd.*

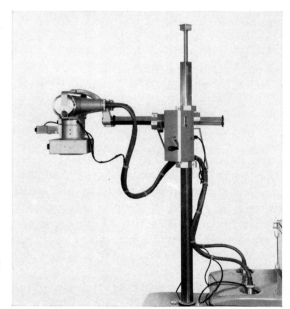

Fig. 9.10 Vertical extension of the tube column of a mobile X-ray set. *By courtesy of Picker International Ltd.*

The tubestand

The base of the unit illustrated is 629 mm wide and 1219 mm long. It has two big wheels at the back and two castor wheels at the front and a steel bumper bar at the sides and front. A strong vertical column mounted on the base supports the cross-arm which carries the X-ray tube. This cross-arm has a telescopic extension (Fig. 9.9) which allows the tube to be positioned at a distance of 1067 mm from the centre of the vertical supporting column. The vertical column also has an extension (Fig. 9.10) so that the X-ray tube can be brought to a height of 2096 mm from the ground. With the X-ray tube brought down the vertical column as near to the floor as it will go and the X-ray beam directed horizontally parallel to the floor, the anode to floor distance is 762 mm.

For transport about the hospital, the X-ray tube can be brought down the vertical column and turned with the cross-arm over the base so that the unit becomes compact and thus can be more easily and safely manoeuvred. Vertical movement of the cross-arm up and down the supporting vertical column is controlled by an electric motor. From the point of view of a radiographer trying to use such a unit in a variety of more or less difficult situations, the ability to position the tube a long way from the floor and a long way from its vertical supporting column is very helpful.

This is one of those mobile sets which is provided with a motor drive which will take it forwards and backwards and up a sloping ramp even with a gradient 1 in 6. The motor drive is powered by two 12 volt batteries which are mounted on the base on each side of the vertical column beneath a fibreglass cover. These batteries have a built-in charger which operates when the unit is connected to the mains, cutting down to a trickle charge if the batteries are nearly fully charged. The charging current is automatically switched off when charging is complete. One charge of the battery will drive the unit for some miles.

Battery maintenance

The 12 volt batteries used to drive this mobile unit are similar to those put in a motor car, but they are larger and are of 'heavy duty' type. Like all batteries they need some simple maintenance if they are to give good service. Well-maintained, these batteries should last for up to two years or more of useful life, and they are guaranteed for 12 months provided that they are kept charged and are attended to with care. If they are not looked after, they may fail after a few months.

The manufacturers of this unit issue simple rules for battery care, as below.

1   The unit should be left connected to the mains every night, at week-ends and at all other times when the unit is idle if it is driven over long distances. This will recharge the batteries. When they are fully charged, charging stops and a neon light on the battery cover glows to indicate that the batteries are fully charged.

2   Naked lights or lighted cigarettes should not be held near the batteries when they are being charged.

3   The acid level in the batteries should be checked every two weeks. The proper level is 6 mm above the plate separators, and if the acid level is below this it should be topped up with distilled water (*nothing else*).

4   The hospital engineer should be asked to check and service the batteries once a month. The recommended specific gravity when the batteries are fully charged is 1·263 to 1·278 at 25°C (77°F).

The high tension generator

The high tension generator gives a maximum output of 300 mA and 125 kVp. It would not be a practical arrangement to attempt to operate an X-ray tube at 300 mA in a self-rectified circuit because of the very high maximum current involved, and the high tension generator includes full-wave rectification provided by means of selenium rectifiers. This gives greater efficiency and results in lower mains current being drawn.

As in the case of static units in the X-ray department, the high tension generator and its rectifiers and the filament transformer for the X-ray tube are enclosed in one oil-filled earthed steel tank. This tank has a fibre-glass cover and is mounted on the base of the unit immediately behind the vertical column and the batteries for the motor drive. The high tension generator in its tank is connected to the X-ray tube by means of high tension cables just as if it were a static unit in the X-ray department. These can be seen in Fig. 9.8 connecting the X-ray tube to the generator tank.

Control unit

The control unit is located under a hinged lid behind the generator tank on the base of the unit. It has the features listed below. The numbers in brackets after any item indicate the page numbers in this chapter where more is said concerning any given control feature.

1   A lever which selects forward or reverse for the motor drive of the equipment.

2   A selector switch which allows additional power to be used when the equipment is taken up a slope.

3   An ON/OFF switch for the drive.

4   An indicator lamp which shows when the set is switched on.

5 A milliamperes selector which allows selection of six different tube currents (see below).

6 A meter which functions as a milliampereseconds meter before the exposure (by means of a pre-reading scale) and as a milliampere meter during the exposure (recording the tube current on another scale).

7 A warning light which indicates when the selected radiographic factors represent an overload of the X-ray tube.

8 A timer with a range from 0·2 second to 5 seconds (page 345).

9 Buttons to control the movement of the X-ray tube up and down the vertical column.

10 Mains ON/OFF switch.

11 Kilovoltage control with 40 steps of selection (see below).

12 A switch so that a bucky grid may be electrically connected into the circuit if the X-ray set is being used in the X-ray department with a static bucky table.

13 Pre-reading kilovolt meter scaled from 0 to 130 kVp (see below).

14 A lamp which indicates that the X-ray exposure is taking place.

15 Line resistance selector switch (page 345). This functions also as a mains ON switch.

16 Brake lever for the motor drive. This cuts the electrical supply to the motor and applies a disc brake.

17 A handswitch carrying the exposure button is at the end of a lead which is 2 metres long and plugs into the control panel (the *Code of Practice* used in the United Kingdom recommends 2 metres).

Tube current (milliamperes) selection

The milliamperes selector allows six different tube currents to be pre-selected. These are 25 mA, 50 mA and 100 mA on the fine focus of the X-ray tube, and 150 mA, 200 mA and 300 mA on the broad focus. The tube current is interlocked with kilovoltage and time so that warning of overload can be given. The X-ray tube can thus be protected against the selection of a combination of factors which is beyond its rating. The tube current selector switch selects also the focal spot which is to be used.

Kilovoltage selection

The kilovoltage selector is a manual control which rotates five times and gives 40 steps of selection, the maximum giving 125 kVp. Before the kilovoltage control is used, the tube current should be selected; the kilovoltage obtained from each chosen position of the kilovoltage selector is then shown on the pre-reading kilovolt meter.

The timer

The exposure time is selected by means of a manual control on the control panel. The timing is electronic and the timer has a range from 0·02 second up to 5 seconds. With a mobile set of high output short times will be used, and the timer is required to be accurate for very short intervals and need not be scaled to give long exposure times. To make another exposure of the same duration it is not necessary to reset the timer.

Radiographic output. Mains requirements

For all portable and mobile equipment but particularly when large primary currents must flow, the resistance of the mains becomes very important. When the exposure begins, the voltage of the mains supply falls (mains voltage drop under load) by the amount necessary to transmit the load current against the mains resistance. Where the load currents and the mains resistance are both high, there will be a big voltage drop. If this drop is greater than 20 per cent of the mains voltage, it may be difficult or impossible to obtain enough power to operate the X-ray set properly. Radiographs may be 'thin' and results of a consistent standard may not be obtained.

Because of the importance of mains resistance, the manufacturers include among the specifications of high-powered mobile sets a statement of maximum line resistance if the set is to be used at its full output satisfactorily. In this case of a 300 mA set the maximum line resistance which can be tolerated is 0·32 ohms when the set is operating on a 240 volts supply. On a lower supply voltage the same tube milliamperage gives rise to bigger primary current and hence bigger voltage drop on a resistance of 0·32 ohms; this is why the manufacturer states the resistance in relation to the supply voltage for at a lower voltage the maximum resistance which can be accepted must be lower too.

Furthermore it is usual to provide a control on the control panel by means of which some adjustment for mains resistance can be achieved. In this particular case the control is called a line resistance adjuster and it has six positions. A mobile set must be used from many different supply points in a hospital, and each supply point may have a different mains resistance associated with it. For example, supply sockets in some wards will have a greater length of cable reaching them than do the supply sockets in others which are nearer the hospital substation. The resistance adjustor enables a series of additional resistances (known as padding resistors) to be included in the primary circuit. The variable resistance from the adjustor *plus* the mains resistance (which varies because of differences in the supply points) together must add up to a certain fixed resistance at the input side of the X-ray set. Where mains resistance is smaller, a greater resistance is selected by means of the switch; where mains resistance is higher, a smaller resistance is selected by means of the switch. With the total resistance at the input side determined, the manufacturer can know how much voltage drop occurs at any given tube load, and in the circuits operating the X-ray tube he can make allowance and compensation for it.

For the particular mobile set illustrated here, the installing engineer fits a numbered plate beside each supply point where the set is to be used. The numbers correspond to the settings on the adjustor and so the right setting for any given outlet point may easily be chosen when the set is used. With some units it is left to the radiographers to adjust a resistance selector switch at each supply point while reading indications on a volt-meter. They can then make the necessary adjustments routinely just before the radiographic exposure; or if they wish they can number the supply sockets for themselves.

It is to be realized that there are two possible situations which may invalidate this system of bringing the input resistance up to a known value. These are as follows.

1   When the mains resistance is so high as already to be *above* the value which it is intended to achieve by means of the padding resistor.

2   When the mobile set is used with an extension lead to lengthen the cable by which it is plugged into the mains. The resistance of the cable from the wall socket to the X-ray set must be included in the calculation of the total resistance at the input side of the unit. However, it is of course possible to estimate the resistance of any given length of extension cable and to take this into account; for example by raising the setting of the line resistance selector switch by one stud when 10 metres of cable are used.

The maximum radiographic factors of a high-powered mobile set such as this cause it to draw very heavy currents from the mains during the X-ray exposure. If such a set is to be used at its full output, a 13 amperes or 15 amperes point of supply is not ideal and it is better if special supply points are arranged. A 30 amperes supply point can be used, but the installation of special 30 amperes supplies to be reserved for X-ray usage only in a number of wards in a hospital may be as costly as purchasing the mobile unit itself; so it is not surprising if hospitals are reluctant to undertake it.

Provided that the resistance of the mains is low enough (and many modern mains are adequately low in resistance), a 300 mA mobile unit can be used from 13 amperes supply points with a special 13 amperes plug which has no fuse and is suitable for wiring to the heavy cable of the set. (The cable is heavy because it must carry the high currents necessary to operate the X-ray set.) This special plug designed for use only with X-ray sets can be combined with a special 'sparkless' switch socket as the outlet from the mains.

These arrangements are satisfactory for high-powered equipments which are being used in the wards of the hospital, for this constitutes 'occasional' use—whatever it may feel like to a busy radiographer who spends a whole day undertaking 'mobile' work in wards and theatres! When a high-powered mobile unit is used in a fixed location in an X-ray room or clinic, it is preferable that a 30 amperes socket and switch should be provided.

At its full output a high-powered mobile set draws current much in excess of 30 amperes. It is unlikely that the maximum kilovoltage and tube current would be used together for a radiographic exposure, but 300 mA even at 80 kVp draws a mains current of about 150 amperes. These heavy currents will not flow for long, since the use of the highest tube current implies also the use of the shortest exposure time. So the high current will flow for only fractions of seconds. The very short time intervals allow the high current to be drawn from the supply point without blowing fuses, provided that the current protection given is in the form of fuses which are the wire or cartridge type and is not an electronic circuit breaker. An electronic circuit breaker opens the circuit instantly when the current for which it is set is exceeded. When longer exposure times are used, the tube current will be lower and the current taken from the mains will be lower too.

CAPACITOR DISCHARGE MOBILE EQUIPMENT

To meet the demands of the radiographer, high X-ray output is a desired feature for mobile equipment. The patients who are to be examined with mobile sets will likely be in states to find full co-operation difficult or impossible. So radiographers need equipment which can provide high milliamperages and thus can allow the use of short exposure times to obtain radiographs. The quality of the radiographic result is a prime requirement in the minds of radiographers when they consider the relative merits of various mobile sets among which purchase is to be made.

The hospital finance authorities who pay the bills have, of course, in *their* minds prime requirements which are wholly different from those of a radiographer. People who authorize the spending of money in public concerns first of all may wish to keep the sums expended as small as possible and secondly require the spending to be highly effective.

High-powered mobile sets of the conventional type, as we have seen, may need special mains installations at every point of use. When these sets are used at their full output, heavy mains currents are drawn and wall sockets should be at least 30 A outlets suitably fused. Such special wiring installations are expensive and the cost can amount to several thousand pounds. The people authorizing this expenditure are bound to ask 'Is this special installation fully used?' To this question the answer must be 'No'. The special wiring is in fact being used only during the short periods of time for which the mains current flows to give the power required for the exposure: that is, during the very short intervals for which radiographic exposures last. So for even a busy department, using the mobile sets many times a day, if all the exposure times were added up the sum would be a very small part indeed of the 24 hours of a day. Financial authorities tend to look askance at such a discrepancy.

The need to resolve such difficulties has led to the development of mobile X-ray sets which use for the exposure energy which has been stored in a capacitor. We describe here some typical features of capacitor discharge units which are now available.

The High-tension Source

The basis of operation of a capacitor discharge X-ray set is the use of a circuit to charge a capacitor up to the kilovoltage required for the exposure. The capacitor then becomes the source of the power for the X-ray exposure: the capacitor is disconnected from its charging circuit and connected to the X-ray tube for the exposure and its discharge through the X-ray tube constitutes the milliampereseconds of the radiographic exposure factors. The arrangements are very simply indicated in Fig. 9.11 which shows a block diagram alongside the handswitch of the X-ray set. When the user presses the button marked *Charge* (in some cases this pushbutton may be on the control panel and not in the handswitch) the capacitor is charged through the high tension source as indicated in the block diagram by connections at G_1 and G_2. When the required value of kilovoltage (which is pre-set through a control) has been reached, the charging is automatically stopped and the pilot lamp associated with the pushbutton indicates *Ready*. To charge the capacitor from zero volts to 60 kV requires about 5 seconds and from zero to 100 kV needs about 15 seconds. After charging has stopped, when the radiographer presses the exposure button (marked *X ray* in Fig. 9.11) the capacitor is connected to the X-ray tube as indicated in the block diagram at X_1 and X_2. It discharges through the tube and thus constitutes the X-ray exposure.

In the circuits for the charging of the capacitors, there are arrangements of solid state rectifiers and capacitors which are such as to allow the capacitors to function both for storing energy and for multiplying voltage. So pace and weight may be saved in this equipment by the absence of the standard high tension transformers by means of which high voltage is provided in conventional mobile sets.

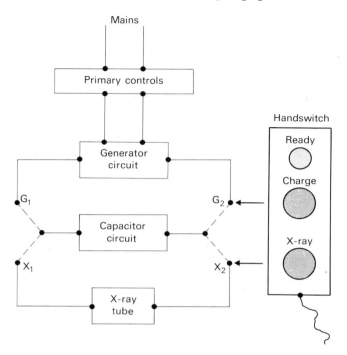

Fig. 9.11

In any capacitor discharge mobile set, the importance of the value of capacitance provided is that greater capacitance results in more charge for a given voltage and more charge is more milliampereseconds for the X-ray exposure. Typical is a capacitance of 1 microfarad and a milliampereseconds range from 0·4 to 50 or from 2·0 to 60; a capacitance of 0·5 microfarad might give a range from 1·0 milliamperesecond to 25 milliampereseconds.

It is obvious that as the capacitor discharges the voltage across it at the beginning of the exposure (that is, the selected kilovoltage) must fall with the loss of charge of the capacitor. For example, a capacitance of 1·0 microfarad charged to 100 kV has 100 mAs as the charge upon it. If the radiographic exposure is 4 mAs, the remanent charge at the end of the exposure is 96 mAs and the voltage corresponding on the capacitor is 96 kV. If the radiographic exposure is 20 mAs, at its termination the charge on the capacitor will have fallen to 80 mAs and the voltage across it then stands at 80 kV. Unless this situation is checked, when a high milliampereseconds load is demanded the last part of the exposure period can find the X-ray tube emitting radiation which has so slight a penetrating power that it contributes nothing to the radiographic result and delivers to the patient a needless dose of useless radiation. It is usual therefore in capacitor discharge equipments to limit the fall in voltage that occurs. For example, it may be limited to a maximum of 35 per cent on a heavy milliampereseconds loading with a long exposure time. This implies that at 100 kV the tube voltage will not fall to lower than 65 kV. At low milliampereseconds loading the fall may be as low as about 5 kV.

Conventional generators used in mobile equipment provide the X-ray tube with a voltage waveform which is pulsating in character and follows the sine wave variations of the a.c. mains supply, varying in the cycle from zero to a maximum and down to zero again. For capacitor discharge sets, the waveform of the voltage across the X-ray tube is not pulsating and it follows the pattern of the falling voltage across a discharging capacitor: its graph has no relationship to the a.c. mains and is a continuous line following an exponential curve as illustrated in Fig. 9.12. In practice, as we have indicated, the fall in voltage is checked so that it does not fall to a value lower than about 65 per cent of the peak value and the important point here is that it is a maintained continuous voltage and is not a pulsating one.

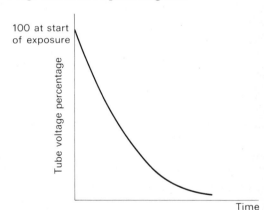

Fig. 9.12

A continuous voltage as opposed to a pulsating one gives high X-ray output for any given exposure settings expressed in milliampereseconds and kilovolts. So a capacitor discharge mobile set in comparison with a conventional generator of the same loading capacity makes more efficient use of electric power in translating it to densities in the final radiographic image: exposure settings can be lowered and this is always an advantage for a radiographer using mobile X-ray equipment.

The X-ray tube

The X-ray tube of a typical capacitor discharge mobile set is a rotating anode tube with a single focal spot of size 1·2 mm and a heat storage capacity of 80 thousand heat units. It is usually grid-controlled: this allows the exposure to be cut off at any given point, providing consistent and precise milliampereseconds values.

The X-ray tube is fitted with a light-beam delineator. In conjunction with this a pair of lead shutters can be arranged so that they are *open only* when the exposure switch is in the *Prepare* and *Expose* positions. At all other times the shutters are fully closed. This feature limits the leakage radiation and allows the capacitor to be discharged after the exposure without the emission of X-rays at a dangerous level (the discharge takes place across the X-ray tube).

The tubestand

The essential features of the tubestand of a capacitor discharge mobile set do not significantly differ from those of mobile sets with conventional generators. Most of these features are recognizable in Figs. 9.13 and 9.14 and are as follows;

1   a strong base with wheels and castors which allow easy movement;
2   a rotatable vertical tube column and extensible tube cross-arm which provide a full range of movements;
3   a tank for the high tension circuitry mounted on the base behind the vertical column;

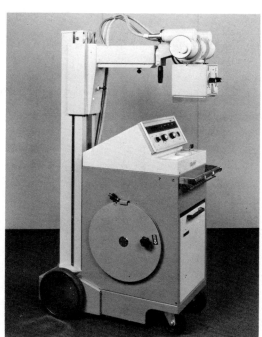

Fig. 9.13   Capacitor discharge mobile set MC 125L–30.
Illustration by courtesy of Medical X-ray Supplies Ltd. and Shimadzu Medical X-ray

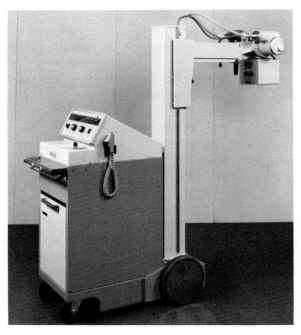

Fig. 9.14 Capacitor discharge mobile set MC 125L–30. *Illustration by courtesy of Medical X-ray Supplies Ltd and Shimadzu Medical X-ray*

4   connections between the high tension circuitry and the X-ray tube by means of high tension cables;
5   a control desk on top of the tank;
6   a separate exposure handswitch on a length of cable which, in accordance with current codes of practice, should be at least 2000 mm in length;
7   there may be batteries to power a motor drive for easy transport and an in-built charger to charge the batteries when the set is left on charge connected to the mains for the purpose.

The control unit

The controls of a capacitor discharge mobile X-ray set provide an automatic charging circuit for the capacitor. The charging process is initiated through a pushbutton which may be on the control desk or on the handswitch. When the voltage across the capacitor has reached the level of the selected kilovoltage, the charging is automatically stopped. If there is a leakage of charge before the exposure and consequently a fall in voltage from the selected value, the charging is renewed to restore the kilovoltage to the needed level.

The kilovoltage selector provides a range from 30 kV or 40 kV up to 100 kV or 125 kV in continously adjustable stages, with display by a meter of the kilovoltage on the charged capacitor. For the set illustrated in Figs. 9.13 and 9.14 the range is from 30 kV to 125 kV with digital indication. If the pre-selected kilovoltage is altered after the charging is complete, the tube voltage is automatically adjusted to the new value which has been set.

The two remaining factors of exposure (milliamperes and time) are not individually set. Instead a single selection (that is, milliampereseconds) is made. For the set shown in Fig. 9.13 and 9.14, the milliampereseconds control has fifteen steps of milliampereseconds: 2, 3, 4, 5, 6, 8, 10, 12, 15, 20, 25, 30, 40, 50 and 60 mAs.

In another capacitor discharge mobile set which is on the market the radiographer does not select a millliampereseconds value for the exposure. Instead of a milliampereseconds control there is a two-position switch which is called a *mode-selector*: the two positions are *Chest* and *Skeleton*. The radiographer simply sets the mode selector and chooses kilovoltage: selecting the kilovoltage automatically sets the X-ray tube current. On the chest mode setting, the time of the exposure is fixed at 40 milliseconds. On the skeleton setting the exposure times are between 40 milliseconds and 60 milliseconds.

The controls of a capacitor discharge mobile set include the usual handswitch with a pushbutton to initiate the exposure. As usual, this is a two-stage procedure. Depression to the half-way position heats the filament of the X-ray tube, starts the rotation of the anode and opens the lead shutters between the portal of the X-ray tube and the light-beam diaphragm.

Other features of the controls of these capacitor discharge mobile sets are: a mains ON indicator; a capacitor charge indicator; an indication that the set is ready for exposure; and an indication that the exposure is taking place. Fig. 9.15 shows a sketch of the control desk of a typical capacitor discharge mobile set which incorporates the features mentioned here.

The radiographic output and
the mains requirements

The radiographic outputs of capacitor discharge mobile sets place them in the *high-powered* category. For example one such set (the one in Figs. 9.13 and 9.14) gives the following:

Radiography rating   30–125 kV
mAs system   2–60 mAs in 15 steps.

The technical data of other mobile sets which may be taken as typical are:

1   300 mA at 50 kV
   150 mA at 100 kV
    30 mAs at 100 kV

2   Kilovoltage range   40–125 kV

Maximum peak milliamperage   500 mA

Milliamperseconds selection   0·5–60 mAs in 17 steps.

The mains requirements are simple since the mains supply is not directly providing the power for the X-ray exposure. It is being used to provide power to the circuitry to charge the capacitor. These sets can therefore be used from any standard mains outlet and they need no special installations. The power requirement for the set illustrated in Fig. 9.13 and Fig. 9.14 is

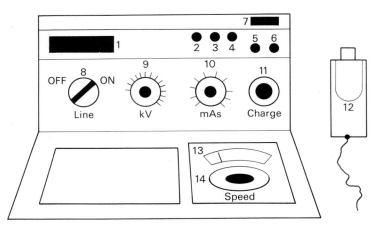

Fig. 9.15

1 Kilovolt meter which gives digital display of the kilovoltage on the charged capacitor

2 Indicator lamp which shows when the line is switched on

3 Indicator lamp which shows when the set is ready for the exposure. This lamp lights up when the exposure switch is pressed into the Prepare position

4 This lamp lights up to indicate 'X rays on' and shows during the exposure. It also shows when the capacitor is discharged with the shutter closed.

5 This lamp indicates when the capacitor is being charged

6 This lamp indicates that charge is present on the capacitor and extinguishes only when there is no residual charge on the capacitor

7 Exposure counter

8 ON/OFF switch

9 Kilovoltage control which preselects the voltage from 30 kV to 125 kV to which the capacitor is to be charged. If it is wished to alter kilovoltage after charging is complete, the tube voltage automatically adjusts to the re-set value.

10 Milliampereseconds control which gives a range from 2 mAs to 60 mAs in 15 steps

11 The charge pushbutton which starts the charging action for the capacitor

12 Handswitch which initiates the exposure

13 Battery voltmeter which monitors the charging of the batteries which provide a drive for the set

14 Switch to select the driving speed for the set and also to connect the battery to its built-in charger. There is a choice of three forward driving speeds and two reverse speeds.

typical and it amounts to only 2 kVA. Even a poor mains supply is not taxed to charge capacitors and mains voltage variations have no effects on the radiographic results which are obtained.

CORDLESS MOBILE EQUIPMENTS

In an earlier section of this chapter we described a high-powered mobile set which used batteries to obtain electric power to drive it from place to place, thus saving someone's physical energy in pushing. This mobile set used electricity from the mains for the X-ray exposure. It is to be distinguished from mains-independent mobile equipment which uses batteries as a source of energy for the X-ray exposure and not for propulsion.

One mains-independent battery-powered mobile equipment uses two 12 volts car batteries as its source of electric power. These batteries give a 24 volts d.c. supply which operates a small rotary converter; this piece of equipment converts the 24 volts d.c. to polyphase a.c. which is fed to a triple autotransformer and hence to a twin three-phase high tension transformer. The a.c. is then rectified by means of twelve solid-state rectifiers and the X-ray tube obtains a rectified six-phase supply (12 pulses).

Another mobile set which is 'cordless' and independent of the mains obtains power from three 40 V nickle-cadmium cell groups. The cells store 10,000 mAs at 100 kV and at lower levels of tube voltage the available milliampereseconds are proportionately greater. The power contained in the cell groups is used not only for the X-ray exposure but also for the drive to transport the mobile set from place to place: it is claimed that repeated exposures at full output may be made even when the unit has been driven up to 0·8 mile before it reaches the patient and is set up for the first exposure.

During the exposure, the voltage waveform across the X-ray tube is a stabilized unidirectional voltage with a slight ripple, the maximum peak value being 110 kVp. This voltage waveform ensures that the tube produces useful X-rays throughout the exposure time and hence it is claimed that a tube current of 100 mA equates in output and hence in the radiographic result with 150 mA from a conventional generator with a pulsating voltage wave-form.

It is unnecessary to re-charge the batteries between exposures. Manufacturers claim, for example, that up to 500 'average' exposures can be made without re-charging the batteries. The battery packs of cordless mobile sets are usually rechargeable through chargers built into them and operable from a 5 A mains: one such battery pack can be recharged to full capacity in eight hours and in shorter times than that if its state of discharge is less.

X-RAY EQUIPMENT FOR THE
OPERATING THEATRE

When X-ray equipment is used in an operating theatre, there are three important hazards to be considered. These are as follows.

1 The risk of taking infection into the theatre with a piece of equipment which may be widely used throughout the hospital and cannot be sterilized efficiently.

2 The risk of explosion where electrical equipment that may produce a spark is used in an atmosphere that may be explosive because of anaesthetic gases. This risk is decreasing because anaesthetic gases which readily ignite or promote ignition are now less often used.

3 The radiation risk to everyone in the theatre.

In order to be helpful with the problems of infection and explosion risk, manufacturers have given their attention to features of design which might be used to make the risks less. The risk of infection can be greatly diminished if there are shielding covers over parts of the equipment where dust could gather and which it might be difficult or impossible to wipe down with antiseptic as a sterilizing measure. It will be noted, for example, that the unit shown in Fig. 9.8 has smooth fibreglass covers on its batteries and high tension transformer tank, and that the control panel is closed over with a hinged lid. Other units have similar features to reduce their ability to collect dust and to make them easy to clean. Such units, however, are not suitable for use with inflammable anaesthetic gases unless special measures to avoid sparking have been taken in their design.

Modern high tension cables have smooth plastic sheaths and these can be cleaned with antiseptic fluid. The cable carrying the stator supply to a rotating anode X-ray tube also has a smooth plastic sheath.

The parts of an X-ray set which may give rise to sparks are the control sections where contacts are being opened and closed through relays and switches. So the explosion risk can be reduced if the control unit of the X-ray set is not in the theatre at all. This has been done in some mobile equipment for theatre use which is divided into two sections. The section for use in the theatre consists of the high tension generator and tubestand mounted on a wheeled base (Fig. 9.16). There is a fibreglass cover over the foot of the tubestand and the high tension generator which comes to within 12·5 mm of the floor. It is therefore easy to wipe down with a sterilizing agent, and the fact that the equipment is used only in the theatre and not for the work in the wards of the hospital is in itself a help in reducing the risk of infection. The control section (Fig. 9.17) is also on a wheeled base and is intended to be placed in an ante-room outside the theatre. It may also

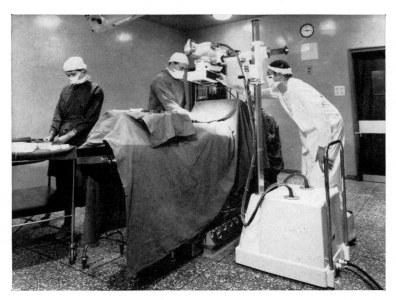

Fig. 9.16 A mobile tubestand with high tension generator in an operating theatre. *By courtesy of Picker International Ltd.*

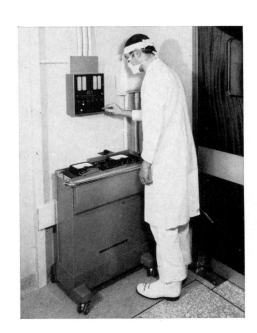

Fig. 9.17
The control unit outside the theatre. *By courtesy of Picker International Ltd.*

control a number of separate tube units being used in various theatres in the same block.

This separation of the control unit can be achieved also by putting into the operating theatre equipment which is not mobile as we have here interpreted the term. Within the theatre the tubestand may be a permanent installation, the control unit being in a fixed site in an ante-room and perhaps serving more than one X-ray tube in more than one theatre. Where a control unit (mobile or not) is used outside the theatre, for efficient use it is necessary to have a team of two radiographers, to work one outside and one inside the theatre with a system of intercommunication.

Quite apart from X-ray equipment, an explosion risk can exist in the theatre through static electricity. Static electricity is electric charge produced by friction applied to insulated bodies. This friction can simply be that given by passage through the air and high electrical potentials can build up. Two objects which have acquired charge in this way may be brought close together and charge is then transferred from the object at higher potential to the one at lower potential. This creates a spark which may be extremely small and yet can be enough to cause an explosion in a flammable atmosphere. To help with this problem, some X-ray equipment is provided with wheels made of special conducting rubber. This prevents the build-up of static electric charge on the mobile unit as there is a continuous conducting path from the X-ray set to the floor. Such wheels are used also on other equipment in the theatre.

To reduce the radiation risk, X-ray equipment in the operating theatre must be used with careful limitation of the beam. The most satisfactory way of doing this is by means of adjustable diaphragms used in conjunction with an 'optical' viewer giving a direct view of what the X-ray tube 'sees'. This is easy to use in a brightly-lit theatre. The viewer gives a visual indication of the field covered and thus makes it easier to use the smallest possible areas for irradiation. The optical viewer does not require an electric circuit to provide it with light as the field is viewed by the theatre illumination; this recommends itself as a safety measure in its elimination of a source of sparks. The viewer is described in Chapter 8 (page 306).

Before leaving the subject of X-ray equipment in the operating theatre, there is another aspect which should be mentioned and that is the need to save time. A patient in the theatre is a patient at risk and all who are concerned with caring for him wish to submit him to anaesthesia and open surgery for the shortest time that is consistent with efficient work. Radiographers must therefore produce their radiographic results as quickly as possible and equipment is designed to enable them to do this. It is not within the scope of this book to consider fully how rapid radiographic results may be obtained in various ways but it is certainly worth looking at X-ray equipment for use in the theatre which is significantly time-saving. This equipment enables fluoroscopy to be done with an image intensifier and it is superceding other special theatre installations.

Mobile image intensifier units

One way of saving time in the use of X-ray control during surgery is to employ a mobile unit for fluoroscopy with an image intensifier.

This reduces to a minimum the number of radiographs which will be taken, and thus time is saved but perhaps with increased radiation dose. The time required by a surgeon to check his procedure by looking at a fluoroscopic image is short in comparison with that needed to produce a radiographic record by even rapid methods. For the sake of radiological safety, the practice of fluoroscopy in situations away from permanent departmental installations should never be undertaken unless it can be done with a special unit which incorporates an image intensifier and is designed to allow fluoroscopy to be mobile and relatively safe.

Furthermore by means of a cone and internal diaphragm the beam is carefully and closely limited to the small field size of the intensifier tube. This is essential for radiation safety.

A television link is added to the equipment so that the X-ray image may be viewed on one or more monitor screens by more than one person. This aids teamwork and should help to shorten the overall time spent on certain procedures.

Radiographers should remember that if they are operating fluoroscopic (or indeed any other) X-ray equipment in the absence of a radiologist, the responsibility for radiation safety is carried inescapably by the radiographer using the equipment. This gives to the radiographer an authoritative voice which should not hesitate to speak and to endeavour to make itself heeded if necessary by even the most senior surgeons, although this is predictably not always easy. If radiation dose to the patient and/or staff appears unreasonably high, the radiographer must call a halt.

The x-ray tube, the image intensifier, the tubestand

Essential features of a mobile unit for fluoroscopy are the X-ray tubehead and the image intensifier mounted so that they are in opposition at the ends of a C arm. This construction is shown clearly in Fig. 9.18. The X-ray tubehead is at the lower end of the C arm in the picture and the image intensifier is at the upper end with its input phosphor facing towards the X-ray tube. At the back of the image intensifier is a television pick-up tube

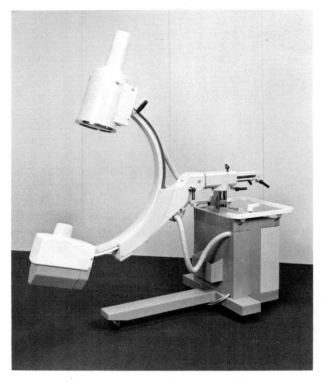

Fig. 9.18 A mobile X-ray generator with image intensifier and television pick-up on C arm construction. This one has a two-frame memory. *Illustration by courtesy of Medical X-ray Supplies and Shimadzu Medical X-ray.*

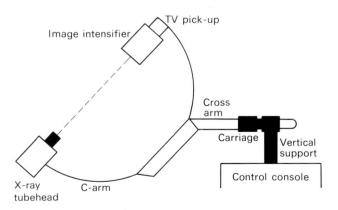

Fig. 9.19

(television camera tube) which might be a 625-line Vidicon or an 875-line Plumbicon. (Image intensifiers and television are explained in Chapter 11.)

The C arm is mounted on a cross-arm which extends from a carriage carried on a vertical support rising from the control console: Fig. 9.19 sketches these arrangements. The control console is on a wheeled base so that the whole apparatus is fully mobile. The X-ray tubehead and the image intensifier are held directly opposite to each other with the X-ray beam permanently centred to the input phosphor of the intensifier and collimated just to cover that field. Thus direction of the X-ray beam to the image intensifier is precise and certain and unalterable. Since the X-ray tube and the intensifier tube are attached to the C arm and move together, movements of the C arm give rapid and easy positioning of the X-ray tube and the intensifier tube about the patient with the beam directed vertically or horizontally or obliquely and remaining central to and at right angles to the input phosphor of the intensifier. Fig. 9.20 sketches some of these possibilities.

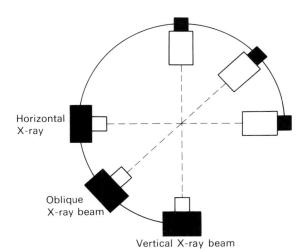

Fig. 9.20

Horizontal X-ray

Oblique X-ray beam

Vertical X-ray beam

The vertical support can be raised and lowered and the cross-arm can be extended through the carriage. The C arm can slide through 90 degrees in its support carrying with it the X-ray tubehead at one end and the image intensifier and television pick-up at the other. The C arm and its support can be rotated about the horizontal axis of the carriage. So the equipment enables a good range of positions and projections to be used without waste of time spent in re-arrangements.

The tubehead houses the X-ray tube. Typical for a modern mobile unit with an image intensifier is an X-ray tube with a stationary anode and two focal spots. For fluoroscopy a small focal spot of size 0·6 mm² is used and a larger focal spot of size 1·8 mm² serves for radiography.

The input phosphor of the image intensifier is caesium iodide which gives an image of good contrast and resolution. A secondary radiation grid which is removable is incorporated in the image intensifier. The grid ratio might be around 5 : 1. Units are available which offer a choice for the field size of the image intensifier tube. Field sizes of 6 inches (150 mm) and 9 inches (230 mm) are available from the manufacturers of such equipment.

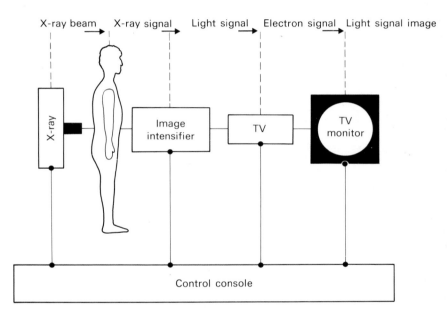

Fig. 9.21

The high tension generator

The X-ray tube and the high tension generator are together in the tubehead as a tank construction. So high tension cables are not required and a multi-cored low tension cable connects the generator to the controls. The high tension generator typically is single phase with full-wave rectification provided by silicon rectifiers: that is, the generator is a two pulse one.

The control console

Fig. 9.21 is a block diagram to show the sequence of transferences that must be controlled in any equipment which embodies fluoroscopy with an image intensifier and television chain. The start of the sequence is the X-ray generator producing an X-ray beam which is passed through the patient: it emerges on the far side as an X-ray pattern made of the varying transmissions and absorptions by the body tissues. This pattern constitutes an X-ray signal. The image intensifier tube receives the X-ray signal and converts it to a light pattern (a visible radiological image). This light pattern or light signal is composed by the varying intensities of light to which the image intensifier has transferred the X-ray signal. This light signal is received by the television pick-up tube (television camera tube). The television tube transfers the light signal to become an electron signal and the varying electron signal is passed to the cathode ray tube which is the television monitor. Here the final transference takes place and the cathode ray tube, receiving a varying electron signal, displays the information as a light signal. This of course is a visible image composed by the varying light intensities to which the varying electron signal has been transferred. As the block diagram shows, there are controls for all the units in the chain—except for the most important one of all who is the patient!

Fig. 9.22 is a sketch to show features of a typical control console for equipment of this sort and the key in the caption identifies the features. Typical for the controls of the X-ray tube settings is a manual selector of kilovoltage for fluoroscopy or for radiography with steps between 50 kV and 105 kV. This is shown at 17 in Fig. 9.22. At 9 is shown a pushbutton to insert an automatic stepless adjustment of kilovoltage during fluoroscopy which is a feature of modern units. This is achieved through an electronic balance which responds to the intensity of the electron signal from the television pick-up tube. The electronic balance gives an output signal through which kilovoltage can be automatically adjusted to a suitable value relative to the radio-absorptiveness of the subject (see also p. 391).

Typical of the milliamperage settings for fluoroscopy is a range from 0·1 to 3·0 mA and a control for this is shown at 15 in Fig. 9.22. For radiography the kilovoltage and the milliamperage settings are linked and the following are typical:

50 mA at 55 kV
40 mA at 80 kV
30 mA at 105 kV

The timer for radiographic exposures is electronic and gives a range from 0·1 to 3·0 seconds. It is seen at 8 in Fig. 9.22. The exposure switching is also electronic on the primary side of the high tension generator and it is phased so that the circuit closes and opens at the zero points of the ac mains cycle. For the television chain the circuitry includes controls which allow the image to be transposed right to left (pushbutton 6 in Fig. 9.22) and inverted top to bottom (pushbutton 7 in Fig. 9.22). Further controls (pushbutton 12 in Fig. 9.22) provide for a memory circuit with two magnetic discs (see also p. 342). This means that image storage is possible. With two television monitors for display it is possible to compare an image from the memory circuit with another one in real time. Another facility available is for pulsed fluoroscopy with an electronic selector allowing choice of programmes: the rates provided vary from 1 flash per second to 1 flash every 5 seconds. This allows an observer to monitor dynamic events without subjecting the patient to continuous irradiation.

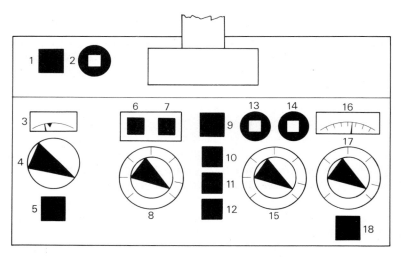

Fig. 9.22

1 Pushbutton to lower whole C arm unit to control console
2 Warning light to indicate overheating of the X-ray tubehead
3 Mains voltage compensator meter
4 ON/OFF switch and mains voltage compensator
5 Pushbutton to zero the fluoroscopic timer
6 Pushbutton to transpose the image right to left
7 Pushbutton to invert the image top and bottom
8 Timer for radiographic exposures
9 Pushbutton to insert automatic adjustment of kilovoltage during fluoroscopy
10 ⎫
11 ⎬ Lifting and lowering pushbuttons
   ⎭
12 Pushbutton to use for the memory circuit
13 Indicator light for X RAYS ON during fluoroscopy
14 Indicator light for X-RAYS ON during radiography
15 Milliamperes selector for fluoroscopy
16 Kilovolt meter
17 Kilovoltage selector switch for fluoroscopy and for radiography
18 Pushbutton for X RAYS ON

Mains requirements

A mobile unit for fluoroscopy with an image intensifier and television chain is suitable for operation at mains outlets from standard wall sockets. The power demand is about 2·5 kW and thus in the United Kingdom the unit can be connected to the phase voltage of the mains with a plug fused for 13 A.

Chapter 10
Fluoroscopy

Nearly every X-ray department possesses equipment for making fluoroscopic examinations. The term *fluoroscopy* implies the use of a fluorescent screen, that is, a sheet of material which fluoresces when X rays strike it. When a patient is placed between a source of X rays and this screen the X-ray image becomes a visible light image and can be observed.

The advantages of the procedure are speed and ease and that it makes possible the study of movement. A radiologist can watch and elucidate any dynamic function as it occurs, such as swallowing, breathing and the opening and closing of valves in the heart. Furthermore, *during* examination a patient can be moved into various positions in order to determine the one which will best show a particular abnormality, for example the profile projection of an ulcer situated somewhere on the posterior wall of the stomach. Fluoroscopy should not be employed except to obtain clinical information which otherwise is unobtainable. This is because the radiation dose to the patient from fluoroscopy can be much greater than from a radiographic procedure. It is important that any doctor who undertakes fluoroscopy—particularly one who is not a radiologist—should be cognizant of the potential radiation dangers of the investigation; and equally so should radiographers be aware.

In order to perform fluoroscopy the bare essentials are an X-ray tube, a patient and a fluorescent screen, together with some means of arranging and supporting the three in appropriate relationship to each other. In practice, modern fluoroscopic equipment is always more elaborate than this. Its sophistications are dictated by: (a) the advantages of being able to make a film (or other) record of screen appearances as they occur; (b) requirements of radiation protection; (c) the concept that—using a single piece of apparatus—one should be able to examine the patient in positions which are feet downwards, head downwards, horizontal and at all stations between. Special fluoroscopic/radiographic tables are required which we shall consider in Chapter 12.

In radiodiagnostic practice, two forms of fluoroscopy are to be recognized. The first of these is described as direct fluoroscopy. In this, the operator faces the fluorescent screen itself and makes immediate observation of the

366

images created on the screen by the attenuations of the X-ray beam.

In much commoner contemporary usage is intensifier fluoroscopy or television fluoroscopy. These descriptions imply the presence of an image intensifier tube and associated equipment which electronically and optically process the immediate fluorescent image in order to brighten it; the brightened image may—or may not—finally be viewed by means of closed circuit television and necessarily is transmitted through an optical system.

DIRECT FLUOROSCOPY

Fluoroscopy enables organs in movement to be studied. This is an unique facility, outweighing certain limitations which are associated with the production of a direct fluoroscopic image and may inhibit its accurate recognition by an observer. These relate to its colour, its sharpness and its contrast.

The colour of fluorescence

Materials which change invisible radiation to luminous radiation are known as *phosphors* and the effect is luminescence. When a substance is luminous only so long as it is irradiated, it is described as being *fluorescent*. (This is in distinction to a *phosphorescent* material, which continues to emit light for a period after the stimulating radiation has been removed.)

In radiodiagnosis, fluorescence is a useful effect which has several applications, perhaps most familiarly in the form of intensifying screens in cassettes for radiography. Just now we are concerned with the production of a fluorescent image to be—not recorded on a film—but displayed immediately to human eyes.

Student radiographers are soon made aware that the colour of fluorescence from an intensifying screen should match the colour-sensitivity of the film to be employed. The human eye is no different from film in this respect: it is more responsive to some—bright—colours than to others which appear to us as 'dark' colours. The phosphor of an irradiated fluoroscopic screen should 'look' bright to the eye. Zinc cadmium sulphide is a material which is used in the manufacture of a simple fluorescent screen because it fluoresces with a yellow-green light, a colour which affords us the greatest visual acuity at low levels of illumination. (Visual acuity refers to our ability to separate or recognize the small details of an image.)

The structure of a fluoroscopic screen

The structure of a screen for direct fluoroscopy is comparatively simple. The phosphor is coated upon an underlying stratum of white pigment, placed on a suitably prepared and finished sheet of cardboard. For mechanical strength, the manufacturer mounts this arrangement on some radioparent material—such as Paxolin—which is attached behind the cardboard base. Over the front of the screen must be put a piece of lead glass of which the purpose is to prevent irradiation of an observer by the primary beam. In the interests of radiation protection, the lead equivalency of this glass is subject to legislation or recommendation by many governments.

When a fluorescent screen of the type under discussion is viewed directly by the eye, the observed image is defective in the respects which have been mentioned (p. 367): relative to the images which we can produce on radiographs, the fluoroscopic image is unsharp, lacks brightness and has poor contrast. These features are considered below.

THE FLUOROSCOPIC IMAGE

The sharpness of the fluoroscopic image

The principles which govern the sharpness of the fluoroscopic image are the same as those which affect its production in a radiograph. A full discussion of them is outside the scope of this book. However, in order to clarify the next few paragraphs for the reader it should be remembered that:

1 the term *intrinsic unsharpness* refers to blurring arising from the nature of the material used to record the image;

2 *geometric unsharpness* is a projection effect and present because in practice we cannot obtain a point source of radiation.

We shall now consider the extent of these factors in relation to the fluoroscopic image.

Intrinsic unsharpness

Like the phosphors employed in the intensifying screens used for radiography, the material of the fluoroscopic screen is crystalline in form. The size of these crystals can be pre-determined in manufacture.

Unfortunately those factors which minimize the intrinsic unsharpness of a fluoroscopic screen—that is, the use of a thin screen composed of small crystals—may be the very ones to limit its brightness. Since the intention of the whole procedure implies observation by the human eye, the production of fine detail becomes irrational if it is achieved at the expense of visibility. In a screen to be used for direct fluoroscopy sensitivity is a more significant and desirable attribute than is the ability to offer high resolution.

It is difficult to measure the unsharpness of a fluorescent screen to absolute standards of accuracy. The unsharpness inherent in simple fluoroscopic screens is said to be of the order of 0·3 mm. This does not compare as unfavourably as one might suppose with the unsharpness of most intensifying screens used in radiography. The fluoroscopic image appears unsharp to a direct observer if its low level of brightness makes him unable to appreciate the small differences in sharpness which would be obvious to him on the examination of a *radiograph* of the same subject. The limiting factor in his perception of the image is not the resolving power of the fluorescent screen.

Geometric unsharpness

Fluoroscopic screens work under conditions which increase geometric unsharpness. These are as follows.

1   The anode-screen distance is usually less than most anode-film distances employed for radiography.

2   The subject-screen distance is greater than the subject-film distance in many radiographic procedures, unless the screen is held closely against the patients at all periods of examination—and in some cases even when the patient is so compressed.

3   In some equipment, fluoroscopy is selected on the smaller focus of a dual-focus tube but in others it occurs on whichever focal spot is chosen for exposure of the associated radiographs; there is a potential likelihood that this will be the larger focus.

The student will know from earlier study of the projection of X-ray images that short anode-film or -screen distances, long subject-film or -screen distances and large tube foci are—separately and collectively—conducive to image unsharpness.

The brightness of the fluoroscopic image

In the case of a simple fluoroscopic screen the brightness of the image is very poor compared with the brightness of a radiograph viewed under normal conditions on an illuminator: the latter has a luminosity at least 50,000 times greater than such a fluoroscopic screen.

There are ways by which in theory the brightness of the fluoroscopic image could be improved.

1   Since the screen's luminance is a direct function of the quantity of X rays reaching it, increasing the intensity of the X-ray beam brightens the fluoroscopic image. However, it is estimated that if this image were to have a brightness equivalent to that of the radiograph it would be necessary to conduct fluoroscopy at tube currents of 400–1600 mA. This is clearly not feasible, not only because such an electrical load on the X-ray tube would be

intolerable in magnitude, but also on account of the very high radiation dose incurred by the patient under these conditions.

2 Since the effect of fluorescence depends upon *absorption* of the X-ray beam, increasing the thickness of the phosphor layer increases the production of luminescence. Pursuing this principle to its logical conclusion, we might say that the optimum thickness of a fluoroscopic screen is the thickness which will absorb all the X rays which fall upon it. However, the theory is not so good as it sounds, since light which is produced in deep layers of the screen cannot penetrate the surface and is invisible to the observer. Consequently the production of light anywhere beyond a certain depth is a profitless exercise.

The contrast of the fluoroscopic image

The contrast of an image—whether it be fluoroscopic or radiographic—is simply the ratio of brightness in contiguous areas. In the case of a radiograph this can be objectively measured and given numerical value, quite apart from the subjective impression made on an observer. In relation to the fluoroscopic image, the subjective effect is perhaps the only one which need be considered; it will enter into our discussion of image perception.

However, it can be said that the contrast of the fluoroscopic image is inherently poor and that one of the reasons for this is the relatively high kilovoltage which must be employed. At low tube tensions, different varieties of tissue differentially absorb the X-ray beam to a much greater extent than in the case of the more penetrating radiation produced at high kilovoltages. Bigger differences of absorption result in bigger differences of brightness and therefore in an image of greater contrast. We might therefore expect the contrast obtainable in fluoroscopy to improve if we were to reduce our working kilovoltage.

This is another theory which breaks down in practice. The intensity of an X-ray beam is significantly influenced by the applied tube tension. Lowering the kilovoltage reduces very rapidly the resultant intensity of radiation; that is, it very rapidly diminishes the brightness of the screen image and consequently diminishes also our ability to perceive it.

The perception of the fluoroscopic image

As we have seen, neither the sharpness nor the contrast of a fluoroscopic image are ideal; nevertheless neither in itself imposes the ultimate limitation on our recognition of the image. The real sinner here is the lack of brightness and the reason for this is found in the physiology of human vision.

The student no doubt will remember that the human retina contains two kinds of light-sensitive cell. These are (a) rods and (b) cones. The cones are sensitive to colour and to white light above a certain intensity. They are numerous in the centre of the retina, the region of keenest vision. The rods on the other hand cannot detect colour and they transmit light to the brain in shades of grey. Their chief function is to recognize light and motion at levels which are below the threshold of cone vision. They have the ability to adapt themselves to darkness and we are all familiar with the fact that when we remain for a while in a darkened room we can see much better after a time than when we first enter it. The increase in sensitivity which the retina develops after a period in darkness is remarkable: after 10 minutes of dark-adaptation the increase is ten-fold; after 18 minutes the increase is a hundred-fold; after 50 minutes the retina is probably 1,000 times more sensitive than it was in the first moments of the experience.

Because of the poor brightness of a fluoroscopic image which has not been processed by any system of intensification, our perception of it depends upon rod vision. Once we lose cone vision we find that two important elements of retinal function become seriously weakened: one of these is visual acuity and the other is intensity discrimination. Visual acuity is the ability of the eye to recognize as separate entities two different light stimuli: that is, it refers to our recognition of detail. Intensity discrimination is the term which describes our ability to recognize differences in brightness; that is, our ability to recognize contrasts.

These physical facts mean that we view the fluoroscopic image with very limited retinal function and that the impairment of our vision is such that we are less able to recognize detail and less able to recognize contrast.

Reference was made earlier to the rod cell's ability to dark-adapt. The increased retinal sensitivity which we can obtain from this results in a reasonable appreciation of the direct fluoroscopic image which we have described. It is the reason why a room for fluoroscopy should be fully darkened during use if no image intensifier is employed. Anyone performing a fluoroscopic examination in these circumstances should not attempt to begin it without first allowing his vision to accommodate to the reduced illumination.

Chapter 11
Image Intensifiers

In the previous chapter we consider the production of an image on a fluorescent screen by means of X rays and the use made of this for fluoroscopy. We saw then that the direct fluoroscopic image is inferior to the radiographic one in respect of:

1 brightness;
2 detail sharpness;
3 contrast.

Because the image lacks brilliance its low levels of sharpness and contrast are aggravated by our use of rod vision—which has no discrimination—in looking at it: if brilliance can be improved other weaknesses in the image may be mitigated. Consequently the development of means to brighten fluoroscopy was a significant advance in radiology and has meant the virtual disappearance, from hospitals in the United Kingdom, of directly viewed fluorescent screens.

The process of brightening the image during fluoroscopy is called image intensification. The use of equipment to do this is associated with two other benefits:

1 potentially lower radiation doses, because lower tube currents may sometimes be employed;
2 the possibility in all instances of displaying the information from a fluorescent screen upon closed circuit television. Used in this way, television has several advantages and a few disadvantages and these will be discussed later in this chapter (see pages 396, 397).

The association of closed circuit television with apparatus for image intensification is virtually universal. Because television is now an inseparable part of image-intensifying equipment and found in almost every X-ray department, radiographers need to know at least a little about television tubes and television monitors.

THE TELEVISION PROCESS

Television contains many detailed elements of technical complexity but—

making the simplest assessment possible—we can say that only two processes are concerned in principle:

1 a visual image, which is a light pattern, is converted to an electron pattern and then to an electric current or voltage which will vary in proportion to the differing light intensities of the original (visual information becomes electrical information);

2 the varying electrical current is converted back to a light pattern which makes a visual impression on an observer similar to the original (electrical information becomes visual information).

The process seems like a sort of photography and it is not surprising that the apparatus used is a television camera. This—like others—has an optical system but the real 'eye' of the instrument is a specialized tube, known as a pick-up tube, which 'looks' at the scene to be televised; in the case of radiology the scene is a fluorescent X-ray image.

The camera tube is not to be confused with the tube which receives the electrical pattern in the television monitor and converts it back to a visual image: this is a cathode ray tube. The two have similarities but in the immediate context it is their differences of function which matter and the television camera or pick-up tube is the one upon which we shall concentrate just now.

The television camera tube

There are several kinds of television camera tube in use for image intensification in medical radiology. They have different qualities which may make one more appropriate in certain circumstances than another. Television camera tubes work on a principle either of photoconductivity or photo-emission. Photo-emissive systems are not in general use at present in X-ray equipment for image intensification and so are to be omitted from the following discussion.

We may obtain a general understanding of a photoconductive system if we consider first the camera tube which is called a vidicon.

The vidicon

The vidicon is depicted diagramatically in Fig. 11.1. It is an evacuated glass tube about 2·5 cm in diameter (1 inch) and about the length of a pencil. It may be considered to have three sections:

1 a target section;
2 an electron gun;
3 a scanning section.

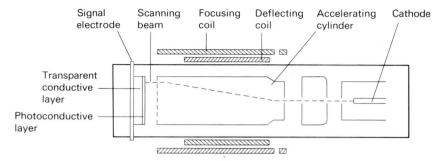

Signal electrode Scanning beam Focusing coil Deflecting coil Accelerating cylinder Cathode

Transparent conductive layer

Photoconductive layer

Fig. 11.1 A vidicon camera tube

The target

The target of a vidicon tube is photoconductive. This description refers to the target's ability to pass electric current when light is falling upon it; and to resist or inhibit electron flow in the absence of light. The stronger is the intensity of light reaching the target, the less is the resistance offered by it and the greater is its conductivity; that is, the higher will be the current caused to flow in an appropriate circuit which includes the target. In the case of a vidicon, the target material is antimony trisulphide.

The target section of the vidicon consists of:

1 at the front of the tube, a glass faceplate;

2 laid down on the back of the glass faceplate, a conductive transparent layer of zinc oxide which allows light to reach the target and forms part of the signal electrode of the vidicon;

3 the target area itself, a layer of antimony trisulphide which is coated thinly upon the presenting surface of the transparent signal plate.

The structure of the target material may be considered as a large number (millions) of minute photoelectric cells and is sometimes described as a mosaic. Varying light intensities, directed upon this mosaic, produce an electrical change which causes each cell to liberate a number of electrons in proportion to the intensity of light reaching the cell. The release of electrons puts a charge on the cell, which effectively becomes a capacitor, having a surplus positive charge (electrons have 'gone') on one plate and a corresponding negative charge on the other.

The next step is to consider how the acquired charges on these capacitors may be converted to a signal current: this is done by means of an electron gun and a scanning beam.

The electron gun and the scanning section

The function of the electron gun is to produce a suitable beam of electrons.

It consists of:

1   a heated cathode, which emits electrons on the same principle as the hot filament of an X-ray tube;

2   a grid (an electrode) which controls the density of electron flow (the value of the beam current), by means of a variable voltage bias;

3   a second grid which accelerates and focuses the stream of electrons in a fine beam as it enters the scanning section of the tube.

Both the quantity of electron flow and the beam's cross section influence the quality of the televised image: too many electrons produce noise (random scintillations) in the final picture; and the smaller the cross section of the beam the more detailed is the image, given that other factors affecting resolution remain the same.

In the scanning section of the tube, externally mounted coils produce an axial electromagnetic field by means of which:

1   the electrons are focused on the target of the vidicon;

2   the beam is moved over the target area in an orderly scanning action.

The required scanning action is similar to the movements of the eye in reading a page: that is, from a beginning at the top left corner, the eye moves in a horizontal line to the right; it then flicks back to the left, a little lower down, and reads the second line. This process is repeated until the bottom of the page is reached.

In the case of the electron beam in the vidicon, a rectangular area known as the raster is thus traced on the target, resulting in one complete picture of electronic information. The number of scanning lines which compose the raster varies with different television systems. In the television systems under discussion, rasters having 625 lines are in general use. Scanning systems are further discussed on p. 382.

Having completed one frame, the electron beam then immediately repeats—and continues to repeat—the scanning process, at an image frequency which synchronises with the frequency of the mains supply. This means that discrete electronic 'pictures' succeed each other at a rate of 50 every second in the United Kingdom (60 every second in the U.S.A.).

Given the circumstances that the faceplate of the vidicon is presented to an optical image (that is, a light image), as the electron beam passes over the mosaic of the target—from one cell to the next and line by line—a partial discharge and then repletion of the charge of each illuminated cell occur. Each depleted element of the mosaic in turn is recharged to its original condition and a continual series of current surges or pulses is produced, whilst the electron beam 'reads' the target. Each such pulse of current is the electrical equivalent of the light coming from a small portion of the original optical image; and every complete scan of the raster represents one optical picture or frame.

The varying video signal current produced in the way described is passed through a resistor. This is called the load resistor and is connected in the input circuit of an amplifier known as the video preamplifier. A varying voltage is produced across the resistor, which is fed to the amplifier: this voltage constitutes the video signal.

Properties of the vidicon

To aid our readers' understanding, the preceding account of a vidicon camera tube has been simplified to some extent. Certain electrical requisites, functionally significant to engineers, have been ignored in the interests of making clearer the operation of the photoconductive target, which gives the vidicon its particular properties and is arguably its most important part.

However, in operation certain practical effects must be considered and these are explained under the headings which follow. They should be considered in conjunction with the fact that X-ray television makes more stringent demands on the vidicon than are encountered during other television. The significant differences in the two circumstances relate particularly to the low contrasts which often are a feature of the X-ray image and to the comparatively low brightness and contrast offered by the image intensifier. A vidicon facing, say, an outdoor daylight scene receives very much more light than one which 'looks' at a fluorescent screen, particularly as there should be concern to keep radiation doses low during television fluoroscopy. To this degree a high performance is consequently required from a vidicon employed for the medical purpose.

Lag

Lag is the conveniently short word which is used to describe retention of an image for some while after cessation of the radiation stimulus which has produced the image.

In relation to the vidicon tube, this means that when an optical image, presented to the faceplate, is suddenly removed the vidicon continues to produce a signal current for a time afterwards, which may persist during several scanning periods. Build-up lag is the term used for the rather similar circumstance, when the faceplate initially is illuminated, that the signal current requires several scanning periods to reach a stable value.

Lag is a characteristic of the vidicon tube which may intrude unduly during television fluoroscopy of a moving subject. For instance, it tends to impede the accurate placing of a cardiac catheter, because the catheter tip appears blurred; but lag would be less significant during an operation for hip pinning, where the subject is considerably less dynamic.

The lag of a vidicon decreases with increased illumination of the faceplate; but we need to remember that when a vidicon is used in conjunction with an image intensifier the required brighter illumination must entail a higher radiation dose for the subject and also a greater load on the X-ray tube. (Readers of this book should be familiar with the implications of both circumstances.) However, it is probably true that modern vidicons react more quickly than those of an early generation.

Sensitivity

The expression of the sensitivity of a vidicon or similar camera tube essentially refers to the amount of illumination required by the photoconductor, if the maximum signal current is to be obtained. It is expressed as the ratio of the signal current to the illumination of the faceplate. Unless radiation doses are to be unacceptably increased, vidicons employed in television fluoroscopy receive less light than is usually specified for their operation. Particularly sensitive vidicons consequently are necessary.

Generally speaking, vidicons are less sensitive than some other camera tubes (orthicons) which are photo-emissive in operation. The sensitivity of a television camera tube should be constant over the whole area of the target or vignetting of the image (see p. 393) will increase.

Dark current

The sensitivity of the vidicon can be increased if the target voltage is raised. The target voltage is the voltage applied to the signal plate of the vidicon and its magnitude is of the order of 20–60 V positive in respect to the cathode.

However, the advantage obtained from an increase of the target voltage carries a disadvantage somewhere else in the system: what is known as the dark current also increases and tends to make more obvious any blemishes or non-uniformity of the target layer. Such defects, which cannot be entirely avoided in manufacture, are responsible for the introduction of anomalous 'spots' to the television image.

Dark current is the name given to a small signal current which flows when the faceplate of the vidicon is not illuminated. When dark current is high, the available range of signal current may be significantly reduced.

Other camera tubes

As well as the vidicon, other television camera tubes of a photoconductive type are in use for television fluoroscopy. Perhaps the best known of these is the plumbicon. In this tube the photoconductor is lead monoxide. Relative to the vidicon, certain characteristics of the plumbicon are listed below.

1 The plumbicon is slightly the larger of the two tubes.

2 It has a faster response, so that less movement blur is seen.

3 It exhibits more quantum noise (see p. 406), which the vidicon's greater lag tends to conceal.

4 The resolution of detail is poorer.

5 Virtually no dark current is present.

Other camera tubes now available for television fluoroscopy are the chalnicon and the newvicon. These have been described as having features which place them in the catalogue somewhere between the vidicon and the plumbicon.

The cathode ray tube

The television receiver or monitor is the apparatus concerned with the process of converting electrical information into visual information; its function is to receive the video signal and reassemble it as a visible image. The monitor consists of a cathode ray tube and its associated circuitry.

The cathode ray tube is a funnel-shaped evacuated glass tube. Its narrow end contains an electrical system designed to emit, accelerate and focus a stream of electrons; the expanded end of the tube forms a special screen which is coated with a material which will fluoresce when electrons strike it. Such a tube is depicted diagrammatically in Fig. 11.2.

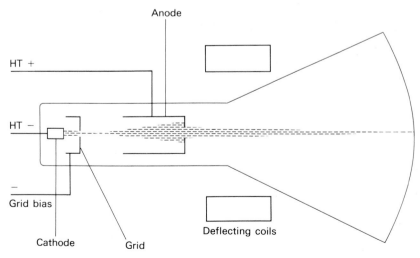

Fig. 11.2 A cathode ray tube.

The electrical system

Like other vacuum tubes known to the student radiographer—the X-ray tube itself and television pick-up tubes—the cathode ray tube contains a heated filament (the cathode) and depends for its function on the emission of electrons from this filament. The electrons so produced are accelerated towards the screen at the other end of the tube by;

1   a potential difference between the cathode and the screen;
2   a high positive voltage on the anodes.

In Fig. 11.2, for the sake of simplicity, only one anode is shown but in practice there are two or more: they are annular in form and, through the central hole in each, electrons pass in a stream towards the other end of the tube.

Fig. 11.2 shows the focusing effect of the control grid. This electrode is negatively biased in relation to the cathode and has a small central aperture which concentrates the electrons to a very narrow beam.

The control grid has an important function not only in its focusing action but because it controls the density of the electron beam. A high negative voltage on the control grid diminishes the electron flow; conversely a low negative voltage on the control grid results in an electron beam of high intensity. Thus, if the video signal is fed to the control grid we obtain a variation in the density of the electrons reaching the screen of the cathode ray tube which corresponds to variations in the video signal itself.

The fluorescent screen

Many substances are known which will fluoresce when electrons strike them. Those employed in cathode ray tubes vary to some extent with the use to which the tube is to be put. Cathode ray tubes are employed in radar, for example, and in this case the colour of the fluorescence is less important than its brightness. For television, on the other hand, the colour must be as near white as possible if the picture is to be black and white.

Zinc phosphates, silicates and sulphides are all examples of phosphors which will fluoresce under electronic bombardment. It is usual to employ one as a base and to add other materials which modify the response of the phosphor. These are:

1   activators, which change the colour of the fluorescence;
2   killers, which affect the duration of image retention in the phosphor.

In the case of the tube in a television monitor the phosphor on the screen should:

1   have maximum sensitivity;
2   have a long life;

3 fluoresce with a white light;
4 exhibit short image retention.

To obtain a white trace from the screen it is usual to combine two or three colours of fluorescence. The screen must be uniformly coated throughout its area. The thickness of the deposited layer is significant, since a thick coating diminishes the brilliance of the screen from the front and too thin a coating reduces the life of the tube. Many modern television tubes have an additional coating of aluminium particles which both increases brilliance and helps to preserve the active material.

The brightness of the spot produced on the screen by the impinging electrons depends on their intensity, assuming a given material and coating weight. A dense electron beam results in strong fluorescence; a sparse flow of electrons produces weak fluorescence. In this way light and shade are created in the picture in relation to the varying signal voltage which is applied to the control grid.

The scanning circuitry

Just as an electron beam scans the target of the pick-up tube line by line, so must it do the same in the cathode ray tube in relation to the fluorescent screen. It builds up the total picture at great speed in a series of small discrete elements and then replaces each completed picture with another, similarly created.

The process works because of the eye's persistence of vision. The retina retains an image for about $1/12$ second and we accept as a continuously moving image what is really a fast recurrence of separate images. In broadcast television in the United Kingdom the electron beam moves from one side of the screen to the other 625 times in $1/50$ second to make one complete picture or frame; in most of Europe and in the U.S.A. the line scans which make one frame are 625 in number and in France 815. Scanning systems are further considered on page 382.

In the cathode ray tube the necessary deflection of the electron beam from side to side and the vertical deviation required to give it a rapid flyback from the bottom to the top of the raster are obtained from either charged deflector plates or electromagnetic coils: some of the latter are shown in Fig. 11.2. In modern television charged deflector plates (electrostatic system) are virtually not used, except in test instruments. Scanning coils (electromagnetic scanning) are the usual method of controlling the electron beam. The fluctuating voltage which is applied to the deflector plates or coils and alters the position of the beam is called the timebase. The timebase circuit is the circuit responsible for varying this voltage: a number of different kinds of such circuits exist.

Other circuitry associated with the cathode ray tube synchronizes the scan of the electron beam in this tube with that of the electron beam in the camera tube: both must be scanning the same picture element at the same time, the camera tube in analysing the scene for transmission and the cathode ray tube in rebuilding it in a logical sequence as a comprehensible image. The synchronizing signal consists of a series of pulses but the generation of these need scarcely concern readers of this book.

Another necessary part of the system provides what are known as blanking pulses. These ensure that the screen is blank during the period of flyback, that is when the scanning spot is returning to its beginning point either from the end of a line or from a complete scan of the raster. The blank interval is naturally so brief that the eye is unaware of the absence of picture information during it.

The television image

The television image is constructed from lines and its qualities and defects are related directly to its linear nature. The larger the number of lines and the smaller the scanning spot used to make a complete picture, the better is image detail.

However, there are limits to the number of lines which can be employed in practice, owing partly to transmission difficulties and ultimately to the finite size of the scanning spot. The greater the number of lines the smaller must be the scanning spot and obviously it cannot be infinitely reduced in size.

The viewing conditions and the number of lines influence each other to some extent. An observer near to a monitor cannot see the whole picture, nor escape its linear structure if the lines are not close enough together: many people incorrectly suppose that they will improve their vision of a television picture by peering at it from a short distance when in fact what they really see better in this way are only the lines. However, for anyone standing far away the picture may become too small. The lines should be sufficiently numerous to be indistinguishable at a comfortable viewing distance, and this is about 1·8 m (6 feet) for a picture of which the diagonal is 30 cm (12 inches). We may reasonably say that the proper distance from which to view a television image is to allow 30 cm (1 foot) for every 5 cm (2 inches) of the screen's diagonal.

At the present time the most common number of lines in use with image intensifiers is 625 per frame. Systems based on 1250 lines are available but of course are more expensive and perhaps their purchase is seldom justifiable.

Scanning systems

Whatever the number of lines on a television system, the information they contain is read by means of the regular motion of an electron beam, to and fro across the target of a camera tube or the screen of a monitor. This scanning movement may follow a sequential pattern or it may be of the kind known as interlaced scanning which reduces flicker.

In each case the reading movement is relatively slow, while the flyback to the beginning of a line is much faster. The terms 'slow' and 'fast' must be understood relatively, since one complete scan of the raster occupies only 1/50 or 1/60 second depending on the frequency of the main supply: it is convenient to govern the frame repetition rate by means of the mains frequency.

The rate of frame repetition is a matter of importance, since if it is too low the observer sees merely separate pictures and not a continuously moving one; consequently the image appears to flicker. To avoid this a minimum repetition rate of about 48 per second is necessary.

Sequential scanning

The sequential method of scanning is the simpler. In this—as we have described earlier—the electron beam begins at the top left corner of the raster; moves horizontally—or with a slight downward inclination—to the right; flies rapidly back to the left and begins another similar trace a little lower than the first. From the bottom right corner the beam takes a diagonal route back to its starting point in order to begins a fresh scan. These movements are depicted in Fig. 11.3.

The disadvantages of the sequential scan are technical and need hardly concern radiographers. They are associated with the fact that the method requires a wide frequency band during transmission unless a low picture repetition rate is acceptable. These problems can be avoided by a system of interlaced scanning.

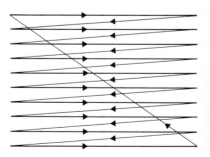

Fig. 11.3 Sequential scanning by an electron beam.

Interlaced scanning

An interlaced scanning system is shown in Fig. 11.4. In this, the electron beams reads only alternate lines in each frame scan. Referring to the diagram the scanning spot begins in the middle of the first line at point A. At the end of this line, fly-back is to the beginning of line 3 and in this manner only the odd numbers of lines are scanned. From the end of the last odd line in the raster, the beam flies back to the starting point of line 2 and goes through all the even lines, finishing at the mid point of the last line at B as indicated in the diagram.

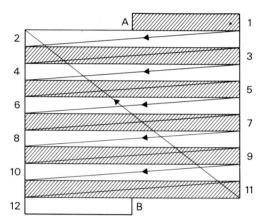

Fig. 11.4 Interlaced scanning. The odd-numbered lines of the raster (striped areas in the diagram) are scanned first, followed then by the even lines (clear areas in the diagram). This system is called double interlaced scanning.

Taking a field of 625 lines as being the one most commonly in use this means that each scan of $312\frac{1}{2}$ lines takes place in 1/50 or 1/60 seconds—depending on the mains frequency—and a complete picture is created in 1/25 or 1/30 second. The frame repetition rate is still 50 or 60 per second from the oberver's point of view but transmission is easier and cheaper because the actual picture frequency is lower.

The system depicted and explained is known as double interlacing : triple interlaced scanning is also used.

X-RAY IMAGE INTENSIFIER TUBE

Principles of operation

Brightness amplification of the fluoroscopic image is obtained by means of an image intensifier tube. The principles of an image intensifier tube are depicted diagrammatically in Fig. 11.5.

The tube provides an evacuated glass envelope at one end of which is a fluorescent screen, the input phosphor. X rays falling upon this screen produce light photons in the expected way. One X-ray photon of high energy may release thousands of light photons. (In accordance with the principle of the conservation of energy, the released light photons will have lower energy.)

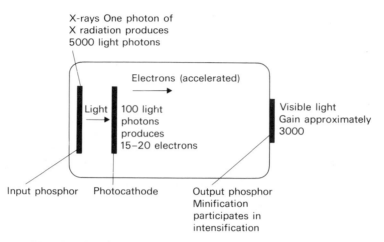

Fig. 11.5 The principles of an image intensifier tube.

Adjacent to the input phosphor of the image intensifier tube is a photocathode which produces electrons when light strikes it in the ratio of one electron for about five absorbed light photons.

In the body of the intensifier tube the electrons are accelerated and focused by means of applied voltages and so reach the output phosphor. This is similar in material to the screen of a cathode ray tube, that is it fluoresces when electrons strike it.

However, the fluorescent image which results on the output phosphor of the intensifier tube is much brighter than the ingoing image by reason of two separate facts:

1 the electron acceleration;
2 the small size of the output phosphor compared with the input phosphor.

Looking at the second of these points a little more closely, we can say that the amplification in brightness is related to the reduction in area. An intensifier tube of which the input phosphor is 13 cm (5 inches) in diameter may have an output phosphor only 1·3 cm (0·5 inches) across. Such a reduction to 1/10 of the original area produces an intensification in brightness of 100 times.

The overall gain from an image intensifier tube of this kind may be several thousandfold, but it is impossible to be exact when experimental conditions are not specified. A statement may be made of the gain factor of an image intensifier but it is meaningless, since this factor compares the brightness of the output phosphor with the brightness of a standard fluorescent screen: and no such universal standard exists. A more reliable indicator is found in the *conversion factor*, which is expressed as the ratio of the luminance of the output phosphor of an image intensifier tube to the input radiation dose rate. The conversion factor necessarily is influenced by radiation quality: experimental conditions—of kilovoltage and beam filtration—have been stated for obtaining it.

Construction and function

Fig. 11.6 illustrates diagrammatically the structure of an image intensifier tube. Its essential constituents are:
1   an evacuated glass—or in some instances metal—envelope;
2   an input screen (input phosphor) which is in intimate contact with a photocathode;
3   an electron focusing and accelerating system (electron lens);
4   an output screen (output phosphor).

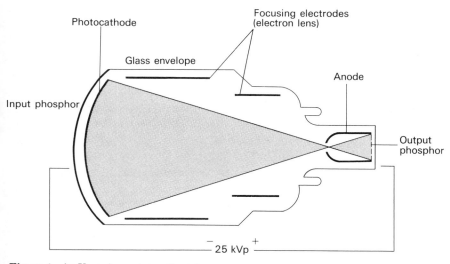

Fig. 11.6   An X-ray image intensifier tube.

The input screen

For electron-optical reasons, the input phosphor is domed: it is described geometrically as the sector of a sphere). It is made by vaporizing sodium-activated caesium iodide on a spherical surface of aluminium; this gives a very thin input screen, having little intrinsic unsharpness.

Overall, the unsharpness from an image intensifier tube depends on:
1 the characteristics of the input and output screens;
2 the characteristics of the electron-optics (the photocathode and the electron-focusing and electron-accelerating electrodes).

Relative to certain other phosphors which have been used, caesium iodide emits a larger number of light photons per X-ray quantum. Its use in the way described improves the sensitivity and resolution of an image intensifier tube.

Image intensifiers are usually described in terms of the diameter of the input phosphor: 12·5 cm (5 inches), 15 cm (6 inches) and 23 cm (9 inches) are commonly available 'sizes' of image intensifier; more recently, a 35 cm (14 inches) intensifier tube has become available. Obviously, the nature of the clinical task is influential in forming a preference for one or another of these intensifier tubes: for instance, generally speaking, gastrointestinal examinations are more easily performed when the input field is large; whilst a smaller intensifier would be happily chosen in the case of a children's hospital. It may be noted, however, that as the size of the input field enlarges, so also do the intensifier's volume and weight; inevitably the equipment becomes more difficult to support and to handle.

The photocathode

The function of the photocathode is to convert the light pattern produced at the input phosphor to a correspondent pattern of electrons. Consequently it is important that the shape of the photocathode should conform intimately to the shape of the input phosphor. If there is not a close association between them, light from the input phosphor will spread before it reaches the photocathode: this will result in blurring and a loss of image detail.

Although a close contact is essential, nevertheless the photocathode must be separated from the input phosphor or the sensitivity of the photocathode will deteriorate with time. The separating layer must be both thin and transparent: it may be glass or an inactive chemical.

The material of the photocathode is a combination of alkalis: antimony, potassium, caesium and sodium. The description *multi-alkali* is sometimes applied to the photocathode as an expression of its compound nature.

The electron lens

The term *electron lens* describes a system of electrodes which influences the velocity and direction of an electron beam. Such a system is found in an X-ray image intensifier tube and is obtained from the effects of an electric field existing between the photocathode and other electrodes within the glass envelope. The electrodes composing the electron lens are:

1 an anode cylinder;
2 a number of annular focusing electrodes placed between the photocathode and the anode.

In Fig. 11.6, two such focusing electrodes are depicted but there may be more than this.

A potential difference of about 25 kV is applied between cathode and anode; the cathode voltage is zero and the anode voltage about 25 kV positive in respect of the cathode. The voltages on the focusing electrodes cannot satisfactorily be quantified here but vary in different instances. To make a general statement, we may say—of two such electrodes depicted in Fig. 11.6—that the voltage on the one nearer to the photocathode might be + 200 V; and on the one nearer the anode might lie between 3 and 8 kV positive; it is apparent that electrodes nearer to the photocathode are associated with lower voltages than those near to the anode.

The output screen

Entering the anode cylinder, the electrons—no longer in a field of electrical stress—diverge towards the output phosphor in the manner indicated in Fig. 11.6. On the output phosphor, which they strike with high kinetic energy, the electrons create a fluorescent image which corresponds in detail to the original but is much brighter for the reasons already discussed. As shown in the diagram, the electrons' lines of travel through the neck of the anode result in the image on the output phosphor being inverted relative to that on the input phosphor.

Light from the output phosphor must be prevented from passing in reverse through the vacuum tube to the photocathode (optical feedback), as additional electrons released in this way would deteriorate the final image. For this reason the output screen is backed by a thin sheet of aluminium.

The material of the output screen is zinc cadmium sulphide activated with silver; the screen is mounted on a thin sheet of glass.

Electron-optical magnification

Many image intensifier tubes offer a facility allowing the operator to obtain a magnified view. The electron-optical system is the agent which achieves this, through an alteration in the potential on the focusing electrodes nearest to the anode cylinder.

The effect is a change in the minification of the image, the minification ratio becoming smaller. Use of only the central area of the input screen (narrow collimation of the X-ray beam) and display of the image over the full area of the output phosphor result in a magnified visible image.

Fig. 11.7 depicts a dual-field image intensifier tube: it illustrates how the action of the electrodes affects the minification ratio and how the collimated X-ray beam is used to obtain an optical magnification at the output phosphor.

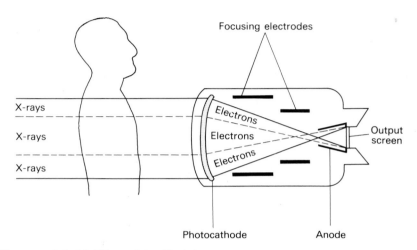

Fig. 11.7   A dual field image intensifier tube.

Press-button switches enable the operator conveniently to select either condition of operation at will, with automatic adjustment of:

1   X-ray beam collimation;

2   radiation intensity in order to maintain a constant brilliance of the output-phosphor (this implies the use of a higher kilovoltage for magnification, as the input phosphor must be more strongly excited);

3   the electron lens.

An example of an image intensifier tube of this kind is one known as the 23/13 cm (9/5 inch). In this tube the full sized field normally displayed is 23 cm (9 inches) in diameter, while the magnified area corresponds to the central 13 cm (5 inches) of the full circle. Similarly we may have a 28/18 cm (11/7 inches) dual-field intensifier tube.

Enclosure

The image intensifier tube normally is enclosed in a metal case or shield, the purpose of which is to provide mechanical, anti-magnetic and radiation protection. The housing must be light-proof but it is important that it should be dry and enclosed as well. It must be enclosed in order to prevent the entry of (a) moisture which could result in sparking and (b) dust which would be attracted by electrostatic forces to the viewing face.

An adaptor plate allows the intensifier to be fitted to the fluoroscopic table on the support which links together the image receptor and the X-ray tube. If the intensifier is over-table, it may be—but is not necessarily—balanced by means of a ceiling suspension bracket. A small image intensifier tube can be mounted opposite an X-ray tube on a C-shaped support and used as a mobile unit (see Chapter 9, p. 359); and readers of this book may encounter in their hospitals the more intricate and subtle mountings devised—and indeed required—for television fluoroscopy of the heart.

Automatic compensation for changes in beam attenuation (ABC)

During most investigations, a patient undergoing fluoroscopy is not a passive, more or less homogeneous subject but offers dynamic attenuations of the X-ray beam. For example, during an examination of the gastrointestinal tract a radiologist may begin with a routine survey of the thorax and may 'follow' the swallowed contrast agent along the alimentary tract, from its first ingestion by the mouth to its passage through the pylorus and the first part of the duodenum. Then, studies of the stomach and duodenal cap may entail rotation of the patient to oblique and even to lateral projections of the region. Thus, in the course of one examination, the subject's radiopacity may change from producing very little absorption to producing a high absorption of the X-ray beam; and may as quickly change again, as the radiologist manipulates the image intensifier and the patient.

Unless compensation is made for these fluctuations, the result must be an unstable brightness of the image, which at one extreme will exhibit dazzle or flare and at the other extreme will appear 'too dim'; in either circumstance, detail cannot be appreciated.

Essentially there are two ways in which a constant image brightness may be obtained for various degrees of X-ray attenuation within a subject. They are:

1   to vary the electric gain in the television channel so that the brightness on the monitor remains uniform, despite variations in the incoming signal;
2   to alter the intensity of the X-ray beam applied to the patient, increasing it as the subject's radioparency decreases, so that the input signal to the intensifier remains virtually constant.

The first of these methods of brightness control entails little circuitry and corresponds to the automatic gain control incorporated in any radio set for the purpose of maintaining the volume of its output against a fading of the input signal. For television fluoroscopy the second method is the more satisfactory, although the more complicated. It is better for several reasons. One of them is that image brightness is maintained without amplification of noise in the system: increasing the gain on a television camera tube must raise both brightness and noise levels at the same time.

When image brightness is controlled by altering the intensity of the X-ray beam, a further advantage lies in the direction of radiation safety. A system which monitors and controls the dose rate at an image intensifier's face is doing likewise in respect of the patient. In theory and provided that the system has been properly set and is without fault, the patient should receive no higher level of dose than is necessary for the required image quality.

Regulation of the dose rate at the image intensifier could be achieved by an energetic radiographer through repeated adjustments of millampere and kilovoltage settings; that is a simple but—in general—not really a practical solution to the problem. Automatic regulation of image brightness is necessary during cine fluorography and is now a required feature of an image intensifier. It is often denoted by the letters ABC which stand for automatic brightness control; perhaps the expression *automatic beam control* may be preferred for the system under discussion since it controls the intensity of X rays reaching the image receptor and is independent of the gain and sensitivity of the television camera tube. Most equipments include a facility which permits reversion to manual control of the X-ray output, if an operator so wishes during examination of a 'thick' subject.

Stabilization of dose rate

The dose rate at the intensifier may be stabilized by any of several means, as follows:

1 automatic control of tube voltage, the value of the tube current (milliamperes) being preset;

2 automatic control of tube current, the tube kilovoltage being preset;

3 automatic control of tube current and tube voltage in proportion to one another;

4 automatic control of tube voltage and tube current in inverse proportion to one another.

The first system is the one which enacts automatically what a radiographer most likely would do during manual operation of a generator's controls. The third system links tube voltage and tube current together over a wide range of values: for example, 0·6 mA at 40 kV might increase to 3·2 mA at 110 kV. This method of brightness stabilization can result in lower image contrast than manual control of the generator might give, since kilovoltage settings are usually a little higher than 'normal'.

The last method of beam control is thought to be particularly suitable for subjects where the differences occurring in the attenuation of the X-ray beam are only slight; that is, where the subject has low contrast, for example the gall bladder. Since the set fluoroscopic kilovoltage is always the lowest that will result in the required image brightness, the fluoroscopic image may be expected to have more contrast than is usually the case.

It will be sufficient for the readers of this book if here we explain more fully just one means of controlling the dose at an image intensifier's face. The means now to be considered is the one which has been listed first: it effects an automatic adjustment of the X-ray tube's kilovoltage, raising this when the dose rate falls and decreasing it when the dose rate at the intensifier rises, in order to maintain an image brightness which is effectively constant.

Automatic control of kilovoltage

Fig. 11.8 indicates schematically an arrangement whereby part (about 5%) of the light from the image intensifier's output screen is fed to a photomultiplier (see p. 185). The photomultiplier produces a current proportional in value to the amount of light reaching it.

The light monitored usually is that originating from the central area of the input phosphor and this area is described as a dominant. When the

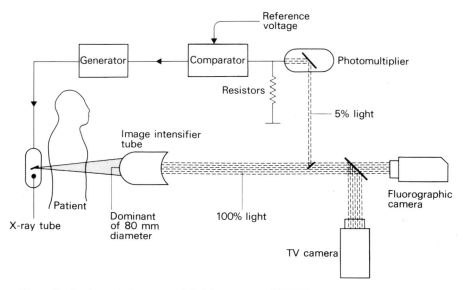

Fig. 11.8 A schematic for automatic brightness control (ABC).

dominant is central the regulating process becomes independent of the effects of high intensity primary radiation which might bypass a subject occupying only part of the intensifier's input field; for example this circumstance might occur—or be allowed to occur—during fluoroscopy of the vertebral column. The proper location of the dominant, which has a diameter of about 80 mm, is as important in this context as in association with automatic timing of the duration of a radiographic exposure.

The current from the anode of the photomultiplier is taken to a number of variable resistors, giving rise to a voltage drop across these. The greater the current flowing through a given resistor, the greater is the associated voltage drop: and so the fall in voltage is proportional to the brightness of light from the dominant.

A comparator compares the voltage drop with a reference or nominal voltage, having a value of perhaps 5 volts. To put this another way, the comparator is comparing a varying voltage with another which is constant in value; and the varying voltage is changing in correspondence with the brightness of the light signal from the intensifier.

If the value of the variable voltage is other than the nominal value, the comparator—operating through a number of control circuits—causes the high tension transformer to drive 'upwards' or 'downwards'; and thus—if image brightness is low—to increase and—if image brightness is high—to decrease the kilovoltage across the X-ray tube. A reader, who is in doubt about the design of a transformer from which the voltage output might be influenced by automatic means, should look again at the reference on p. 82 to a motor-driven sledge, which can move a contact over a stripped section of the windings of a transformer, under the influence of a control circuit. The same principle is relevant here.

Selection of dose rate

Many equipments with automatic brightness controls give the operator push button selection of one of two dose rates: these are designated by the relative terms 'high' and 'low' and their selection operates so long as ABC is the chosen mode. (Should the fluoroscopist decide to employ manual control of tube kilovoltage and current, this must obviate the use of a preselected dose rate.) In the case of the ABC system described in the previous paragraphs, a change in the dose rate can be affected by alteration of the reference voltage in the comparison stage.

It is important in practice to recognize that selection of the higher dose rate does not increase the brightness of the image on the intensifier. Image quality will be improved because quantum noise is reduced. In the interests of keeping radiation doses to acceptable minima, fluoroscopists should reserve selection of the higher dose rate to instances of diagnostic difficulty.

Aberrations of image intensifier tubes

Images which are put to technical use should reproduce a subject truthfully and in detail: but—like many other image-makers—an X-ray image intensifier tube has certain characteristics which entail departure from the truth. Three of these are briefly described below.

Distortion

An aberration, which in optics is described as a pin-cushion distortion, occurs in an X-ray image intensifier tube because there is a change in the minification ratio over the full area of the image: the ratio becomes smaller towards the periphery. The minification ratio of an intensifier tube is simply the ratio of the diameter of its input fluorescent screen to the diameter of the image projected upon the output phosphor. Because of geometric and electron-optical effects, the ratio is not constant over the entire field: there is greater reduction in detail size at the centre of the output field than occurs on its periphery. This alteration in scale causes straight lines on the periphery to appear as curves which are convex toward the centre of the field; the nearer are lines to the margins of the field, the more marked is the effect. In practice this is not usually an introducer of diagnostic error, but care should be taken—perhaps especially so during orthopaedic surgery—to keep the area of clinical interest always in the centre of the scene.

Vignetting

Vignetting is an optical aberration which occurs in all compound lenses and results in a lens transmitting less light at its periphery than at its centre. Consequently, the central region is the brightest part of the image. In the case of image intensifiers, the term describes—as might be expected—an appearance that the image of an irradiated homogeneous subject is darker at the edges than at the centre.

There are three reasons for the property of vignetting by an intensifier tube:

1 an X-ray beam does not have a uniform distribution of energy;

2 the domed shape of the input phosphor puts the periphery of the screen further from the source of radiation than is the centre; thus radiation intensity is less at the periphery relative to the intensity measurable at the centre;

3   the minification ratio is smaller at the periphery; this ratio governs the gain and conversion factor of the intensifier tube, these being reduced as the ratio becomes smaller.

Drop in resolving power

Statements of the resolving power of an image-making system express the system's ability to carry information of the smallest details of a subject. During television fluoroscopy the properties of the image intensifier tube are not the only parameters of resolution. Others, more influential in practice, include: the size of the focal spot of the X-ray tube; quantum noise and the signal to noise ratio; low dose rate and output brightness; low contrast in the subject.

So far as the image intensifier tube itself is concerned, the feature to be noticed here is that—for electron optical reasons—the resolving power at the centre is higher than at the periphery of the image field.

The intensifier's resolving power can be manipulated through selection of the potentials applied to the electron lens and usually a compromise is sought: settings are made which give a little less than optimum resolution at the centre, in order to 'even out' the resolution obtainable over most of the field and ensure that only at the extreme periphery is it likely that the lowered resolving power will be perceptible to the majority of observers.

In the case of a dual-field image intensifier tube, during those times when only the central part of the input screen is utilized, resolution is uniform over the entire area of the projected image.

Viewing the intensified image

The output phosphor of the image intensifier tube has a diameter of perhaps 1·25–2·5 cm (0·5 to 1 inch), and this of course is much too small for an observer to appreciate detail by looking at it directly. In any case, owing to the cross-over of the electrons' lines of travel, the image is upside-down. Both these effects mean that a magnifying optical system is necessary at the output phosphor before the image can be viewed.

The objective lens

In front of the output phosphor of the image intensifier tube is mounted a basic objective lens collimated to infinity, that is the lens gives a parallel beam of light. An objective lens is by definition one which forms an image of an original object: it produces an image of whatever is under observation.

In this case the function of the objective lens is to form an image of the appearances on the output phosphor of the intensifier tube and to introduce the light into an optical system, which will transmit it to a viewing optic or a vidicon camera, usually the latter. The lens of the viewing and recording system and the objective lens, although they are separately designed, together make what is known as a tandem optical system. The coupling of two lenses in a one-to-one tandem arrangement both conveys more light and readily allows the beam to be split for the introduction of a cine camera or a serial fluorographic camera. Fig. 11.9 schematically indicates such an optical system for an X-ray image intensifier.

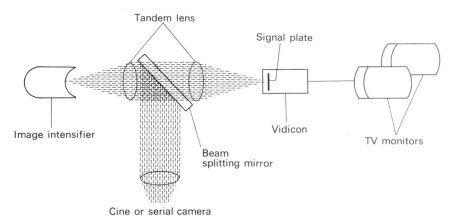

Fig. 11.9   A schematic of the optical system of an X-ray image intensifier tube.

The cone of light emitted by the optical system is called the *exit pupil*. In the case of direct viewing the observer must place his eye in this beam in order to see the image. Most people prefer the exit pupil to be wide enough in diameter to cover both eyes. If it is not, the image cannot be displayed on an open mirror and the operator must view the screen monocularly, in the way in which a telescope or microscope is used. It then becomes more difficult to keep the image continuously under observation, as anyone will know who has used a telescope. Slight head movements, or motion of the subject observed, easily cause the watcher to lose sight of whatever is being studied.

Direct vision with a mirror

An open mirror placed to reflect the light from the optical system provides the most satisfactory method of viewing the intensified image by direct vision. The mirror can be rotated and thus altered to different positions which are appropriate for viewing an erect patient when the fluoroscopic table is upright or one who is recumbent upon the table.

The image distributor

A gadget known as an image distributor or light splitter is usually fitted which provides channels for up to three viewing or recording systems.

The image distributor consists of three mirrors mounted on a common spindle. The spindle is motor driven by a movement designed to maintain stability in the mirrors' position. The mirrors are beam-splitting in type; that is, they partially reflect and partially transmit light, the light in this case being that from the objective lens. Two of the mirrors may reflect 90 per cent of the beam and transmit 10 per cent: the third mirror does the reverse.

The effect of the image distributor is to split the light from the objective lens into two out of a possible three parts. We might suppose, for example, that the three possibilities consist of a viewing mirror, a cine camera and a serial camera. By means of pre-set controls the apparatus would permit the following procedures.

1 Fluoroscopy, the observer receiving 90 per cent of the beam and the remaining 10 per cent being lost.

2 Cinefluorography, the cine camera receiving 90 per cent of the beam, while the observer has 10 per cent in the viewing mirror to enable him to watch the phenomena he is filming. (This small portion is not so inadequate as it sounds: it is 10 per cent of the tube current when it is boosted from a fluoroscopic value to the higher milliamperes needed for radiography.)

3 Serial radiography, when similarly the associated camera receives 90 per cent of the light and the observer has 10 per cent in the viewing mirror as a monitoring channel.

The image distributor provides a total of six possible combinations, one of which is to feed all the light to a television system.

A two-way mirror viewer for direct vision is another option. This device enables two or more people to observe the fluoroscopic appearances together in separate mirrors and could be helpful during, for example, cardiac catheterization if closed circuit television were unavailable.

The recording of the intensified image will be further considered in the next section of this chapter.

Closed circuit television

The use of closed circuit television to view the intensified image—as opposed to direct vision of the output phosphor—has several self-evident advantages.

1 Almost any number of people can study the image at the same time.

Monitors may be situated not only in the X-ray room but elsewhere in the department or in the hospital, wherever there is need of such a demonstration for teaching or consultative purposes.

2 The monitor or monitors in the X-ray room can be placed in any convenient locality: for example, one may be ceiling-mounted and on a pivot allowing it to face anywhere about the room, while another, smaller one is in the radiographer's control cubicle. The radiologist is not restricted in position at the fluoroscopic table.

3 The monitor can be satisfactorily viewed in a room shaded only from direct sunlight. This makes any necessary surgical procedure—for example, that involved in placing a catheter—easier and safer to undertake.

4 The monitor provides an additional, independent means of varying the brightness and contrast of the intensified image.

There are some disadvantages to viewing by closed circuit television which are mainly associated with recording the intensified image (see below). However, apart from this, television inevitably deteriorates detail, because it is an indirect method of viewing. Some loss of sharpness occurs in every optical or electron-optical system through which an image is passed.

The arrangements for television pick-up of the image from the output phosphor of the intensifier tube are indicated in Fig. 11.9. The television camera tube associated with the image intensifier tube is photoconductive in type, for instance a vidicon (see p. 373). The scanning system has 625 lines.

RECORDING THE INTENSIFIED IMAGE

The process of photographing the image from a fluorescent screen is called fluorography. The fluorescent appearances with which we are concerned are those produced by image intensifying equipment and it is useful to consider now the reasons why—although we have brightened it—the image is not ideally sharp.

The resolution of the intensified image

Resolution is the process by which something is separated into its component parts: in an image, resolution refers to the amount of detail which is observable. Whenever images are formed and recorded, detail is present to a greater or less extent, depending upon certain characteristics of the image-forming and image-recording systems. We speak of the resolving power of such systems. (In medical radiography significant characteristics begin with the size of the focal spot of the X-ray tube and the geometry of image projection.)

Tests can be made which will discover resolving power and give it meaningful expression. It may be formulated as the number of pairs of black and white lines which an image-forming or image-recording device can demonstrate in a length of 1 mm. With decreasing separation between a series of parallel lines on a chart, increasing optical refinement is needed to show that they are separate.

The visible image

The human eye itself is an image-recording instrument and we know from everyday experience how limited its resolving power sometimes is. When we look at a test chart, the edges of thin lines placed very close together soon merge one into the other and we become unable to distinguish each individually at normal viewing distances.

The quality of an image is dependent on the amount of information of a subject which the image conveys to an observer and it is significantly influenced by the resolution obtainable from the system producing the image. Unfortunately when an image must pass through a number of stages in a system, resolution is lost at each successive stage: detail becomes poorer the more complex we make the chain of processes.

In medical radiography with high definition intensifying screens the maximum resolution obtainable is estimated at about 5 line pairs per millimetre. This is an example of a 'short' image-forming chain, having few 'links' or stages. In fluoroscopy, the resolution of the image seen by an observer using closed circuit television necessarily is worse because detail is lost within an extended image-formulating system. This loss of detail affects not only observation of the fluorescent image but also its recording. Such recording includes usage of a suitable camera, several being available.

Fluorographic cameras

A camera introduced to an image intensifying system, for the purpose of recording fluoroscopic appearances, may do so from either of two situations.
1 The camera may be linked one-to-one to a suitable television monitor and thus record an image present on the monitor screen.
2 The camera may be inserted between the image intensifier tube and the television pick-up tube; by means of a light-splitting mirror, the camera then receives the image directly from the output screen of the image intensifier tube, in the manner indicated in Fig. 11.9. Its lens should be as close as is feasible to the objective lens of the intensifier's optical system.

A little thought may demonstrate that the second method of procedure is generally preferred. There are several reasons for this.

1 The camera's position at the intensifier by-passes the television link in the optical and electron-optical chain and thus image resolution should be higher.

2 Television monitors—especially inexpensive ones—are readily affected by voltage variations. (X-ray departments generally are ill advised to economise on the purchase price of television monitors.) When the light reaching the television camera is relatively poor—as it is in the case of an image intensifier tube—the monitor screen may exhibit a variability of brightness which can spoil a film record of the appearances (through causing random variations in film blackening).

3 Television is a line-scanning process and may produce line patterns on a film.

4 If cinefluorography is the procedure in hand, the recording speed (number of frames per second) of a camera placed in the television system is limited by the framing speed of the television system itself.

The cameras used for fluorography are either cine cameras or serial cameras which will make a single exposure or a short sequence of exposures at a maximum rate of 6 per second, or perhaps 12 per second.

Cinefluorography

Cinefluorography puts heavy electrical loads on an X-ray tube and generator. It necessitates rapid rates of exposure (frames per second): 16 f.p.s. is the minimum number if the images are to be appreciated as a continuous dynamic record.

The record is made usually on 35 mm (roll) film, although 16 mm cameras have been used; these can run at higher speeds but the images are much smaller.

Cinefluorographic equipment often is pulsed in operation. This means that the X-ray tube, which is grid controlled, is not continuously energized during filming but passes current only during those periods when the camera shutter is open. The alternating periods, in which the film is moved through the camera to obtained the next frame, naturally require the shutter to be closed. To continue to energize the tube during these intervals is to produce X rays which cannot affect the film and merely administer an unnecessary dose to the subject of the examination. The non-pulsed and the pulsed methods of operation are diagrammatically summarized in Fig. 11.10.

Serial fluorography

Cameras for single shot and serial operation use either cut film (100 × 100 mm) or roll film (70 mm or 105 mm). The larger film formats are

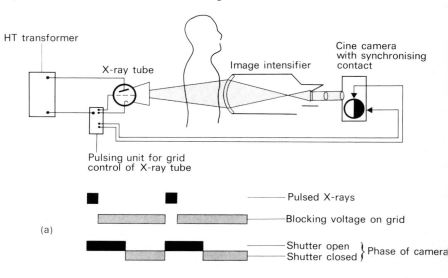

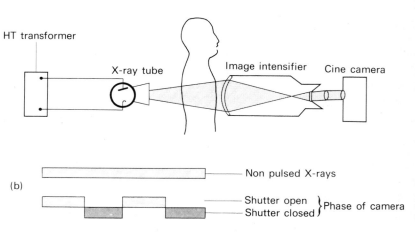

Fig. 11.10 (a) A schematic to show how a grid-controlled X-ray tube can be synchronized with a cine camera's shutter so that X rays are emitted only when the shutter is open.

(b) Cinefluorography when the X-ray tube is continuously energized, whether the camera shutter is open or closed.

readable by the majority of observers without magnification. Since it is mechanically more difficult to move separate sheets of film than to wind a roll, the 100 mm cameras are slower.

It is a required characteristic of both types of fluorographic camera that any exposed single film or short length of roll film may be removed easily from the camera as a daylight operation at any time. This is to enable a particular patient's fluorographs to be extracted immediately for processing and examination. In the case of the 100 mm camera, extraction of the exposed film involves simple withdrawal of a receiving magazine; in the case of a roll film camera, it is necessary to operate a blade which cuts the film before the magazine (reel) can be removed.

Video tape recording

The appearance of the intensified image can be recorded on video tape. This is a process of magnetic recording, similar to what is done with sound on a tape recorder although it is more complex. The recording apparatus—as one might expect—looks like a big tape recorder. It has two large recording heads and similar control features for record, standby, play back, rewind and fast forward. A tape index enables any portion of the tape to be found quickly.

Video tape is a 2·5 cm (1 inch) or 1·25 cm (0·5 inch) tape, along the upper edge of which can be two audio channels. These can be used for synchronous recording of—for example—the patient's speech or heart sounds, together with a commentary which may be made either simultaneously with the video signals or independently later. The audio and video tracks can be erased, again either simultaneously or independently. At the lower edge of the tape there is a single track on which synchronizing pulses are registered. The width of the tape affects resolution: greater width means improved detail.

In operation, the video signal from the X-ray television chain is fed to the tape recorder by means of cables. The recorder does not necessarily have to stand close to the X-ray table as it can be remotely controlled from the table side. Afterwards the tape can be played back—at once or at any later time—either on the existing monitors for the X-ray set or on any other monitor anywhere else, for example in a radiological reporting room or a lecture theatre.

The advantages of making the record on video tape as opposed to cine film are several.

1 No special projection equipment is needed.
2 No processing is required. The image can be viewed immediately.
3 The system entails a smaller radiation dose for the subject than does an equivalent record on film. This is because the tube factors chosen for fluoroscopy require no alteration for video tape.
4 Video tape can be used again and again if the image is first erased. The

tape is expensive but each reel provides virtually one hour's running time. The image is satisfactory for retention as a permanent record.

5   The contrast and brightness of the taped image can be varied to suit the tastes of individual observers by means of the corresponding controls on the viewing monitor.

The simplicity with which it is obtained and the immediate availability of the video record make this an excellent form of preliminary survey during such radiological procedures as angiocardiography. For diagnostic purposes a cine film is usually preferred, mainly because of the higher resolution of the image.

Video image storage

A video disc recorder may be used to provide storage capacity (a 'memory') for the output from the television camera tube during television fluoroscopy. The disc is magnetic and about 10–15 cm in diameter; it carries a variable number of tracks from 1 to 4 and is capable of storing several hundred images more or less indefinitely.

The disc recorder may be manually operated but very often its mode is automatic. In clinical practice its main application is to provide a 'freeze' and 'recall' facility during use of a mobile image intensifier for the X-ray control of orthopaedic surgery (see page 364). This means that interfacing circuitry in the equipment prevents the continuation of a fluoroscopic exposure for longer than is necessary to record the video image (2 seconds or less). An immediate and automatic play-back of the stored image then appears on the television monitor: the operator is provided, thus, with still or 'frozen' picture which can be studied for any length of time without further irradiation of the patient concerned.

Through manually operated push-button control, it is possible also to store any single television fluoroscopic image and to recall it subsequently. If a second television monitor is available, the stored image may be displayed simultaneously with visualization of the real-time image. This would allow a surgeon, during a hip-pinning for example, to study anteroposterior and lateral projections together.

A PANEL-TYPE IMAGE INTENSIFIER

In the field of image brightening, a different type of image intensifier has been developed which offers some advantage in certain situations. At its heart is a two-stage panel-type intensifier tube, the flat design of which has two consequences of practical significance:

1   the intensifier can replace a standard fluorescent screen on a conventional fluoroscopic/radiographic table and does not inconveniently increase the weight of the equipment;

2   the intensifier becomes particularly suitable for fitting in small or low ceilinged radiodiagnostic rooms which may have occasional usage for gastrointestinal fluoroscopy but are structurally unsuitable for the installation of larger intensifiers.

Relative to the systems for television fluoroscopy described elsewhere in this chapter, the panel-type intensifier requires about 2 to 3 times the dose rate, if a sufficiently bright image is to be obtained in dimmed room-light. It is limited to direct viewing and cannot be extended to include a television display or any other indirect technique. Any recording of the image must be by direct radiography.

Fig. 11.11 illustrates the functional principles of the two-stage intensifier. Like others, it is a vacuum and has a caesium iodide input screen. This is about 200 mm in diameter and in intimate contact with it is a photocathode (photocathode 1 in the diagram).

The expected energy conversions occur, as in other intensifier tubes: X-ray quanta on the input screen are converted to light photons and these produce an emission of electrons from photocathode 1. Under the influence of an applied potential difference, these electrons are accelerated in straight lines to the first fluorescent screen, creating on this a brighter (intermediate) image.

The associated photocathode (2) performs a second transition of energy from light photons to electrons; these are accelerated through another potential difference (of approximately 20 kV) to reach a second fluorescent screen, which is the output or viewing screen. This screen emits a green light.

The sequence of events just described has brightened the output image in two stages of electron acceleration. There is no further image-processing and—since input and output screens are the same size—the recording ratio is 1:1. In Fig. 11.11, the reader will see a fibreoptic coupling between the first fluorescent screen and the second photocathode. The fibreoptic's function is to 'clean up' the image, that is to enhance visible resolution which is of the order of 2 line-pairs per millimetre and should be optimum over the whole field (see p. 394 for an explanation of why an image intensifier tube may not be employed at its optimum resolving power in many instances).

The two-stage intensifier just described is simple and relatively inexpensive. It should be free of both optical distortion and the artefacts arising from electromagnetic and electrical fluctuations; but inevitably its applications are limited.

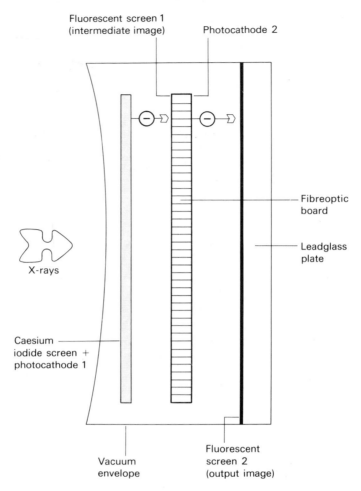

Fig. 11.11 A two-stage panel-type image intensifier tube.

GLOSSARY OF TERMS

The following glossary of television and allied terms is not a dictionary. It is intended to provide the meanings of the more commonly met technical expressions, so that radiographers and electronic engineers can talk to each other about intensifying equipment in the department in a jargon which both understand. Some of the terms included in the following list have been more fully explained in the preceding chapter: others appear here for the first time.

Aspect ratio The proportion of length to height of the raster.

Audio signal see **Signal.**

Beam current The electron current of the beam reaching the screen of a cathode ray tube.

Conversion factor The accepted method of describing the gain of an image intensifier tube in terms of output luminance against input dose rate.

Dark current The current which flows through the photoconductive layer of a television camera tube when no light is falling on it.

Exit pupil The cone of light emitted by the optical system of an image intensifier tube.

Field see **Frame** and **Scanning field.**

Fly-back The name given to the rapid return of the scanning spot (see below) either from the end of a line to the point at which it will begin the next line, or at the end of a frame to the zero point from which it begins a fresh scan. When the brilliance control of a monitor is advanced flyback lines may be apparent.

Frame The area of the picture on the monitor screen. Similarly, the separate exposures or still pictures which succeed each other to give the illusion of continuous movement in cinematography.

Gas spot A bright spot on the output phosphor of a vacuum intensifier tube. It is due to ionization of residual gas molecules in the tube as a result of a high concentration of electrons: such concentrations occur at the cross-over point where electrons converge and then diverge at the anode focus.

Getter A device present in an image intensifying tube for the purpose of eliminating the gas spot (see above). It collects gas molecules from within the tube envelope and may or may not be activated from outside. In either case the process is automatic and the getter consequently makes little impact on the user of the equipment.

Grid An electrode which controls the flow of electrons.

Noise Variations in the video signal caused by extraneously varying currents in any of a number of components. Electronic noise appears as random scintillations on the screen which detract from the picture' quality. See also **Quantum noise.**

Picture element The very small section of a scene at which the electron beam of a television camera tube 'looks' at any one time and which determines the instantaneous values of the signal current: the smallest fragment of picture information. The movement of the beam from one picture element to the next in a series of lines covers the whole field and is so rapid that the eye believes the picture to be continuous. In one frame there may be 50,000 to 100,000 picture elements.

Quantum noise A grainy, mottled appearance in the image on an intensifier tube which is caused by the number of X-ray photons striking the input phosphor being insufficient to create a clear image. It is apparent when— in the conviction that radiation dose reduction is supremely important— fluoroscopy is attempted at too low a level of X-ray tube current. There must be sufficient X rays present to form the picture : detail perceptibility is very dependent on the number of absorbed X-ray quanta.

Raster The rectangular picture area traced by the scanning spot.

Re-trace see **Fly-back.**

Scanning The process of analysing a scene into picture elements in a camera tube, or of building an image from picture elements in a cathode ray tube.

Scanning field The area explored by the scanning beam in either a camera tube or cathode ray tube.

Scanning spot The small electronic spot which sweeps continuously over every part of the scene or image to be televised and splits these into separate picture elements. Other things being equal, the smaller the scanning spot the finer the detail produced.

Signal Electronic information. This may relate to vision (video signal) or to sound (audio signal).

Timebase The fluctuating voltage which is used to vary the lateral position of the scanning spot. As the scanning process is zigzag in character, the motion may be described as saw-tooth and the voltage which produces it as saw-tooth waveform.

Video signal see **Signal.**

Chapter 12
Fluoroscopic/Radiographic Tables

Many X-ray tables are made having the primary purpose of fluoroscopy of the gastrointestinal tract, but combining such a facility with the characteristics of a general radiographic bucky table. In a small radiodiagnostic department, which has only one X-ray room, a fluoroscopic/radiographic table of this kind may be the department's only X-ray table. Such tables are usually well designed for their dual role and no doubt readers of this book will have made a practical acquaintance with one or another of them already; because they are multi-purpose, they are sometimes called combination or universal tables.

Like cars, cameras and much other technical equipment, fluoroscopic/ radiographic tables show various differences from each other: these differences may amount to a number of ways of doing the same thing, depending on the table's manufacturer, or they may reflect the sophistication of the table's performance. It is intended now to describe the main features of certain typical fluoroscopic/radiographic tables: the reader should try to relate these descriptions to equipment with which some practical familiarity has been gained. A table at the end of this chapter (see p. 433) categorizes fluoroscopic/radiographic tables in six groups and indicates the relevance of each group to the workloads of radiodiagnostic departments.

A STANDARD FLUOROSCOPIC TABLE

The fluoroscopic table now to be considered is of a standard conventional pattern: this description means that an X-ray tube is situated beneath the table, whilst the image receptor—commonly an image intensifier but alternatively a fluorescent screen—occupies a position above the table.

When the table is used for general radiography, a separate X-ray tube is associated with it as a rule. This second X-ray tube is mounted in the room by one or other of the usual means, a floor-ceiling tubestand or a ceiling hanger (see Chapter 7). In certain simple equipment, the fitting of the undertable X-ray tube may be such that it can be manoeuvred from this position and applied to general radiography, though this may be limited to the use of only a horizontal beam. Such virtuosity is economical, since purchasing costs and pre-installation requirements are both reduced, but it is not handy. To transfer the X-ray tube from the one to the other position entails a degree of inconvenience to the radiographer and may lose time on an examination; and for fluoroscopic investigations the table has only a very limited scope. This is not typical fluoroscopic equipment and no further reference need be made to it in the present context.

General features of a fluoroscopic/radiographic table

Important general features of a standard fluoroscopic/radiographic table include:

1 a drive of some variety, capable of moving the table, so that it may be used in a horizontal, or other angular position;

2 an apparatus called the *serial changer* or *spot film device* or *explorator* which permits radiographs of the fluoroscopic appearances to be taken during the fluoroscopic examination;

3 a bucky tray and mechanism in the accustomed place immediately beneath the table top.

The bucky and its mechanisms (see Chapter 8) we need not further consider at this point as they are not concerned with the fluoroscopic uses of the table.

Fig. 12.1 represents a typical universal table, shown in the horizontal position. The table base is a heavy structure. It must support the weight of the body of the table, the undertable tube, the image receptor and the serial changer, together with the counterweight systems associated with the movements of these; also of course the bucky and its counterweights. The base provides pivot points on which the body of the table can tilt and it often houses the motor drive.

Within limits, the dimensions of these tables vary between different models. The following are typical:

width, 710–740 mm (28–29 inches);
length, 1880–2280 mm (74–90 inches);
height, 800–875 mm (32–34·5 inches).

As it is more easily accessible, a low table is advantageous to the patient.

The sides of the table are enclosed with panels of sheet steel and these are finished in stove enamel for protection and ease of cleaning. The material of the table top is necessarily radioparent, for example laminated paper-base bakelite.

A footpiece on which the patient may stand is provided with every tilting table. It is adjustable in height and can be removed altogether when the table is used in the horizontal position for radiography.

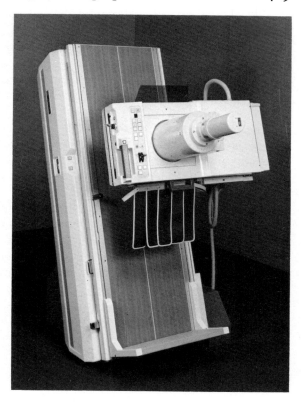

Fig. 12.1 A fluoroscopic/
radiographic table. *By
courtesy of Shimadzu
Medical X-ray.*

Other accessories for the security of the patient are available usually; for instance handgrips and shoulder rests. These are fitted when required by means of rails on the table sides: a DIN standard specifies such rails in order that accessories shall refer equally well to a number of tables.

The table drive and table movements

The table-tilt drive may be from an electric motor—sometimes two motors— or an electro-hydraulic mechanism. A movement of the table through 90 degrees in 20–25 seconds is customary. Some motors are two-speed so that the table may be tilted more slowly if required: this would be desirable during myelography for instance. In this case the table requires approximately twice as long to travel through the same angle. The electro-hydraulic mechanism, however, is variable in speed and—if the operator wishes—can be slowed down until the motion is barely perceptible. In many examples automatic acceleration and deceleration occur at the extremes of the movement.

The range of tilt available in a tilting table is described as being from the vertical to, say, 55 degrees *adverse*. This means that it is possible to move the table so that the patient can be brought from the upright through the horizontal to a position in which his head is 55 degrees below the horizontal. The adverse tilt may alternatively be described as the Trendelenburg tilt: this term is of surgical origin and denotes an operating position in which the patient's head is at a lower level than his pelvis. Fig. 12.2 illustrates these positions of a fluoroscopic tilting table.

For gastrointestinal radiology a maximum adverse tilt of at least 10–15 degrees is desirable. For myelography a much greater adverse tilt is usually necessary and tables are available which provide Trendelenburg angles of 65 degrees and even 90 degrees; that is, the patient can be turned completely upside down.

At the end of this chapter an attempt is made (see Table 12.1) to categorise the characteristics of different groups of fluoroscopic tables and to show the purposes to which each group may be appropriate.

In those instances where a steep adverse tilt is—or may be—used it is obviously necessary to support the patient and accessories to do this are

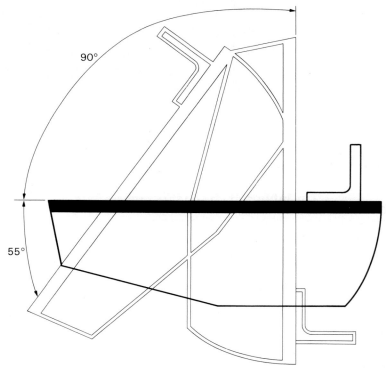

Fig. 12.2 *By courtesy of Picker International Ltd.*

normally supplied with the table. Devices for this purpose include a shoulder rest, hand grips and various kinds of harness. It is to be emphasized that any radiographer preparing to use these must make certain that they are in good order and correctly fitted to the table before the patient has to depend upon them. Immediate attention must be given to any patient who says he is slipping on the table, even if the radiographer privately believes that the statement has been inspired by a natural alarm over his experiences and is therefore disinclined to take it seriously. If the patient is right and the radiographer wrong, a very grave accident may occur.

The table will stop automatically in the maximum Trendelenburg and vertical positions. In some examples it will automatically stop or pause at the horizontal as well. In this case a switch is usually provided to allow it to drive to the Trendelenburg without interruption if the operator wishes. In all models, motion of the table can be arrested at any intermediate position.

If they are mishandled, tilting tables can be dangerous occupants of the X-ray department. A risk to the patient has already been mentioned. There are risks too to the equipment itself and to other equipment which may be in the room. Damage can easily occur if the radiographer or anyone else attempts to tilt the table without first making sure that its way is clear. Cables can be pulled from supports or junctions, while cast-iron components—such as the sides of the footrest—fracture readily if they meet obstruction. The writers have known two such footpieces broken within a month because a chair—which was of wood and not considered to be very strong!—was twice left under the end of the tilting table when it was moving from the horizontal to the vertical.

In order to prevent damage in this kind of accident—especially to the X-ray tube—manufacturers often include switches in series with the motor: these break the supply when the tube approaches an obstruction or at positions of the table and X-ray tube such that the tube is very close to the floor. There is also a measure of safety in making the switches which normally operate the table-drive of a self-cancelling type; that is, they flick back to their 'off' position as soon as finger- or foot-pressure is removed. This at least prevents anyone leaving a tilting table in motion without attention.

In addition to the table-tilt drive, most apparatus now provides a power-driven movement of the table-top on the base longitudinally (as shown in Fig. 12.3) and in many cases transversely as well. The facility assists easy positioning of a patient. In the vertical position of the table, with the patient standing on the footrest, longitudinal travel of the table-top can be employed to raise a short adult or a child to a height convenient for examination. It also makes the table adaptable for use with a rapid film- or cassette-changer (see Chapter 14) as the patient can be screened and then driven over the

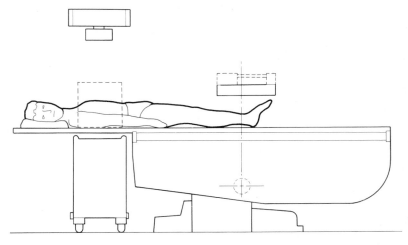

Fig. 12.3 A table with longitudinal movement of the top, enabling a patient to be moved without lifting him. Here the patient has been moved over a rapid film changer. *By courtesy of Picker International Ltd.*

changer placed at one end of the table, without the necessity of any movement by the patient himself. This is the situation depicted in Fig. 12.3.

The extent of the table-top travel varies between different examples. In the case of one table it may be 1000 mm (40 inches) all told; another provides 1000 mm (40 inches) at the head end and 700 mm (28 inches) at the foot end. When the table is tilted, such an excursion naturally becomes restricted because of the likelihood of collision with the floor and manufacturers normally interlock the two movements. Indeed a table is sometimes so well integrated that it does not merely stop tilting when the extended end nears the floor: it continues to tilt, while at the same time sliding its endangered part upwards into a safe position.

Features of the tube carriage

The X-ray tube is fitted under the table on a carriage which permits the tube to move longitudinally for most of the length of the table and to make a transverse excursion which covers the width of the table. This carriage supports also the image receptor (either an image intensifier tube with its accoutrements or a simple fluorescent screen). It should be of such a design that the X-ray tube and the image receptor—upon which the central X-ray beam is orientated—cannot be moved independently of each other. The purpose of this construction is to ensure that always there will be a visual indication—from the image receptor—of the presence of X rays when the tube is activated, whatever position the tube may occupy: it is a measure towards radiation protection.

However, this provision by itself goes only part of the way towards controlling radiation risks. Fig. 12.4 depicts X rays emanating from an X-ray tube of fixed aperture. When the image receptor is in position A the primary beam is fully included within the area of the receptor. However, the next patient is stouter than his predecessor and the image receptor is moved to B. Part of the beam then falls beyond the borders of the receptor and may irradiate the observer as shown.

To prevent the situation just described it is mandatory for the tube aperture to be such that the primary beam is included within the area of the image receptor, even when the latter is at its maximum distance from the

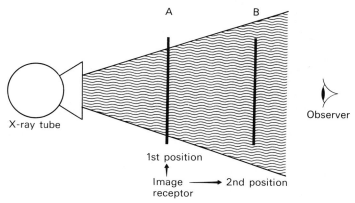

Fig. 12.4

tube. The beam should be limited by an automatic adjustment of the diaphragm system which will restrict the area of the aperture as the image receptor is pulled further from the tube and open it again as the tube receptor distance is decreased. Some further points related to radiation protection and fluoroscopic equipment will be mentioned in a later section of the chapter (see page 429).

The undertable tube is fitted with adjustable diaphragms similar to those associated with the light-beam delineator of the overtable tube (see Chapter 8); in this case of course there is no need for a lamp and centre-indicator. These diaphragms must be of a design which permits them to be fully closed. They are now usually electrically operated from switches on the receptor's carriage: in simple equipment a mechanical transmission by means of Bowden cables may be seen.

The carriage couples together the X-ray tube and the image receptor in a manner which is sketched in Fig 12.5. The distance between the table-top and the tube is fixed and is of the order of 380–510 mm (15–20 inches). The distance from the table-top to the receptor is necessarily variable, between approximately 180 mm (7 inches) and 535 mm (21 inches). This means of course that the anode-receptor distance is not constant and will vary to some extent, depending upon the thickness of the subject examined. We may compare, for example, the very different distances which may obtain when the subject is a young baby and when an obese adult is examined. It is doubtful if radiographers recognize these alterations in anode-film distance (the cassette being at image receptor level) when selecting exposure factors for radiographs taken at fluoroscopy. Indeed they probably do not need to

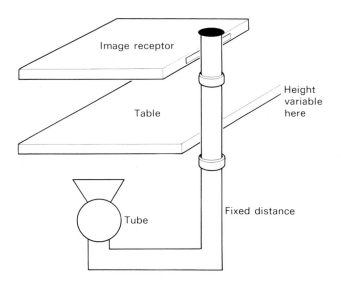

Fig. 12.5

do so, since in normal practice between one adult and another the change in distance is not great enough in proportion to make the radiograph unacceptably under- or over-exposed.

The image receptor can be moved in three directions relative to the table:

1   towards and away from the tube as already described;
2   with the X-ray tube across the table from side to side;
3   similarly lengthwise along the table.

At any selected point the carriage can be locked in position by electro-magnetic brakes operated by switches on the carriage; (1) is usually described as compression, (2) as lateral or transverse movement and (3) as longitudinal movement.

In order that repeated manipulations of the apparatus shall be less tiring, these movements are in all but very simple tables either fully motorized or assisted by a servo motor. In some cases all the movements of the carriage are motor-driven, but often only one—longitudinal movement—has this benefit.

The use of a motor-drive, whether on the movement of the table top (see previous section) or on that of the tube carriage, could involve the patient in hurt and possibly injury if at the same time the image receptor were firmly compressed. To avoid this risk the circuitry of the table should include switches which—as soon as either motor-drive operates—automatically override the on/off switch of the compression brake, irrespective of the switch position. For the same reason, if the compression movement is positively driven, the motor-drive should have a slipping clutch which will prevent extremes of pressure from being accidentally applied to a patient.

In addition to the features just described, the carriage includes the mechanisms and switches of the serial changer (explorator). These will be described more fully in the next section.

For the purpose of protecting the observer from radiation scattered by the patient's body a lead-rubber apron is attached to the carriage so that it will hang below the image receptor when the table is vertical. It is mobile and normally can be fitted to the left or 'open' side of the tube carriage (the side where the operator will stand) whenever fluoroscopy is performed with the table horizontal.

Manufacturers have evolved a number of ingenious and simple devices by which the apron can be changed in position quickly and without effort. It is important that they should have done this, since in gastrointestinal examinations every patient is studied in both erect and supine positions: in the course of the average fluoroscopic session the apron has to be moved many times.

In order to ensure that it provides radiation protection of an approved standard, the form and structure of this apron may be specified in international recommendations, or national codes of practice, which refer to diagnostic radiology. In the United Kingdom, these matters of the safety of equipment's design are the concern of the Health and Safety Commission and the National Radiological Protection Board; publications of the British Standards Institution and the International Electrotechnical Commission also may be relevant.

In general X-ray departments, fluoroscopic tables of the kind described may spend about half of their time in use for ordinary radiography. On this account manufacturers give considerable thought to the retracted or parked position of the image-receptor. It is desirable to leave a clear working surface which is readily accessible to the patient, the radiographer, the bucky tray and the overtable X-ray tube, whether floor- or ceiling-mounted. Students will see in their own departments a number of methods of parking the image receptor and serial changer.

Usually they can be pushed crosswise to one side of the table, when a catch or lock on the carriage is operated. If it is a ceiling-supported image intensifier, this is often removable from its place on the carriage and may be conveyed to another part of the room where it is out of the way of the 'traffic'.

Preference for a particular parking facility is a matter of personal opinion and influenced to some extent by the space available in the X-ray room concerned and the nature of the work for which the room and equipment are to be used.

However, a practical point of which radiographers who operate these units should be aware is that in some examples it may not be advisable to tilt the table to the vertical when the image receptor is in the parked position. Anyone who manipulates a table in this manner should be sure that the usage is appropriate.

In order to prevent damage from mistreatment of this kind the manufacturer may fit a special microswitch in the motor circuit. This switch is open circuit when the image receptor is parked and closed circuit when it is in the working position. Failure to lock the carriage properly may result in the microswitch not operating and can be a reason for the table not tilting when required. The switch should be checked before urgent messages are sent for the services of an engineer.

The serial changer (spot film device)

The purpose of the serial changer or spot film device is to allow films of fluoroscopic appearances to be exposed quickly; this is an important aspect of gastrointestinal radiology particularly, for such appearances are often transient. The name *serial changer* which is used in the United Kingdom and Europe is strictly incorrect; the term *serial* implies exposures made at predetermined intervals and at a faster rate than one per second.

The serial changer essentially is a lead-lined recess constructed as an integral part of the carriage for the undertable tube and the image receptor. It is situated to the right of the mount for the image receptor, with which it forms a continuous lead-protected tunnel.

The serial changer contains a conveyer which accepts cassettes by a variety of means in different examples and in a variety of sizes. A cassette is placed in the conveyer and the latter is either automatically or manually driven into a position for exposure between the patient and the image receptor. The exposure is made from a switch placed near at hand with other controls on the carriage. On completion of the exposure the cassette is returned by the same drive to its protected standby point. It can then be removed for processing of the film and a fresh cassette placed in the conveyer to wait until it is required. In various examples, unloading and reloading are done from the right or from the left or from either side.

The serial device is a relatively sophisticated piece of apparatus since it normally provides for a number of 'programmes': the operator is able to expose a cassette using any of several formats. These formats vary, from a single exposure of the cassette's full area, to a series of exposures each on a different part of the film. Fig. 12.6 shows the provisions of a typical serial changer.

Students will readily become familiar with the systems made available by the equipment in their own departments.

The multiple exposure techniques—in distinction to a single exposure utilizing the full area of a film—are often described as spot films or 'spots', A programme-selector placed with the other controls on the carriage allows the operator to choose any of these procedures at will.

The student will meet a variety of designs in the serial changers of different fluoroscopic tables and in the ways in which they index, control and effect the movement of cassettes. Those which are unfamiliar often look complicated, yet practice in their use endears most of them to us. Certain features are present in all serial changers.

1 A secondary radiation grid. This can be moved to and from the exposure field as the operator wishes—usually by means of a lever and a simple manual control knob, sometimes by motor-drive. The grid may be stationary or of the oscillating type (see Chapter 8) in which case it will be set in motion automatically before each exposure. It is often a fine-line grid (see Chapter 8).

2 A lead mask or slide which is introduced into the exposure field when films are to be 'split' into vertical halves: that is, it provides an aperture about 10–12 cm (4–5 inches) in width.

3 A compression cone. This device is curiously misnamed. It is not cone-shaped at all but really is a rectangular or circular 'box' of a substance transparent to radiation. Like the other accessories it can be moved to and from the exposure field as the operator wishes. Its purpose is to provide abdominal compression as this enhances—for example—visualization of the gastric and duodenal mucosae or the duodenal cap. Very often two different sizes of cone are available and either can be fitted to the coneslide according to preference.

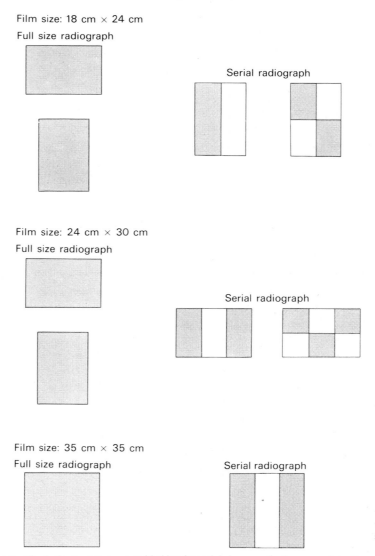

Fig. 12.6 Typical programmes provided by the serial changer of a fluoroscopic/radiographic table.

The operation of the serial changer

When a radiograph is to be taken during fluoroscopy, not only is it necessary to move the cassette quickly into the exposure field but a number of other events associated with the X-ray tube and generator must automatically occur before the film may be exposed. These are as follows.

1   Fluoroscopy must be switched off.

2   If the tube anode is not normally rotating during fluoroscopy it must be set in motion and brought to full speed for radiography.

3   The tube filament current (see Chapter 2) must be boosted to the higher value required for a tube current of 200–300 mA as distinct from fluoroscopic settings of 1–3 mA.

4   If fluoroscopy normally occurs on a very small focus, for example 0·3 mm (see Chapter 7), then a changeover must be made to the larger focus needed for heavy tube currents and short intervals of exposure.

5   When the exposure (time × milliamperes × kilovoltage) occurs it must be in accordance with factors which are pre-set on the generator, in order to avoid repetitive and delaying alteration of controls between fluoroscopy and radiography.

This is really an impressive series of electrical events about which radiologists and radiographers probably seldom think—although student radiographers may be obliged to do so. The adjustments and changes occur automatically on pressing the radiographic exposure switch on the serial changer; there is usually a switch on the generator which must be pre-set in an appropriate position (for example at 'serial' or 'remote') in order to by-pass the normal exposure handswitch of the unit.

Although these events take place without our attention, they are bound to require a certain interval of time. The slowest in effect is the acceleration of the tube anode, which usually occurs in 0·8 seconds (see Chapter 7). Because of all this we find that when we press the exposure switch and the cassette moves into the exposure area, there is an interval of approximately 0·8 second before we see the exposure made. There is a bonus in this small delay since it stabilizes the cassette if the rapid travel should lead to vibration.

As a further deterrent to the production of movement unsharpness, in some serial changers use of the exposure switch applies the brakes, irrespective of switch positions. Generally speaking, serial changers have a dual-action exposure switch. Light pressure prepares the system for radiography and then the exposure can be made immediately at any time afterwards with continued heavier pressure from the finger.

A table for myelography

Myelography is not necessarily infeasible on the tilting tables used for gastrointestinal and other fluoroscopic examinations: but it may be inconvenient, necessitating difficult movements of the patient and awkward arrangements for radiography during the procedure. In departments where the demand for myelography is high, there is justification for the purchase of tables having attributes of design which render them especially suitable for myelography; these features do not exclude the use of the table for other fluoroscopy. The following characteristics are found to a variable degree in tilting tables which are designed for myelography.

1   A wide range of tilt; that is not less than 65 degrees adverse tilt. Some tables are designed to give 90 degrees adverse tilt. The ability to provide a steep adverse tilt is the single most significant feature which distinguishes a myelography table from others.

2   A variable speed on the table-tilt drive. (Common on other tables.)

3   A power-driven table-top. (Common on other tables.)

4   A means of linking the overtable tube to the undertable tube carriage, so that both tubes are simultaneously centred. This is helpful because essential to myelography are lateral radiographs which are taken while the patient is prone and consequently require horizontal projection of the (overtable) X-ray beam. A lateral cassette-holder is an essential accessory.

5   An efficient system for harnessing and supporting the patient. In some instances the patient-support system may be elaborated to comprise a rotating cradle.

6   A facility for bi-plane fluoroscopy.

This description refers to the possibility of fitting another image-receptor (a small image intensifier) to the left side of the table. Energised by the second X-ray tube, such an intensifier permits fluoroscopy of a recumbent patient by means of a horizontal beam. Associated with the intensifier is a transport system for introducing a cassette within the X-ray beam and thus obtaining a record of fluoroscopic appearances in this projection. Both the intensifier and the cassette-transport system can be brought close to the patient across the top of the table and can be motorised in either direction along the length of the table: the first of these measures improves detail sharpness in video and radiographic images; and the second allows an operator to follow the flow of a contrast agent over the spinal contours as a patient is tilted.

This equipment is both costly and specialised. It is rarely installed in other than regional or similar large neurological centres.

REMOTE CONTROL (TELECOMMAND)

Manufacturers of X-ray equipment have developed the principle of remote control—otherwise described as telecommand—of a fluoroscopic table: that is, the fluoroscopist is not constrained to stand beside the patient whilst making the examination but can be elsewhere in the room, in a lead-protected cubicle, or even in another room. Such equipment has implications of both advantage and disadvantage; but of more immediate concern to us now are the implications of design. Among these, the following are significant points.

1 An image intensifier and a closed circuit television system for viewing become essential.

2 All movements of the table, the image-intensifier/X-ray tube combination and the serial changer are motorised of necessity.

3 In almost all instances of a remote control facility, the conventional arrangement of undertable tube and overtable image receptor is reversed: an integral tube-support links an overtable X-ray tube to an undertable image intensifier.

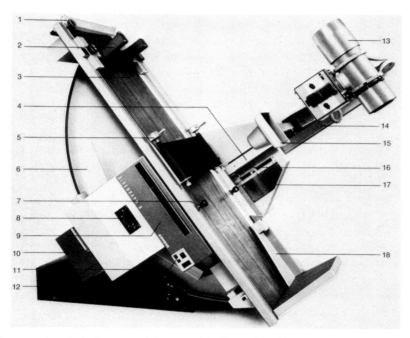

Fig. 12.7 A typical telecommand fluoroscopic/radiographic table.

1 Protective strip
2 Shoulder supports, adjustable longitudinally and transversely
3 Floating table top
4 Attachment for tomography
5 Compression band
6 Curved segment of table
7 Handgrips for patient
8 Angle indicator, showing degree of tilt
9 Undertable spot film device with intensifier and TV camera
10 100 mm fluorographic serial camera
11 Control panel for table-side operation
12 Base of the table
13 X-ray tube with collimator
14 Support column for X-ray tube assembly
15 Removable compression cone
16 Angle indicator for central X-ray beam angulation
17 Tomographic height indicator (fulcrum)
18 Footrest with height adjustment

By courtesy of Siemens-Elema AB

The third point above—if the reader will think about it for a moment—embodies a construction which is totally different from a 'conventional' fluoroscopic/radiographic table. We shall consider it in essential form, before referring briefly to more elaborate remotely controlled tables.

General features of a telecommand table

Fig. 12.7 depicts a typical universal table offering the facility of remote control. The overtable X-ray tube is mounted on an integral tube support coupled to an image intensifier (underneath the table), with which it moves in unison. Thus, the overtable tube is used for all examinations made with the table, whether the required mode is fluoroscopy, general radiography, or procedures such as tomography or peripheral angiography. Some of these tables possess great versatility and are suitable for so many radiodiagnostic applications that the description 'universal' is not altogether undeserved, though should not be taken literally! (There is no connection with space travel!)

An arguably significant advantage from the overtable position of the X-ray tube, during both fluoroscopy and any direct radiography, or fluorography, associated with it, refers to the relatively great anode-to-image-receptor distance (for example, 120 cm) and the relatively small distance from the table-top (or subject) to the film or to the input phosphor of the intensifier; for instance, this distance might be 7 cm.

These are good features of an imaging system, if geometric unsharpness is to be minimal. As we have seen (p. 369), an undertable position of the X-ray tube offers a rather unfavourable geometry of projection: the source-to-subject distance is small (for example, about 50–60 cm), whilst the subject-to-film distance is variable and may be quite large. (This will be so, if the radiologist does not compress the serial changer firmly; or if the patient is a small baby who has been placed directly on the table-top and whose body thickness is less than the extent of the serial changer's closest approach to the table. Such circumstances can result in a significant loss of detail.)

In some examples of remotely controlled tables, the anode-film distance can be varied and preselected from a range such as 110 cm to 150 cm; push-button selection of the anode-film distance in three steps (115–135–150 cm) is another typical arrangement.

It may be noted that in some examples the height of the table also can be altered and this may be advantageous when moving infirm patients.

Movements of the table

Telecommand tables, like other fluoroscopic/radiographic tables, must be capable of tilting from the vertical, through the horizontal, to a Trendelenburg angulation. Generally speaking, their capabilities for adverse tilt come within the range o deg to − 45 deg, although some available tables have the scope for a 90 deg Trendelenburg position.

Movement of the table top is required in both longitudinal and transverse directions and usually is quite extensive. A typical series of values is:

—headwards 860 mm

—footwards 440 mm

—transversely 350 mm (+ 180 mm/ − 170 mm).

The speed of the movement is about 45 mm/sec. A telecommand design sometimes facilitates the use of a panning technique in tracking the flow of a contrast agent fluoroscopically: when the coupled intensifier and X-ray tube are moved to the limit of travel—footwards or headwards—the table top will drive in the opposite direction and so extend the scope of an operator's uninterrupted observation. Alternatively, when the table top and the intensifier/X-ray tube combination are driven simultaneously in the same direction, the effect is of an increased scanning speed.

For the patient's comfort and calm, it is essential that the motions described above should occur smoothly. Their control is achieved usually by means of a joystick—sometimes more than one—on the remote console. Such a joystick sometimes may be operated to combine transverse and longitudinal movements in a motion which is oblique in direction.

The control console

For a conventionally planned fluoroscopic/radiographic table, all the controls significant to the operation of the serial changer are placed to hand on the serial changer. However, for easy positioning of a patient during general radiographic usage, those controls which effect movement of the table top may be duplicated in a mounting which is situated accessibly on the radiographer's side of the table. A remotely controlled table must have a separate control console but in this case, too, a table-side control panel should repeat those controls which are needed by a radiographer working at the table.

The number of functions included in such an auxiliary panel varies between different examples and the four below are probably the minimum:

1 transverse and longitudinal movements of the table top;
2 inward/outward movement of the cassette tray for loading and unloading purposes (see also p. 427);
3 angulation of the tube column;
4 longitudinal movement of the tube column.

Additional local controls and indications which may be thought desirable include the following:

5   opening and closing of the X-ray beam collimator;
6   selection of the fulcrum height during tomography;
7   tilting of the table.

The control console, which of course stands separate from the table, must provide means to control every function of the table and its accessories and make relevant indications when these are appropriate. This means that in the case of even a 'simple' example of a remote control facility the console carries many more switches, selector buttons and monitor lamps than does the control panel of a conventional serial changer or spot film unit: there may be 35 or more different devices on such a console. The additional operations and indications which may be needed from these telecommand consoles include the following: application of the compression cone; angle indication during oblique projections of the X-ray beam; variation of the source-image (focus-film) distance; and others.

Because of their numbers and refinement it is essential—if the equipment is to be easily used—that the many controls and indicators necessary to a remote console be arranged in orderly groups. Clearly, not every designer and every operator have the same plan for ideal dispositions of these tools. Perhaps personal experience to date will have convinced readers of this book already that some equipment, with which each may be familiar, is 'good' or 'bad' in this respect. The layout suggested in Fig. 12.8 is not a proposal for perfection but depicts a representative arrangement of a telecommand console which is reasonably favourable and not illogical in its approach.

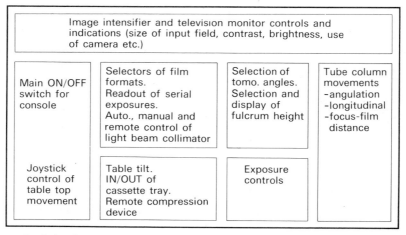

Fig. 12.8   A sketched layout for a telecommand console.

The control console sometimes is on a floor-fixed pedestal or may be of a design that it can be moved to the desire of the examiner

Palpation and compression

One of the controls for the table which deserves special notice—it is peculiar to the principle of telecommand—is the means which enables the fluoroscopist to palpate a patient who is not within arm's reach.

On the table itself, the integrated tube column includes a motor driven carriage for a swingout compression cone, palpating spoon or alternative device (sometimes two such instruments are provided and are interchangeable). Although positioning of the palpator on the patient's abdominal wall and also its subsequent parking movement are motor-operated from the control console, it is most important that the actual compression movement be sensitive to the hand, so that the examiner is aware of the amount of pressure applied and the patient's resistance to it.

Not every telecommand table is fully commendable in this respect (nor, indeed, fully commandable, perhaps!). Typically, the operator uses a large handle, prominently placed on the control console, to obtain compression. A direct link—perhaps partly mechanical and partly hydraulic—between this handle and the compression device reproduces the pressure applied to the patient and allows the radiologist to control it. The operator should not be able to move the table top whilst compression is applied and often an interlock is fitted to ensure that this is so.

In a few instances, compression is obtained by motoring a carriage towards the patient. Such a system should be associated with a slipping clutch, but the operator cannot judge the amount of compression and the arrangement may be dangerous; it contravenes certain safety recommendations in the United Kingdom. Sometimes such a table is provided with a safety measure which ensures that a given maximum pressure cannot be exceeded.

Location of the control console

The best position for the control console, whether in the X-ray room or elsewhere, is a matter for practical decision by the users. Factors which participate in such decisions include features of departmental and room design, as well as individual preferences for a particular way of working.

To put the control console close to the table is to lose some of the advantages of telecommand and may entail increased radiation dosage; but, on the other hand, many radiologists—certainly within the United Kingdom—would accept only with great reluctance, or would refuse to accept, an examining position which put them in another room from their patients for fluoroscopy.

A frequently convenient arrangement is to position the table's control console near to the X-ray generator's control, where both may share the radiation protection afforded by the lead screen which is standard provision in a radiodiagnostic room.

Wherever the radiologist's working station is situated, it should satisfy two important requirements:

1 an occupant of the table must be within the fluoroscopist's sight continuously;

2 the fluoroscopist must easily be heard by—and be able to hear—a patient who is under examination on the table.

A lead glass window is the usual means of meeting the first of these considerations. Such a window must be of adequate size to allow someone seated at the control console to have a full view of the X-ray table.

If the radiologist and the patient are to hear each other without having to shout across a room, microphones and speakers are usually necessary. Such a provision is not technically difficult but perhaps its requirement might be accounted a disadvantage of remotely controlled equipment: there are sure to be certain patients who respond unhappily to a microphone-processed 'voice from the air', issuing questions and instructions. (On the other hand, it has been shown that some patients talk more readily to a computer than to a doctor!)

The spot film unit

A fluoroscopic table which has the image intensifier beneath it must have the spot film unit, or serial changer for direct radiography, similarly placed. Thus the one unit combines the functions of serial changer (when the table is employed for fluoroscopy) and bucky, whenever the table is used for radiographic examinations. This means that the multiple cassette pro-gramme (see p. 418) which a serial changer should offer to the fluoroscopist is available advantageously to the radiographer for other procedures. Time is saved and fatigue and the film bill possibly are reduced when—for example—a 24 cm × 30 cm cassette is quartered by the spot-film system and includes all four standard projections of the temporomandibular articulation; or a 30 cm × 40 cm cassette may be divided lengthwise for the purposes of the anteroposterior and lateral views of thoracic or lumbar vertebrae.

Another inherent feature of a combined spot film/bucky unit is the possibility of monitoring difficult radiographic positioning by a few seconds' fluoroscopy. The change-over from the one mode to the other can be made very quickly and such a check might be appropriate if an experienced operator wished to avoid an error of projection entailing a 'repeat' film.

The combined serial changer/bucky features a cassette tray which usually automatically centres a cassette placed in it, for instance by means of four sliding clamps in the tray. An automatic sensing of the cassette's size is associated with a corresponding collimation of the X-ray beam to accord with the required radiographic field (for exposure either of the full format or of one of its subdivisions, depending on the programme selected).

However, beam collimation is not effected solely by this automated sensing system. The control console usually provides an over-ride, which enables a fluoroscopist to make the radiation field smaller than the area of the selected film format (but never larger, for obvious reasons of radiation safety). This over-ride may be dual in nature and a manual mode obtained through operation of one or other of two buttons on the control console:

1 a 'manual button' (possibly indicated by the symbol of a hand), which gives a radiographer local control of collimation at the light beam diaphragm itself;

2 a 'remote button' (sometimes marked TC) which allows an operator to use a typical slider on the remote console and alter the position of the diaphragm blades, with direct visual supervision.

If the controls include the means to select 'manual' as in (1) above, the button should be interlocked to prevent inadvertent retention during fluoroscopy of a large radiation field (larger than the input phosphor of the image intensifier).

The cassette tray has three positions, as follows:

1 a **loading** position, when the tray is 'out'—like a drawer—at the side of the table and able to receive a cassette;

2 a **ready** position, when the cassette is under the table but not within the X-ray beam (it remains here during fluoroscopy);

3 an **exposure** position, when the cassette has travelled along the table to lie within the X-ray beam. (This movement occurs when the radiographic exposure switch is put at its 'prepare' station and occupies a period of about one second.)

On completion of the radiographic exposure (either a single exposure or a series upon one film), the cassette should return to the 'ready' position, from where it now often provides a visual signal that it requires attention: for example, an appropriate push button on the control console will become illuminated or its light will flash. Radiographers, using the table for radiographic examinations, appreciate a capability to activate this button from the table-side as well as from the control console.

Cassette loading of the combined spot film/bucky unit can be made only from the left, of course; but in other respects the equipment is similar to its serial-changer counterpart on a conventionally designed fluoroscopic/radiographic table in having:

1 a secondary radiation grid, usually of the oscillating type and motored to and from the radiation field;

2   a digital display of the state of the selected cassette programme, that is a record of the number of exposures which have been made on the cassette, as an *aide memoire* to the operator;

3   an interlocking system of some degree, to prevent incorrect usage by an operator (for example, further exposure becomes impossible when the last in any series on one cassette has been made).

In some examples, the spot film unit is capable of providing an electronically controlled rapid series of exposures. These are made upon one cassette at speeds of 2–3 frames per second, given that the cassette is appropriately divided and there is no intervening fluoroscopy.

Elaborations of the telecommand table

Readers of this book may meet, in use in their training departments, telecommand tables which possess much more sophistication than those described in the course of the last few pages. For instance, some tables may offer cassetteless film-changing by means of magazines (see Chapter 16); but the main difference between these tables and their simpler fellows is in the much greater range of movements which they are able to achieve, both of the tube/image intensifier assembly and of the patient.

Typically, the patient is supported in a cradle, which may be available in a variety of sizes to fit adults and younger subjects. This cradle can be turned through a complete revolution around the patient's long axis (− 180 deg to + 180 deg). At the same time, the X-ray beam may be rotated ± 90 deg around the rolling patient, at any angulation of the table.

There is, thus, a wholly free selection of the direction of the incident X-ray beam, which is obtained without a patient having to make an effort to move himself. Any telecommand table permits fluoroscopy with a cranio-caudad angulation of the beam, thus assisting the elucidation of overlapping images (for instance of loops of bowel during a barium enema examination); but these more elaborate multidirectional systems greatly increase the scope of the fluoroscopist in this respect and enhance radiological precision. However, a large clinical demand for specialised fluoroscopic procedures and a consequently heavy workload are prerequisite to the full utilisation of such equipment, the expense of which may be hardly justified in other circumstances. Some tables of this more sophisticated type are planned particularly for paediatric patients.

Advantages and disadvantages of remote control

Certain advantages have been acknowledged in the use of a telecommand table which refer not only to the remote control facility but to the overtable situation of the X-ray tube. Some of these advantages are stated below.

1   Potentially lower radiation dosage to staff.
This applies only if the table is operated remotely; otherwise, radiation risks to the staff may be greater.
2   A longer—and variable—anode-film distance.
3   Better acceptance by nervous patients, especially children and old people. This occurs because there is no confining structure in front of the patient and he is not visually deprived in his strange situation: he can see what is going on around him.
We may note that this visual gain affects both protagonists: the fluoroscopist correspondingly may more easily see the whole of the patient.
4   The ability to undertake fluoroscopy with an angulation of the X-ray beam.
5   The facility for tomography.
6   The X-ray room may not require a separate, ceiling supported—or otherwise supported—X-ray tube. Most tables allow the integral X-ray tube to perform some off-table radiography with a horizontal beam, additionally to its appropriateness to on-table bucky radiography.
7   Reduction in fatigue. This of course is a subjective finding and derived from the reactions more probably of fluoroscopists than of radiographers associated with the examinations in question. Whether, because of the claimed decrease in fatigue, the workload of a radiodiagnostic room effectively may be increased is not substantiated by available evidence in the United Kingdom.

Naturally, telecommand tables have some disadvantages, too. These follow the general lines indicated below.

1   Certain radiologists simply do not like to operate remotely from a patient. There may be several reasons for this: for instance such practice may constitute a significant departure from an individual's previous clinical training; or the deterrent may lie with the relative ineffectiveness of mechanical devices for manipulation and palpation, compared with the subtlety of the human hand.
2   The greater mechanical complexity of the undertable spot film unit may entail slower movement of a cassette; effectively this means that the fluoroscopist must accept a longer delay in exposing 'spots'.
3   Changes in the viewed area of patient—for instance when barium sulphate is 'followed' down the oesophagus—may be made less quickly through remote control, especially in examples of such equipment which do not offer longitudinal drive of the X-ray tube/intensifier column and motor only the table top. In these instances we should remember, too, that to follow the flow of a contrast agent 'downwards' (cranio-caudally) may result in a patient being raised above floor level to a height which feels insecure, may unnerve him and is potentially dangerous if he is unsupported.

4   These tables often are more expensive and need larger radiodiagnostic rooms.

RADIATION PROTECTION

The standard of radiological protection required in fluoroscopic equipment has been a matter of special study and is included in the recommendations of the International Commission on Radiological Protection. Following the Euratom Directive (1976) on radiation protection, regulations made under the Health and Safety at Work Act, 1974, require the standards of the Commission to be observed in the United Kingdom; in many other places, similar legislation and approved codes of practice—which provide supporting information—obtain.

Broadly speaking, there are two main classes of people involved in the medical use of ionizing radiations: one of these is the user and the other the person on whom they are used, that is the patient. Recommendations referring to diagnostic X-ray equipment are concerned with the well-being of each; some recommendations apply to the safety of one group, some affect the safety of the other and some are relevant to both.

In relation to protective measures in fluoroscopy, distinction is made between (a) features of the fluoroscopic equipment itself and (b) the actual conduct of the fluoroscopic procedure. The latter is outside the scope of this book. In this section we will consider some parts in the design of fluoroscopic equipment which are intended to provide protection from radiation.

Cumulative fluoroscopic timer

The fluoroscopic timer is a timing device which indicates the total period of irradiation of the patient. It operates only when the fluoroscopic switch is operated and it provides a means both of recording the period of fluoroscopy and of limiting it if desired.

The mechanism of the timer is a synchronous motor which is equipped with appropriate gearing, a clutch and the ability to start rapidly. A typical timer has two scales, each of which is calibrated from zero to 8 minutes. They are mounted round the circumference of the timer: the inner scale is on a rotating disc which carries a pointer at zero and the outer one is on a stationary ring. A movable stop overlies the outer time scale and this can be put in any desired position on the scale; for example, let us suppose that it is set at 5 minutes.

Before fluoroscopy begins the rotating disc is turned until the pointer strikes the stop. When the fluoroscopic switch is closed the pointer begins to return towards zero on the outer scale and the inner scale shows for how long fluoroscopy has proceeded. Whenever the fluoroscopic switch is opened the pointer stops; whenever fluoroscopy begins again the pointer renews its motion.

If the examination is continued until the pointer has completed its return to zero, any or all of three events can be made to happen:

1   the timer breaks the fluoroscopic circuit and prevents its further use until the timer has been reset;

2   it operates a buzzer which will ring when the fluoroscopic switch is closed, that is when the operator continues to try to use the unit for fluoroscopy;

3   it causes a signal lamp to light which provides visual reminder that the patient has been irradiated for the selected period of 5 minutes.

This timer may be mounted on the wall of the X-ray room, near the control console and preferably within sight of the fluoroscopist's positions; usually it is on the console. No doubt it becomes familiar to student radiographers quite early in their training and the reader is advised to study the above description in conjunction with examination of the timer in actuality.

Such a fluoroscopic timer is exclusively for the protection of the patient. It is not a device intended for the protection of staff. Even if no patient is screened for longer than the selected pre-set period, a note can be made in the patient's records of the length of time for which he was examined on any occasion and this may influence subsequent fluoroscopy of him.

Lead aprons, shields and diaphragms

Lead aprons

Reference was made earlier in this chapter (page 413) to the provision of a lead apron on the serial-changer carriage of a fluoroscopic table for the purpose of protecting the operator from scattered radiation. In the United Kingdom the specification of this apron requires it to be not less than 45 cm wide and 45 cm long and to have a lead equivalent which is not less than 0·5 mm. It must be capable of being moved from the lower edge of the screen when the table is vertical to the operator's side when the table is horizontal. In the USA the *National Bureau of Standards Handbook* does not specify the dimensions of the apron: it stipulates a lead equivalent of 0·25 mm and states that this apron shall not substitute for the operator's wearing a lead apron during fluoroscopy.

Shields

Radiation scattered laterally through the bucky slot of a fluoroscopic/ radiographic table may endanger personnel who stand at the side of the

Table 12.1   Table of fluoroscopic/radiographic tables

General type	Movements of table	Spot film unit	Applications
Simple: X-ray tube under table.	0 deg to 90 deg; adverse tilt 10 deg to 30 deg range. Motorised longitudinal movement of top.	Mechanical programme selection. Manual control of diaphragm shutters etc. Restricted range of cassette sizes.	Gastrointestinal examinations in departments with small workload.
More sophisticated versions of above. I	0 deg to 90 deg; adverse in range 10 deg to 30 deg. Motorised longitudinal movement of top.	Preselection of film formats and automatic operation. Automatic collimation of beam to cassette size. Motorised positioning of masks, compression cone etc. Full range of cassette sizes and possibly facility to load from left and right.	Gastrointestinal examinations where there is a large workload. Can be made suitable for abdominal and peripheral angiography.
II (Possibly has facility to attach a rotating cradle.)	0 deg to 90 deg; adverse in range 65 deg to 90 deg.	Similar to I above.	Special demand for myelography but remarks on I above also apply.
Telecommand with integrated tube-support linked to under-table image intensifier. A	0 deg to 90 deg adverse in range 10 deg to 30 deg. Motorised movement to table top.	Motorised movement of tube/image intensifier combination. Characteristics are similar to I above, but cassette loading is from the left.	All procedures.
B	0 deg to 90 deg; adverse in range 65 deg to 90 deg (otherwise similar to A).	Similar to A.	Specially suitable for myelography because of greater adverse tilt.
C Very sophisticated telecommand, having a patient-support and potential for almost any viewing projection.	90 deg–0 deg–90 deg.	Wide range of movements of image intensifier/X-ray tube assembly combined with patient's support. May offer some anatomical programming.	Relevant to very large X-ray departments with demand for a wide range of fluoroscopic examinations.

table. Consequently it is usual to provide a means to close the bucky slot. This protection takes various forms: it might be a hinged lateral panel which can be raised. Sometimes closure of the slot occurs automatically, from the action of moving the bucky to the foot end of the table (in order to avoid interference with the beam from an undertable X-ray tube).

Protection against scatter at floor level is sometimes provided on the footswitch which is used for fluoroscopy. The structure of the switch is such that the operator places his foot within a metal housing; this housing is recommended to have a lead equivalent of 0·5 mm.

Both these devices and the lead apron are items which are intended for the protection of users of the equipment and not of the patient.

Diaphragms

In an earlier section of this chapter (page 413) reference was made to some features which limit the area of the X-ray beam. A properly designed fluoroscopic table should have the following characteristics of this kind:

1 a tube aperture of such dimensions that the area of the primary beam is *always* included within the area of the image receptor;
2 provision of a system of adjustable diaphragms which (a) are capable of being fully closed and (b) maintain automatically the selected beam area, irrespective of distance;
3 a scatter cone within which the adjustable diaphragms are mounted and which provides a protective enclosure against the lateral escape of radiation;
4 the diaphragm system and its housing so mounted that they move together;
5 a standard of protection from the diaphragm material equal to that provided by the tube housing (see Chapter 7);
6 the diaphragm system situated as close as possible to the underside of the table top, in the case of an undertable tube.

With reference to 6 the student should note that though the diaphragm system must come close to the table panel, this does not refer to the X-ray tube itself: the anode/table-panel distance should not be less than 45 cm (18 inches) and the American *National Bureau of Standards Handbook* further stipulates that it shall not be less than 12 inches.

It is easily recognized that all the above features—each of which is related to control of the primary beam—participate in the provision of radiological protection for both the patient and users of the equipment.

Chapter 13
Tomographic Equipment

In this chapter we shall consider more apparatus which is intended for a particular radiographic purpose, that is for tomography. In order to employ effectively the specialized—sometimes highly specialized—equipment which is designed for tomography, radiographers should know what the apparatus has to do and should understand the processes which they are to control. Because of this, we are opening this chapter with a necessary theoretical discussion.

THEORY OF TOMOGRAPHY

Everyday life makes us familiar with the fact that when a photograph is taken the aspect of the subject which is nearer the camera and the film is the aspect recorded. However, this is not true of a radiograph.

In the same anteroposterior projection of the abdomen, for example, there may be visualized the pubic bones, gas in the transverse colon, an opaque stone in the biliary tract, the renal outlines and the vertebral bodies. If our photographic analogy were applicable to the radiograph, among the structures listed we should see probably only the last two, since they are posteriorly situated in the body and were nearest to the film when the exposure was made. In fact a radiograph presents a composite image which includes any number of structures in the line of the primary X-ray beam.

Tomography is a procedure which allows us to record on a radiograph only selected structures, free from the superimposed shadows of other organs and tissue. The advantages of this in producing clearer visualization are immediately obvious: for example, the gall bladder may be separated from intestinal gas; the lung hila distinguished in the pulmonary vasculature; the larger cranial bones prevented from overshadowing the minute architecture of the inner ear.

To understand this we should consider the patient as a number of anatomical layers. At any one time tomography makes a single layer sharp on a film, while the layers above and below it are indistinguishable because their detail is blurred. This blurring is motional unsharpness: it is produced by movement of the X-ray tube and film during the exposure.

434

Figure 13.1 depicts a patient in whom two anatomical structures, Y and A, are situated in line with each other. The X-ray tube is at T_1 and on the film placed beneath the patient the shadow of Y is recorded at X and the shadow of A at B_1. As we face the diagram, B_1 is seen to lie to the right of X which happens to be at the centre of the film.

In Fig. 13.2, the X-ray tube has moved to T_2; the film too has moved in a similar excursion but in the opposite direction. The image of Y is still—in two senses of the word—in the centre of the film at X but the image of A at B_2 has changed places and is now in another situation altogether, to the left of X.

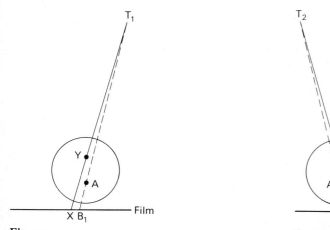

Fig. 13.1

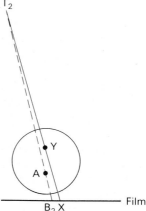

Fig. 13.2

Figure 13.3 is a combination of the previous two diagrams and summarizes the position, as we can now summarize it in words.

1   During exposure of the film, the focus of the X-ray tube moves in a straight line between T_1 and T_2.

2   The film moves in a parallel straight line in the opposite direction.

3   The fulcrum or turning point of these movements is at Y.

4   The X-ray tube, the fulcrum and the film do not alter their relative positions in any way.

5   Therefore the projection of Y on the film is theoretically as sharp as on an ordinary radiograph.

6   This is true not only of Y but of other points in the same horizontal plane.

7   Structures (for example A) which are not in the same plane as Y—they may be either above or below it—are recorded as a blur because the tube focus and the film are moving in their respect.

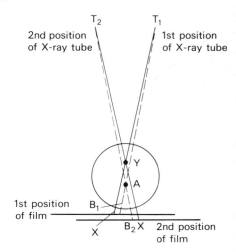

Fig. 13.3

If we content ourselves for the moment with the above simple statement of the conditions of tomography, we can at once appreciate a few of the requirements of apparatus designed to perform it. Such apparatus must have:

1 a means of moving the X-ray tube in a controlled direction;

2 a means of linking the X-ray tube to the bucky tray, so that a film placed in the latter will be simultaneously driven an equal excursion in the opposite direction;

3 a means of altering the height of the fulcrum or turning point of the movement, so that different anatomical levels in the patient may be examined at will;

4 mechanical stability, to prevent unsharpness arising in the fulcrum plane as the result of tube or cassette vibration.

The thickness of the tomographic section

So far we have considered—and have used diagrams to show—a fulcrum point at Y: we have said that the theory must be true also of other points in the same horizontal plane as Y. However, in practice the plane which is recorded on the radiograph will have definite dimensions; that is, it will have certain thickness and is not a surface but a section or layer which is sharp.

This is because there is a lower limit to the sharpness perceivable by the eye. The eye accepts as sharp an image which in fact contains a small element of blur and even if the blur were reduced the eye could not recognize any improvement. We can therefore say that within certain strict limits, details which are slightly above and below Y will be sharply recorded on the film even though they are not exactly in the fulcrum plane: in theory blur is present but it is acceptable because it is not perceivable.

Once we have understood that tomography is concerned with a layer, rather than a plane, we are bound to ask ourselves about the dimensions of this layer. Is the section which appears sharp on the radiograph a thick, or a thin strip?

In Fig. 13.4 there is again depicted the movement of an X-ray tube and film about a fulcrum at Y. Let us suppose that in the line CD (or for that matter in EF, since the two are equal), we have the maximum amount of movement which can be present without the eye perceiving that the image is blurred. Then it follows that the whole of the shaded section in the figure will appear sharp.

In Fig. 13.5 the only change made is a wider swing of the X-ray tube.

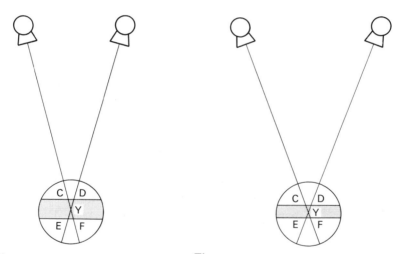

Fig. 13.4   **Fig. 13.5**

CD and EF again define the maximum permissible blur. This time, however, these lines are seen to come much nearer to the fulcrum and the shaded 'in-focus' section is narrower.

In Fig. 13.6 the anode-film distance has been decreased relative to Fig. 13.4 but the movement of the X-ray tube is the same. Again CD and EF represent the limits of acceptable blur. The shaded layer is narrower than it was in the first instance—although not so narrow as it is in Fig. 13.5.

In Fig. 13.7 we have to consider two separate tomographic sections. The first examination is made with the fulcrum at Y_1 near to the film. The second 'cut' is taken with the fulcrum at Y_2, much further removed from the film.

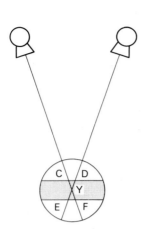

Fig. 13.6   **Fig. 13.7**

The 'in-focus' layer has been shaded in the diagram in each case and we can see that in the second circumstance it is narrower than in the first.

From the foregoing observations we can now accept certain conclusions.
1   A tomographic plane is in fact a layer of some definite thickness.
2   The thickness of the layer is not a constant in all circumstances.
3   Increasing the angle of tube-swing decreases the thickness of the layer.
4   At shorter anode-film distances the thickness of the layer is again decreased.
5   When the distance between the layer and film is great, the layer is thinner than when it is near to the film.

In practice both 4 and 5 above may be disregarded as methods of controlling the thickness of the tomographic layer. Altering the distance between the selected layer and the film results in only small variations and the use of a short anode-film distance in order to obtain a thinner 'cut' would imply some loss of fine detail owing to increased geometric blur. We find, therefore, that satisfactory apparatus for tomography includes a means of altering the angle through which the X-ray tube moves, so that by extending or diminishing its excursion the radiographer can alter the thickness of the selected tomographic layer to suit the requirements of particular examinations.

The ability to alter the thickness of the layer which forms a sharp image is advantageous radiographically simply because there is not uniformity between the dimensions of different body structures. The thinner the layer which is sharp the more selective tomography becomes. It is unnecessary and not helpful for it to be highly selective in examinations of the lung, for example; this is partly because the pulmonary lesions sought are not likely to be less than millimetres in extent and partly because contrast diminishes with decreasing thickness of layer. In the inner ear, on the other hand, the structures to be visualized are very small. It is necessary to be able to look at a number of sections placed not more than 2 mm apart; each section is consequently required to be a very thin 'slice'.

We may notice at this point that professional jargon sometimes refers to the layer which is sharp as a 'cut': we say in tomography that we are intending to take a cut at a certain level to show certain structures. It is a useful short-hand but perhaps the phrase should not be employed without caution. A radiographer once explaining tomography to a student in the presence of a patient on the X-ray table was surprised to find that the patient put a literal meaning on the word and waited in a condition of understandable nervous tension for the touch of the knife.

The student may well ask what *is* the thickness of a layer in any particular tomographic examination. Its thickness is difficult to specify because there is no absolute standard for the measurement of sharpness: we cannot precisely define a boundary for the amount of blur which makes an image either sharp or unsharp. However, for practical purposes one may assume a certain limit and this enables assessments of layer thickness to be made. It varies—depending upon the sophistication of the apparatus and the operating conditions—from a thickness of about 7 mm down to 0·7 mm. Manufacturers' publications about their equipment may include estimates of layer thickness in different circumstances and the student is advised to have a look at these: a knowledge of the layer thickness likely to be obtained in a particular set of conditions is helpful in making the fullest use of specialized and costly machinery.

The tomographic movement

Movement is fundamental to tomography and we must now consider the effects inherent in it. The plane of movement, its direction, its speed and the length of the tube trajectory all influence the results obtained.

The plane of movement

When earlier we said that tomography required the X-ray tube and film to move equally in similar planes of opposite direction, we depicted these planes as being parallel and horizontal. This is the simplest tomographic arrangement, though it is not the only one possible. We will consider it a little further in the section below.

Horizontal planes

Figure 13.8 illustrates movement of the X-ray tube and film in horizontal planes. The student should notice that at the extremities of travel the X-ray tube is rotated on its axis in order to obtain correct beam direction. Nevertheless the vertical height of the anode above the level of the film—represented by the dotted line AF—remains the same. It is evident that the lines AAA (focal spot of the X-ray tube) and FFF (film) are both parallel and horizontal.

The intensity of radiation incident on the line of the film's travel is not the same along the full length of the excursion, because of the increasing obliquity of the line between the anode of the X-ray tube and the film, as

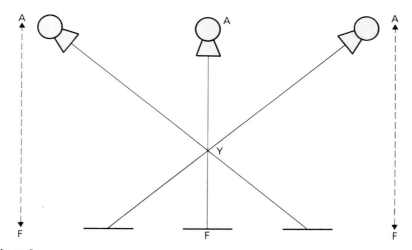

Fig. 13.8

each moves oppositely away from the centre. The obliquity of these lines gives the impression that the geometry of projection has altered, which would result in a changed magnification—and therefore in unsharpness—of the image.

However, this is not really true. As the completed line AF becomes longer, so also does AY. It is this ratio between AF and AY which influences geometry and is significant for magnification and maintained image-sharpness during the movement. AF and AY grow proportionally longer together; that is, their ratio is a constant.

A rectilinear system of this kind is the simplest method of tomography and is often in use. In its practical form, the equipment may offer some risk of vibration, especially as its parts become worn.

Arcuate planes

Although horizontal planes are easier to achieve mechanically, tomography has been described with apparatus which moves the X-ray tube and the film through arcs of circles. This is depicted in Fig. 13.9. Here, the length of the vertical lever AYF is the same as the lengths of the oblique levers A_1YF_1 and A_2YF_2. During the exposure, the height of the X-ray tube above the patient and the distance below him of the film manifestly change; but the ratio which we have discussed in the previous section does not. Putting this in words, the ratio of anode-film distance to anode-fulcrum distance remains the same through tube and film travel. This constancy implies a constancy of image magnification and therefore no loss of sharpness from this cause is

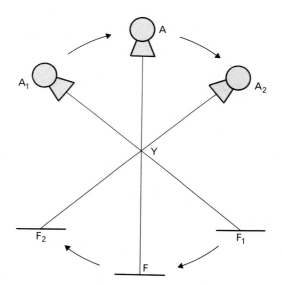

Fig. 13.9

present. The student should note that though the firm's plane of movement is arcuate, the plane of the film itself is horizontal and remains parallel to the selected tomographic plane.

The arc-to-arc tomographic movement is considered to have certain advantages compared with the rectilinear system previously described. Radiation intensity is more evenly distributed throughout the film's excursion and the equipment is less prone to either misalignment or vibration. Subject-film distances are likely to be greater but perhaps this matters very little in practice, provided that the equipment offers a sufficiently long anode-film distance and that other sources of unsharpness can be kept small.

It is possible that the student will meet apparatus which relies on a combination of the two movements described: the X-ray tube travels in an arc, while the film is moved on one horizontal line. In such equipment there is a theoretical failure. While anode-film and anode-fulcrum distances visibly and demonstrably vary, the fulcrum-film distance does not. The important ratios are not constant and consequently neither is the degree of magnification present in the image: the image is bound to be unsharp to some extent.

However, it is to be admitted that such equipment undoubtedly works. One may suppose that it does so because the human eye is not an accurate recording instrument and accepts as being sharp unsharpness within certain limits.

The direction of movement

So far we have laid emphasis on the importance of sharpness in the selected tomographic plane. However, the unsharpness of unselected structures is equally vital to the success of tomography. Clearly we need all structures above and below the selected plane to be blurred to the maximum extent, for if they are not then their shadows will tend to obscure detail in the selected plane.

A large influence on the efficacy of the blurring movement lies in the direction of the tube's swing in relation to the architecture of those structures which it is desired to blur. Let us suppose that some feature which we wish to blur has a linear shape, for example the clavicle.

Figs. 13.10(a) and 13.10(b) are tomographs of a clavicle taken with a linear tube travel such as we have already described. In Fig. 13.10(a) the tube is moving in a direction parallel to the long axis of the bone; in Fig. 13.10(b) the tube is moving at right angles to the general line of the clavicle. Both radiographs were taken under the same conditions of exposure and with the fulcrum of movement at a level 2 cm above the highest part of the specimen. It is obvious which of the two directions results in the most effective blurring. In the first case the tube movement simply elongates the clavicle's shadow and indeed it is to be noticed not only how easily recognized is the identity of the subject but that the bone architecture can be perceived to a limited extent. From Fig. 13.10(b), however, it would be more difficult to say with certainty at what we were looking if we did not previously know the history of the experiment.

From this it is a reasonable conclusion that from any tomographic system we shall obtain maximum blur of structures which are at right angles to the line of section and that we shall be less fortunate in respect of anatomical features of which the main patterns are parallel to the direction of the movement.

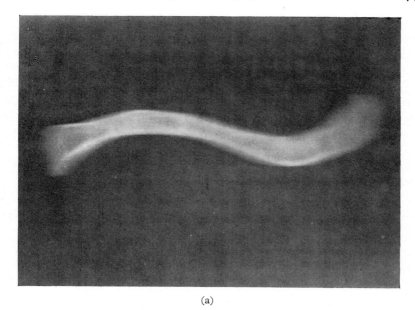

(a)

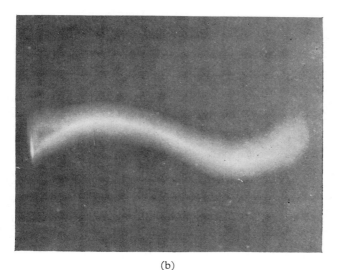

(b)

Fig. 13.10   Tomographs of a clavicle.

There would be no problem in this if human anatomy presented only conveniently placed linear designs which allowed us so to dispose the patient in relation to the apparatus that the tomographic excursion always occurred crosswise. However, of course this is not so. The structures of the body are not simple and linear but complex and subtle in their detail: when the X-ray tube moves linearly there are bound to be some structural outlines to which the motion is parallel and of which the blur is not so complete as we would wish.

Because of these facts apparatus was devised for tomography in which the excursions of the X-ray tube and the film are not the simple straight lines which we have so far considered. The student is asked to remember that however the movements may be elaborated, they will be consistent with the theory of tomography as we have discussed it, provided that the X-ray tube and the film are both doing the same thing but in opposite directions to each other.

Figure 13.11 illustrates some tomographic trajectories which may be provided by sophisticated equipment. They are listed below with some brief annotations.

Linear

This is the classical trajectory which we have earlier considered. It is the one employed in all simple apparatus of the kind which comprises a number of

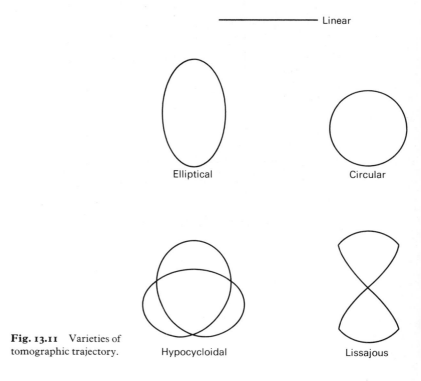

Fig. 13.11 Varieties of tomographic trajectory.

attachments fitted to a standard radiographic table and tubestand or ceiling tube support. This movement undoubtedly is the one most often used. It is particularly suitable for tomography of the thorax where there are no bony structures lying parallel with the tube/film trajectory.

Elliptical

In this the X-ray tube and the film make elliptical excursions parallel with the table-top. The angle of swing—that is the control on the thickness of the tomographic layer—is fixed at 40 degrees. Elliptical movement is perhaps the first obvious variation of a simple straight line and is a step towards the multidirectional movements which result in maximum blur.

Circular

In this arrangement the X-ray tube and the film each describe a circle in parallel planes above and below the table. The angle of swing is controlled by altering the radius of the circle; for example a choice of two radii is provided, resulting in angles of 29 and 36 degrees.

Hypocycloidal

The hypocycloidal movement is the most complex trajectory available and results in highly effective blurring. It is sometimes described as a clover-leaf. This avoids a complicated name and the three segments of the movement do appear to form a trefoil.

It is truthfully said of the hypocycloidal movement that it has no dominant direction: it is not longitudinal in any respect and consequently cannot elongate linear anatomical patterns found in structures which it is desired to blur. The hypocycloidal movement is especially suitable for the tomography of bone and in particular for examining very small bony elements, such as exist in the skull.

The angle of swing during the hypocycloidal movement is fixed at 48 degrees, resulting in a minimum layer thickness of the order of 1 mm. This is extremely selective tomography which is appropriate—and indeed necessary—if the examination refers to small structures, for example the auditory ossicles and the temporomandibular joints.

The Lissajous figure

The Lissajous figure, which is roughly a figure of 8, is another multidirectional trajectory offered by certain equipment. The travel of the X-ray tube and film may be through the whole figure or through only a part of it: for example, through either the lower or the upper ovoid; or through the X formation immediately at the centre; or along either of the sinuous lines which run obliquely through the centre.

By way of summary we can say that basically there are two categories of tomographic movement (a) linear and (b) a group described as multidirectional. The linear movement is simple, technically easy to obtain and sufficiently selective in its effect to be satisfactory for many kinds of examination. The multi-directional group require complex, specialized machinery but their influence is towards the production of fuller blurring and better detail separation. However, the radiographs may be lower in contrast.

A further aspect of tube movement which may be significant is the effect which its direction has on a radiographic appearance often described as *spurious contours* or *interference shadowing*. These appearances are sharp outlines formed by absorption boundaries in tissues outside the tomographic layer. As these distracting shadows are unavoidable in tomography it is important that the interpreter should recognize them and consequently that they should be easily recognizable (perhaps this is the fundamental professional purpose of any diagnostic radiographer: making things *easy* to see on a radiograph). In the case of linear and hypocycloidal trajectories these spurious contours have characteristic forms, long and trailing in the one case and of double outline in the other. When the tube travels in an ellipse or a circle recognition is said to be more difficult.

The speed of movement and length of trajectory

Effect on exposure time

The speed at which the tube moves during tomography controls radiographic exposure time: fairly obviously, the faster the tube movement the shorter is the interval of exposure.

Another factor in the time obtainable is the angle of exposure; that is, the angle of swing through which the tube moves. When the tube describes a wide angle, exposure times are necessarily longer than when the angle is small. Taking as typical the chart relating to a particular apparatus, we find—for example—that at an angle of swing of 44 degrees the minimum exposure time is 1 second. If we accept an angle of 20 degrees of movement of the X-ray tube we can reduce the exposure interval to 0·4 second.

In a similar way the length of the tube trajectory influences the radiographic exposure. A straight line is well known as the shortest distance between two points: consequently, in terms of tube travel, it represents the shortest exposure time obtainable. When the X-ray tube makes any excursion other than a straight line it is bound to take longer and consequently this puts a higher limit on the minimum exposure interval which may be used.

Effect on detail perception

In theory, with a given selection of milliamperes, faster tube travel should mean better visibility of detail, this being more readily perceived in the sharp layer because the shadows of other structures are 'underexposed' to a greater degree when motion is rapid. However, experiment seems to show that in practice the eye finds little difference in tomograms taken over a range of tube speeds. The point is evidently of slight significance to radiographers.

In an allied manner, a long tube trajectory implies increased efficacy of blurring because unwanted shadows are 'spread' over a greater area and are therefore less intrusive.

Summary

A tomogram consists of:

1 the sharp image of a selected layer in the body;
2 unsharp densities due to movement blur in layers above and below the selected one.

Tomography is performed as follows:

1 the X-ray tube and the film are moved through equal and opposite excursions;
2 there is a fulcrum about which this movement must revolve and which does not itself move in relation to the tube and the film;
3 the fulcrum in theory is a point but in practice determines a layer which appears radiographically sharp.

Tomographic equipment is devised so that:

1 the height of the fulcrum layer above the film can be pre-selected between about zero and 20 cm;
2 the thickness of the fulcrum layer can be altered within limits by the use of different angles of tube swing;

3   the movement of the tube may be linear (simple apparatus) or multi-directional (technically complex apparatus);
4   the speed of travel is variable to give a range of exposure times.

If tomography is to be successful it is important that throughout the movements of the tube and the film (a) the film remains parallel with the selected layer in the body and (b) image magnification is constant: this depends upon a constant ratio between the anode-film and anode-fulcrum distances.

MULTISECTION RADIOGRAPHY

Multisection or multilayer radiography is the name given to tomography of a number of body layers simultaneously, each layer being recorded on a separate film. It has a number of advantages.

1   Radiation dosage to the patient is reduced, since a number of separate radiographs are obtained at the cost of a single exposure.
2   Each of these radiographs is taken at exactly the same moment in the respiratory or other physiological phase.
3   Thus, it is the only way in which rapidly transient phenomena—such as vascular fillings in angiography—can be satisfactorily tomographed.
4   It saves time both for the patient and for the X-ray department.
5   It lessens the exposure load on the X-ray tube.

However, it is generally considered that good sequential tomographs—that is, one section at a time—offer finer detail than may be obtainable from even the best multisection procedure.

In Fig. 13.12(a) we depict the familiar arrangement of an X-ray tube (T) linked to a film (F) by a lever which causes them to rotate in opposite directions about a fulcrum (Y). The dotted line joins possible positions of the tube and the film at the end of one such excursion and we have earlier argued to show that a plane through Y is sharply recorded on the film because relatively there is no movement of Y in respect of T and F. The student is asked to notice that in this case the film is depicted as being in a position coincident with the end of the lever which links it to the X-ray tube.

Figure 13.12(b) depicts a different situation in which we have used a box to put a second film (F_2) below the first one (F_1): its position naturally is *not* coincident with the end of the lever which connects them both to the X-ray tube and moves them in its respect. We can see from the drawing that we have created a second fulcrum at Y_2 which is the point of rotation for the X-ray tube and the second film; this records a plane parallel to the one through Y but at a lower level. Any other number of films which we may arrange below the first similarly create their own points of rotation and record their

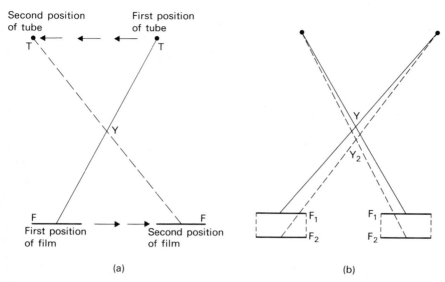

Fig. 13.12

own associated layers; so also will any films placed *above* F_1 but in this case the planes recorded are higher than Y.

Putting this in terms of a general principle, we can say that in tomography the layer recorded on a film is at the level of the fulcrum of the lever concerned, provided that the position of the film coincides with the film-moving point on the lever: films situated above and below this point record layers above and below the lever's fulcrum.

The multisection cassette

Our diagram in Fig. 13.12(b) depicts two films put one above the other with a certain space between them and we have referred to the possibility of arranging several films in a similar relationship. This is the function of the multisection cassette.

The cassette is a metal box up to 7·5 cm (3 inches) deep depending upon the number of films which it is to contain and the spacing between them. A variety of models are available holding 3, 4, 5 or 7 films. Some of these—for example a box for 4 films spaced 5 mm apart—look merely like a rather deep version of a standard cassette and can be placed in a bucky tray. The deeper cassettes, however, need a special support tray or drawer which replaces the usual tray under the bucky diaphragm.

The intensifying screens and separators

A useful arrangement is to fasten the intensifying screens and spacing material together and mount them in the form of a book; the films are then inserted between its 'leaves'. This has practical advantages in that incorrect placing of the films is impossible: they cannot be put other than between the appropriate screens.

The student should note that from any multisection cassette the radiographs would show unequal density if all the screens were of similar speed. As the X-ray beam traverses the box it is progressively attenuated by absorption in the successive layers of the 'sandwich'—particularly by absorption in the screens as opposed to film base and emulsion. This means that the amount of radiation reaching the lowest film in the box is appreciably less than the quantity incident on the uppermost film. If the two radiographs are to be of comparable density—and this they must be for the success of the procedure—then the last intensifying screens have to be greater in speed than those nearer to the X-ray tube.

Implicit in these facts are certain conclusions of practical significance.

1 There is a right and wrong aspect of the 'book' relative to the X-ray tube and usually clear identification is provided. If the assembly of screens, separators and films inadvertently is put into the cassette back to front when the cassette is loaded in the darkroom, then radiographic chaos will follow for sure.

2 A multisection system is photographically slower than the same film used in a standard cassette: this is inevitable since it is a complex in which the faster materials have to be used in circumstances reducing their photographic effect. Radiographic exposures for use with multisection cassettes are usually determined on a trial-and-error basis; it is very difficult for a manufacturer to give reliable guidance in view of the variety of screen/film combinations normally found in use in any sample group of X-ray departments. Available figures suggest kilovoltage increases varying from 8 kVp to as much as 19 kVp and a multiplication of milliampere-seconds values ranging from 1·6 to 2·5. Such figures in themselves are not particularly helpful. A radiographer using a multisection cassette for the first time should recognize that it is likely to be at least 4 or 5 times 'slower' than conventional cassettes employed in the department. Experiments with a step wedge are the best basis for accurate exposure selection.

In a multisection cassette the material used for the separators is significant in that it should not appreciably absorb X radiation and must be free from artefacts. At present it is usually a plastic foam layer either 5 mm or 10 mm in thickness. In some examinations it may be necessary to take radiographs even closer together—say at 1 mm separation.

This can be done easily if the separators and intensifying screens are not fixed together as earlier described. The films are placed on top of each other, with only the appropriate intensifying screens between them, and the spacers used in the back of the cassette to maintain the films and screens in good contact; or a felt pad can be used for the same purpose.

Localization of planes

In sequential tomography the operator knows that the layer recorded on the film is one which is the same height above the table as the pre-selected level of the fulcrum. In multisection radiography, however, the position is more complicated because several layers are recorded simultaneously. We need to know the situation of each in relation to the fulcrum, as it is the fulcrum point which we fix on the equipment.

Most commonly, the top film in a box—the one nearest the X-ray tube—records the fulcrum level. The other films then record layers nearer to the table surface than is the fulcrum point, the exact levels of these being influenced by the distance between films. Although in theory the two quantities are not equal, for practical purposes we can equate them: we can say that when the spacing material and screens separate two films by 5 mm then the planes recorded on these films are virtually 5 mm apart. Care should be taken when multisection radiography is done to see that the fulcrum is set at such a level that each film does in fact record a body layer; failure in this respect has produced tomographs of the X-ray table before now. When tomographic equipment is installed, tests should be made to determine that fulcrum levels are accurately indicated (see Chapter 17, page 616).

It is obviously of first importance for the operator to know which film in the cassette is associated with the fulcrum level. It is not always the top one: it may be the middle film of 3 or 5; and there is a 4-film cassette available in which one pair of films are above the fulcrum level and the other pair below it. The manufacturers provide the relevant information in each case.

EQUIPMENT FOR TOMOGRAPHY

X-ray equipment for the production of tomographs comes in one or other of two categories:

1 accessory apparatus which enables a standard radiographic table and tube support to be used for tomography;

2 specialized tables intended primarily for tomography.

Whatever its type, the accuracy of tomographic equipment is dependent on the quality of its engineering: a rigid structure is essentially important.

Layer radiographic attachments

Accessories used to convert standard equipment to a tomographic function are collectively described as attachments for layer radiography. There are many differences in the detail of such attachments but they have in common the feature that they can all readily—perhaps some more readily than others—be assembled on the X-ray installation for which they are designed and after use can be detached and stored in some convenient place until required for another examination. Tomographic equipment of this variety is attractive when the demand for tomography is low compared with the amount of other radiographic work to be done in the X-ray room concerned.

The components of such equipment are:

1 a linkage mechanism;
2 a pivot unit;
3 a mechanical drive;
4 a drive control, usually a separate wall-mounted unit.

The linkage mechanism

The link assembly, which is seen in Fig. 13.13 is a long telescopic steel rod which couples together the X-ray tube and the bucky carriage by means of clamps and locking handles. In linking them, the rod must allow the X-ray tube and the bucky carriage to be further apart at the beginning and the end of their excursions (see the oblique lines in Fig. 13.8), than they are when the X-ray tube has moved some of the way through its angle of swing and is directly above the film. To achieve this, the link rod may have a telescopic structure. However, its rigidity also is essential and many link rods are not extensible: the X-ray tube is allowed to move along such a rod—which thus effectively is extended—by the nature of the coupling between them. The end of the rod which is attached to the tube carriage may be so designed that when the rod is in position it is impossible to tighten the lock which prevents rotation of the X-ray tube. This ensures that the tube is free to rotate on its axis at the extremities of its travel in the manner sketched in Fig. 13.8: it is a precaution against a human error which could considerably damage the equipment.

A radiographer who assembles layer radiographic attachments before use should always make sure that those parts of the equipment, which require to move, *can* move; and that those parts of the equipment, which should not move, do not do so. Thus, the following brakes should be released or OFF: tube rotation; bucky carriage; 'longitudinal' movement of the X-ray tube. The following brakes should be ON: transverse or lateral movement of the X-ray tube; vertical movement of the X-ray tube; table-top brakes,

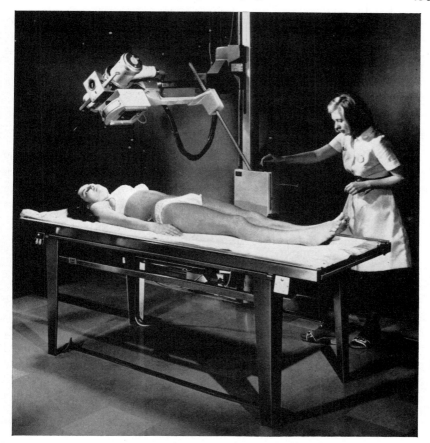

Fig. 13.13 Attachments for layer radiography fitted to a floor-ceiling tubestand and a plain bucky table. The linkage arm is in place and the radiographer is selecting the height of the fulcrum point on the pivot unit. *By courtesy of Picker International Ltd.*

if the top is of the 'floating' type. Some of these effects may be so interlocked that they occur automatically upon correct selection of the tomographic mode; but this is not possible in the case of a mechanically operated brake, of which manual release is always necessary. In all instances, the manufacturer's instructions for fitting tomographic attachments should be followed in detail.

The physical dimensions of the link-rod prevent completely free selection of the anode-film distance. Even when abbreviated to the minimum it necessarily prohibits the use of short distances and equally the arm cannot extend beyond certain bounds. In this connection it is to be remembered that the maximum demand on the length of the tube-film link occurs at the extremities of travel. The length required by the full excursion of the X-ray tube must always be available for it and this places an upper limit on the selection of anode-film distance. In practice the anode-film distance is adjustable on most apparatus between about 92–107 cm (36–42 inches). However, the agent most likely to restrict the selection of anode-film distances is the focused secondary radiation grid (see Chapter 8, page 316).

The pivot unit

The pivot unit, which also is seen in Fig. 13.13, can best be described by saying that it is a turret-like structure—and sometimes is called the fulcrum tower—about 30–38 cm high (12–15 inches). This is fitted to the edge of the X-ray table which is nearer to the tubestand and linkage arm; the latter passes through a pivoting sleeve on the side of the tower.

The functions of this part of the equipment are to provide:
1   a pivot for the opposite movements of the X-ray tube and the bucky tray;
2   a means to alter the height of the pivot point.

The second of these is achieved through a worm screw which can be hand-turned by means of a wheel or large knob. The pivotal assembly travels up or down this worm-drive and the range of movement offered is usually 0·5 cm intervals from 0 to 20 cm above the table surface. In a sophisticated form of this equipment one revolution of the hand-wheel moves the pivot point 1 cm. A scale mounted on an adjacent aspect of the tower is calibrated in centimetres or inches—sometimes both—and the position of the pivot is shown on the scale by means of a suitable indicator (a pointer or line).

The fulcrum tower includes the switch assembly which effects the X-ray exposure. During its excursion from one side of the tower to the other the linkage arm operates primarily two sets of contacts; the first of these initiates the X-ray exposure and the second terminates exposure.

The value of the exposure interval thus obtained is dependent upon the period of time required by the linkage arm to travel between these two stations and this in turn depends upon the speed and angle of the tube movement. It is normal practice for manufacturers to provide information with their equipment about the exposure intervals which result from various combinations of speed and angle. The operator must ensure that the main radiographic timer is set for a period in excess of the tomographic exposure, since whichever timing mechanism provides the shorter interval becomes the dominant agent in terminating the X-ray exposure.

The mechanical drive

Travel of the X-ray tube during the exposure can be achieved by a variety of means. Tomography is not impossible if the only method of moving the tube is by hand but considerations of radiation safety would make this extremely undesirable, quite apart from the difficulty of standardizing such propulsion. For these reasons some form of mechanical drive is invariably employed in current practice and usually is provided by a small motor. If the tube is ceiling-suspended this motor may be the one which effects normal longitudinal movements of the X-ray tube (see Chapter 7, page 292). It is an advantage of ceiling suspension that the tomographic drive is more direct and therefore more efficient when taken from such suspension than from a floor mounting.

When the tube is supported by means of a floor/ceiling stand (see Chapter 7, page 286) the motor may form an integral part of the tube-stand's base or it may be attached to the base and engaged by a lever mechanism with a separate floor-track, alongside the one for the X-ray tube. Students no doubt will notice minor differences of design in such motors in use in their own departments. It is customary for the speed of the motor to be variable by means of a remote control unit. In some instances the exposure can be made during only one direction of tube travel.

The drive control

The control unit for the tube drive is often in a separate wall-mounted box. This usually has switches which permit:

1 selection of the tube's speed of travel;
2 selection of the angle of exposure;
3 trial runs of the apparatus to be made without X-ray exposure.

In some cases a warning lamp is included which indicates when the equipment is energized.

Various sophistications of control are to be found in different examples of attachments for layer radiography. For example, some equipment may provide only 3 or 4 speeds of travel while another gives a choice between as many as 10 or 11. One equipment may offer only two alternative angles of exposure—for example 22 and 44 degrees—while in another it is even possible individually to adjust the angles on either side of the vertical, so that the complete arc of travel is not necessarily symmetrically disposed about the vertical; this could be useful in avoiding rib patterns when tomographing the upper abdomen. A typical angular range found in most equipment is perhaps four or five values, giving exposure angles from 30 to 60 degrees.

Tomographic Tables

Tomographic tables are those planned especially for tomography, although they may allow general radiography to be performed. As a rule, the more dedicated to tomography is the design of the table, the less felicitous is its capability for other X-ray examinations. Few radiodiagnostic rooms can be reserved exclusively for tomography and readers of this book are likely to find the most sophisticated versions of these tomographic tables only in large radiodiagnostic departments, where there is a significant demand for specialised tomography; for instance, of complex cranial structures, such as the petrous bone and temporomandibular articulations.

Tomographic tables of various capability are offered by many manufacturers and cannot here be described in detail. All are alike in the structural feature that the tube support is integrated with the table and can move the X-ray tube and a film through such excursions as we have described in principle in earlier parts of this chapter. Tomographic tables can be categorised in three general groups which are set down below in ascending order of elaboration and do not include two well known tomographic equipments of another nature: these—which are described elsewhere in this book (see p. 458 and p. 525)—are the equipment for computerised axial tomography and that for rotational tomography of the jaws and face.

With reference to the tables within the three groups which follow, the necessary controls of the tomographic function are provided through a separate programme console (or a section of one) which is specific to this purpose. For convenience in use, these controls may be partly or wholly duplicated in a mounting at the table side.

Group I

A tomographic table in this first group characteristically is a simple bucky table for radiography, having a floating top and the particular feature of an integrated tubestand suitable for tomography. Many of the tables in this group provide only a linear tomographic trajectory.

If the table and its X-ray room are to be useful for general radiographic examinations, two facilities are especially important. These are: (1) an ability to rotate the tube column round its vertical axis (preferably through 360 deg) so that the X-ray tube can be positioned for an 'off-the-table' examination, of a patient lying on a stretcher for instance; (2) the possibility of obtaining a horizontal beam projection towards a patient, who may be either on the table or not (for example, he might be standing at a vertical cassette-stand). Limitations in these two respects are certain to affect the table's usefulness, if it is part of an installation catering for a high workload of both tomography and general radiography.

A typical example of a tomographic table in this group possesses the following attributes.

1 Linear trajectory of the X-ray tube and film.
2 A choice of three angles of tube swing: 40 deg., 20 deg., 8 deg.
3 A choice of two speeds at each angle of exposure, as follows:
>   40 deg.   1 sec., 3 sec.
>   20 deg.   0·5 sec., 1·5 sec.
>   8 deg.   0·2 sec., 0·6 sec.
>   (Zonography).

In each case, the tube's speed is greater at the centre of its excursion than it is either at the beginning or at the end. This helps to reduce vibration and to maintain the exposure dose during parts of the cycle when the X-ray source and the film are furthest from each other. (See the oblique lines in Fig. 13.8.) Such speed differentials are not an uncommon feature of equipment design.
4 Layer-height adjustment from 1 to 25 cm in increments of 0·5 cm. The movement of the fulcrum is motorised and under pushbutton control. Its height is visualised by means of a beam of light projected upon the patient's body.
5 Automatic indication—by means of a lighted lamp—of the correct anode-film distance for tomography: this is 1 metre. Selection of any other distance (possible with this particular table) switches off both the monitor lamp and the power supply to the motorised tubestand. This feature is a safety provision, which stops any inadvertent attempt to conduct tomography at a distance which is physically incompatible with the structure of the tube-film linkage.
6 A scan facility, motorising the tube-column in forward and reverse directions longitudinally. This allows a demonstration—without X-ray exposure—of the tomographic movement. A patient who is experiencing tomography for the first time should be warned that the equipment will move; he may imagine that it is falling on him and attempt to leave his dangerous situation. The ability to make a trial run is a helpful feature of any tomographic system.

Group 2

Tomographic tables in this group differ from those in the first mainly in providing a circular or elliptical movement, or both, in addition to a linear trajectory. Whilst these tables may allow conventional 'on-table' radiography and often 'off-table' examinations as well (by means of suitable angulation of the X-ray tube), nevertheless they tend to have less convenience for general radiography and greater dedication to a tomographic function. Their characteristics, in respect of variable angles, variable speeds and motorised adjustment of layer-height, are similar to—and certainly will not be less than—those listed for the simple tomographic table already described.

Group 3

Tomographic tables in the third group are highly specialised. Their design subordinates any other radiographic function to that of tomography, for which alone may the table be considered suitable. The range of tomographic movements which equipment in this group may offer encompasses the following: linear; circular or elliptical or both; hypocycloidal or spiral or both. In addition to the provision of multidirectional excursions of the X-ray tube, the table may have facilities (a) to tilt or rotate the patient, or do both, and (b) for television fluoroscopy.

Students, examining any specialised tomographic tables in their training departments, should be able to determine the group to which the equipment belongs. For special notice are the following variables of the equipment and the means employed for their selection, control and indication:

1   the direction of the tube trajectory—linear or multidirectional;
2   the speed of the tube movement;
3   the angle of exposure;
4   the duration of the exposure;
5   the height of the pivot point;
6   the thickness of the tomographic layer.

As we have seen, each of these factors is significant in tomography. Their materialisation in specific tomographic equipment of any kind strongly affects the versatility of the equipment and its appropriateness to the X-ray examinations which it is expected to perform.

COMPUTED TOMOGRAPHY

Computed tomography is a special form of tomography in which a computer is used to make a mathematical reconstruction of a tomographic plane or slice. Computed tomography is now properly known by the capital letters CT; but others have been employed and in the United Kingdom perhaps the most familiar of these notations is CAT scanning. CAT may stand for computer aided tomography; but equally for computerised axial tomography. Inclusion of the word *axial* serves at least to remind students of the subject that a distinctive feature of computerised tomography is the cross-sectional direction of the tomographic plane.

A distinction has to be made between transmission tomography (TCAT) and emission tomography (ECAT). The latter is performed with a gamma camera following the administration, to a patient, of a diagnostic dose of a radionuclide. During ECAT the patient becomes a temporary source of emitted radiation. TCAT, on the other hand, is no different from any other X-ray examination in depending upon the attenuations of an X-ray beam, when this—emitted from an X-ray tube—passes through the body of a patient to a sensitive recorder. The patient is a transmitter—but not the origin—of the radiation concerned. The uses of radionuclides are not the business of this book and so it is transmission tomography (CT scanning) which we have now to consider.

The scanning principle

During conventional tomography, as we have considered it, the recorded tomographic planes have been longitudinal in the body and parallel to the film; they are coronal in direction when the patient faces towards or away from the X-ray tube; they are sagittal in direction when the patient occupies the lateral decubitus.

During computed tomography, a different geometry applies. This is sketched in its simplest form in Fig. 13.14 and significant features to be noted are:

1 the X-ray beam is strictly collimated, being described as a pencil beam;
2 the X-ray tube is rigidly coupled to radiation detectors which receive the beam leaving from the interposed tissues of the patient;
3 a collimator, to eliminate unwanted scatter, is placed immediately in front of the detectors.

If the tube/detector assembly is moved across the patient (say, from his left to his right side), the intensity of X-rays, reaching the detectors and constituting the *signal* from the system, will depend on the beam's absorption by intervening tissue and will not be constant. The variations occurring depend only upon the quantity of X-rays absorbed.

The intensity differences in the signal represent modifications of the X-ray beam (due to varying amounts of attenuation) considered in the direction taken by the X-ray tube/detector combination. Thus, the identified plane of interest is a transverse section through the body; the aspect of this plane is inferosuperior, the observer effectively looking upwards through the soles of the subject's feet.

A movement of the equipment across the patient, without any change in angulation of the beam, is technically described as a *translation*; and the data obtained from the sequence of measured transmissions constitute an *absorption profile* or projection. A movement of the equipment round the patient, without translation, is described as *rotation*. Equipments with both movements are said to be translate/rotate systems. Others, which have only a rotational movement, are called rotate systems and these are considered later in this chapter (see p. 483).

In the case of translate/rotate systems and following the movement of translation, the tube/detector assembly rotates and then makes another scan,

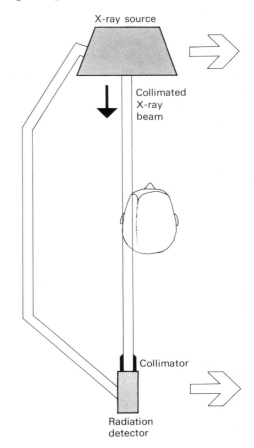

X-ray source

Collimated
X-ray
beam

Collimator

Fig. 13.14 The principle of scanning
during computed tomography.

Radiation
detector

similar to the first, from a new angle. It repeats this process through a series
of angles; as an example, in the case of very early equipment, rotation occurred at 1 deg intervals from 0 deg to 180 deg. Each linear scan
constitutes a *view* in computed tomography. More realistically—because
this shortens the time required for a scan—translate/rotate systems now
rotate through intervals of approximately $7\frac{1}{2}$ deg. Scan times are further
considered on p. 382.

In this manner, several hundred absorption profiles are obtained which
can be stored in a computer and subsequently processed. Fig. 13.15 is a
sketch which illustrates the scanning principle of translation and rotation,
depicting three angles of rotation.

It is to be understood by the reader that the above—referring to a pencil
X-ray beam and a single detector—is an explanation of a simple scanning
procedure, suitable for the acquirement of multiple items of information

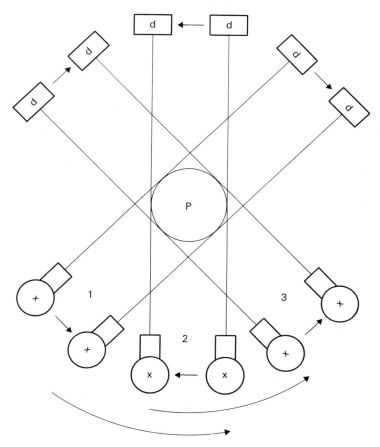

Fig. 13.15 A translate–rotate scanning system.

about absorption (and attenuation) occurrences within an X-ray beam, as it passes through tissue. Practically, equipments have been developed which use similar principles more elaborately and these will be considered later (see p. 382).

At this point it is easy to understand that what has been obtained from the equipment is a large number of measurements of the intensity of an X-ray beam as it leaves different parts of a subject. The exiting intensities may be compared easily with the incident intensities, as these are both externally made measurements. The next step is to consider how—from such acquired data—the essential purpose of all X-ray examinations is to be achieved, which is to determine the internal structure of the subject.

In computed tomography, the subject is a particular 'slice' of tissue, illustrated in Fig. 13.16.; its thickness is established essentially by the width of the X-ray beam We need to know the inner nature of this 'slice' of tissue. As a homely example, the reader may like to think of two articles of food which are commonly sliced in kitchens: these are a loaf of bread and a pork pie which has an egg in its middle. In the first case, the slice of bread is homogenous (or should be!) and external examination provides a fairly reliable guide as to what the inside of the loaf is like. The case of the pork pie is otherwise: any external assessment fails to inform us of the egg's presence and when we cut the pie we find that the slice is not homogeneous but is

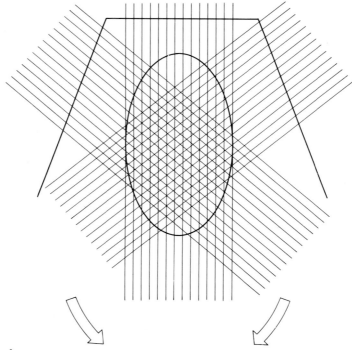

Fig. 13.16

composed of a number of different materials. The task of a CT system is to identify and reveal the egg and other structures within the pie; this part of the process is described as a *reconstruction*. Finally, the system must provide a 2-dimensional visual display of the reconstruction made.

Reconstruction of the image

To construct a detailed image, from certain measured transmissions of an X-ray beam leaving an absorber, involves a practice of mathematics. A large number of mathematical manipulations are required and these are very quickly performed by a computer; they could be realised by a human calculator, but not within an acceptable period of time.

Readers of this book are not expected to know how to handle advanced mathematics (nor are its authors, we hope): but radiographers are creators of images and we should understand their nature. It is necessary now both to identify the problem involved in constructing a CT image and to appreciate the appropriateness of its mathematical solution.

When an X-ray beam passes through a human subject, it is traversing not a single volume of homogeneous material but a succession of volumes of different kinds of tissue (in effect, the pork pie already mentioned). Depending upon the nature of its composition, each successive volume may differently reduce the number of incident photons. Thus, the number of photons arriving at an exit point—that is, the number measured by the CT system—is the sum of a series of fractionations of the beam which have occurred within the irradiated volume. If the internal structure of that volume is to be accurately determined, in order to create a detailed image of it, we must be able to evaluate separately the various fractionations of the incident beam. Fig. 13.17 may help to illustrate this point.

Fig. 13.17a depicts the irradiation of a piece of material which is uniform in density and composed of three conjoined blocks. To each of the blocks a value of 3 has been assigned, resulting in an emergent value of 9 (3+3+3). Fig. 13.17b depicts a similar 'beam sum' obtained from a similar volume of material, but in this case the material is not uniform in density: the three blocks are seen to have each a different value (4+3+2 = 9).

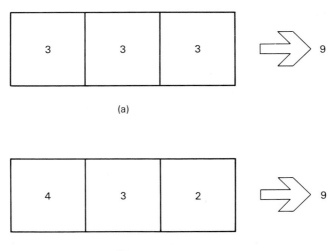

(a)

(b)

Fig. 13.17

In Fig. 13.17, nines are the transmissions measured by the CT scanner. In practice they are the only values known, since they are obtained from a comparison between two directly measurable quantities, the number of incident X-ray photons and the number of emergent photons. In the diagram, the sum 9 expresses a quantity which is the total absorption-value of the irradiated tissue and is the only information that we can derive from directing a fixed X-ray beam through tissue, towards a detector which also is fixed in position. The problem is to determine the several quantities which are summed by each 9 in Fig. 13.17: that is, to compute a value for each separate 'block' within an irradiated material. Only then have we differentiated one tissue from another during a CT scan of a human subject.

For the purpose of this exercise, the scanned 'slice' of tissue must be considered as comprising a large number of small blocks or volumes. This can be done by imposing a grid on the slice (see Fig. 13.18).

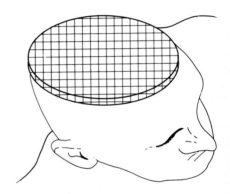

Fig. 13.18

Commonly, each square of the slice might be 1·5 mm × 1·5 mm. The thickness of the slice is approximately 10 mm (determined primarily by the width of the X-ray beam which in this case is assessed as a constant). Thus, each volume element (which is treated as though it were uniform in composition) has a capacity of about 22·5 mm³.

Of course, there is a convenient jargon which ascribes a shorter name to these small anatomical volume-elements. One volume-element is a *voxel* and it is the basic unit of CT reconstruction. When voxels are represented 2-dimensionally on a video display monitor another word is needed for the corresponding elements of the picture. This shorthand word is the *pixel*: it is an abbreviated term for picture element cell and at least avoids a tongue-wrenching twist of English. Even newcomers to computer language should not find it hard to remember that a pixel is a 'pic' and a voxel is a 'vol'.

The essential task during computed tomography is to assign to each pixel a number which represents the attenuation coefficient of the corresponding voxel. The values of these attenuation coefficients are not obtained directly as measured transmissions during a scan: they must therefore be calculated mathematically by the computer. The computer programmer must solve the puzzle and, to do so, must have an organised and systematic approach.

The structure which we have described, consisting of numeric data in a 2-dimensional grid pattern (rows and columns of figures), is called a *matrix*. Fig. 13.19 represents a very simple matrix which consists of a 2 × 2 arrangement of voxels. Each element in this matrix has a different value; putting it in other terms, each voxel has a different attenuation coefficient. We do not know these values, but an X-ray beam—passed in two directions through this subject—would yield four values which are arithmetical

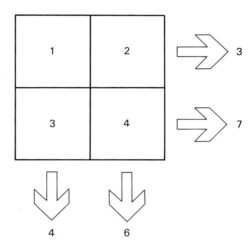

Fig. 13.19   A simple matrix.

additions of the blocks. Thus, the top row has a sum of 3; the lower row a sum of 7; the left-hand column has a sum of 4; and the right-hand column a sum of 6. The computer's task—in principle, not difficult—is to calculate the individual value of each block from these four data.

A number of mathematical methods are available, any of which should yield the four unknown quantities in the problem. With the particular procedure of these methods, readers of this book need not be closely concerned (else, what is a computer for?). However, it is helpful to have a nodding acquaintance with these mathematical schemes (in computer language called *algorithms*), so that we may recognise certain advantages and disadvantages in their application to computed tomography.

The algorithm provides the computer's coherent approach to the problem to be solved. There are several such systematic approaches, each of which can yield a correct result; just as swimmers may use different strokes to drive themselves through water; and competitors in dressage ride horses in a style different from flat-race jockeys. So here there are a number of algorithms applicable to the same problem: they are briefly described below.

1. Iterative reconstruction

An iterative method of calculation was the one employed by early CT systems. Essentially it is a process of trial and error, in which a number of 'guesses' of the individual transmission values within a matrix are made, in order to find a distribution of values which accords with the total or measured transmissions from the various exit points.

Unless the number of CT views is very small, a large number of such estimations is entailed. Consequently, the method is slow and can be an exacting order even for a computer, particularly when a large matrix—greater than 128×128 blocks—is concerned. The use of an iterative reconstruction may mean a delay of several minutes before an image is visualised upon completion of a scan. Consequently, this method is not employed in commercially available machines at this time.

2. Back projection

Back projection has been described as a simplified method of reconstruction; and possibly the performance of it is more simple than the explanation. Keywords in this method are that it uses a repeated 'backwards addition' of ray sums. It is an elementary method which was first employed for medical imaging during the 1960's by Khul, in an application to nuclear medicine.

Referring again to the simple 2×2 matrix in Fig. 13.19, there are two 'horizontal' ray sums (3 and 7) which would result from two horizontal irradiations of the subject by an X-ray beam; these are shown by the horizontal arrows in Fig. 13.20. The first estimation would allot the value of

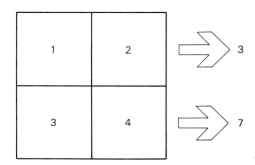

Fig. 13.20

the ray sum in each case to each of the pixels in the row. These estimated pixel values are shown in Fig. 13.21. Vertical irradiations of the subject yield two more ray sums: 4 for the left column and 6 for the column on the right, as shown in Fig. 13.22.

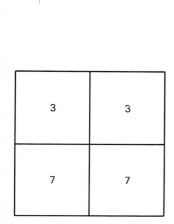

Fig. 13.21

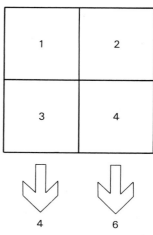

Fig. 13.22

These values also are back projected on the matrix and the new estimations give a matrix which is like the one in Fig. 13.23. The process continues with a similar 'backwards' addition of other ray sums, resulting from diagonal irradiations of the subject. Thus, from the matrix under consideration, a diagonal irradiation upwards and to the right would produce the ray sums shown in Fig. 13.24. These 'diagonal' sums are added

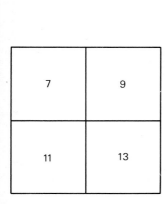

Fig. 13.23

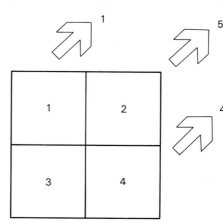

Fig. 13.24

to the sums in Fig. 13.23 and the resultant quantities are depicted in Fig. 13.25.

The same manoeuvres applied to a diagonal irradiation upwards and to the left result first in the ray sums shown in Fig. 13.26 and then in the

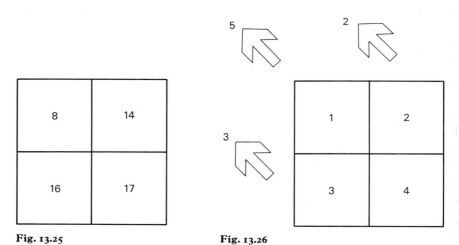

Fig. 13.25   Fig. 13.26

computations shown in Fig. 13.27. All the values depicted in the matrix in Fig. 13.27 have a common 'background' of 10: this constant value can be subtracted, with the results shown in Fig. 13.28. Division by 3 then brings the pixels to their simplest ratios (see Fig. 13.29).

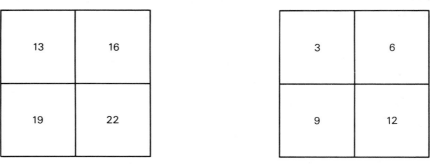

Fig. 13.27   Fig. 13.28

Non-survivors of the last few pages who do not recognize the matrix in Fig. 13.29 should compare it with the original in Fig. 13.19. We may summarise the situation with a statement that finally the value assigned to any one pixel is the sum of all the rays passing through it. All these assigned

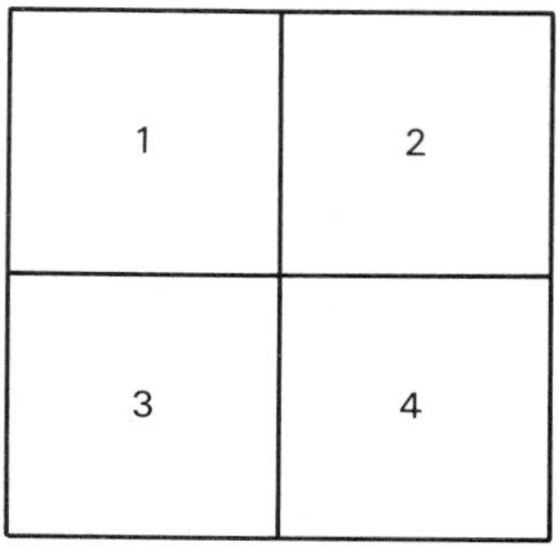

Fig. 13.29

values may be greater than the 'real' radiation transmissions from which they are derived but—if so–there is a proportional correspondence between them; the inter-pixel ratios remain correct and an image of faithfully related densities can be constructed.

However, images reconstructed by means of simple back projection suffer from an artefact which is described as a star pattern. The name is self-explanatory and refers to the fact that a point—considered to be a true circle—in the image is rendered as a star. The effect is a blurred reconstruction. Compensation for this blur is obtained if the transmitted signal is modulated by the computer before it is back projected: such modification endows the method with the names of *filtered back-projection* and *convolution*.

The accuracy of convolution makes this a method of image reconstruction which is widely employed by CT scanners at present. One of its advantages is that each absorption profile is processed as it is measured and there is virtually no waiting period for the image following completion of a scan.

3. Analytical reconstruction

Methods of image reconstruction which come under the heading of *analytical reconstruction* include convolution, which has been described above. It is not intended here to explain the mathematics of the filtering process by which the computer modulates each transmission value. Any such account in this text is unlikely to be appreciated by its readers (even if the authors were competent to write it). It is more important that we recognize the need for this further stage of mathematical analysis, if a blurring inherent in a reconstruction by simple back projection is to be avoided.

Another analytical method of image reconstruction applicable to computed tomography is one known as *fast Fourier transform*. The theory of Fourier analysis is that any fluctuation can be converted to a sine wave and thus be described and compared with other fluctuations in terms of the frequencies and phase relationships of waves. It is a mathematical process of changing the description of a function by giving its value in terms of its frequency components, instead of its spatial coordinates.

The use of the Fourier concept in computed tomography means that the coordinates of each CT projection, the series of transmission magnitudes in 'real' space, are converted to a series of component frequencies, arranged in 'frequency space'. In essence, information which we can understand readily in one language is translated to another, of which most of us do not possess a wide comprehension. At the end of the process, the function's spatial description must be recovered, if the reconstruction is to be clinically appreciated. An advantage of the Fourier scheme during computed tomography is that it replaces with simple multiplication the more complicated mathematic manoeuvres of convolution; but it can be slow.

Analytical methods of image reconstruction have a difficulty when adjacent voxels are very disparate in radiolucency; that is, when there is a sharp interface between the structures examined, for instance between bone and soft tissue. Failure to compensate for such an interface occurs for complicated reasons in physics, mathematics and the present state of the electronic arts. An iterative reconstruction is not so handicapped, but compensation for sharp edges requires a longer time from the computer.

Of the analytical methods which we have considered, convolution is more widely employed than Fourier transform. The latter is relatively slower and less able to provide a reconstruction of only part of a picture, should this be required.

Storing the image

By whatever mathematics the computer may make its calculations, their end is a file in the computer's memory. As we have seen, every file consists of a large number of discrete elements, each of which represents the absorption value of a small volume of tissue. These will be used to compose a picture.

Whilst it is not necessary for the pixels numerically to equal the elements of a CT matrix, there is often a one-to-one relationship between them, which we shall now assume.

Typically, matrixes might be 128 × 128, or 256 × 256. The first matrix gives some 16,400 pixels for one picture; and in the second case the number of pixels is approximately 65,600. The size of these numbers brings understanding of how necessary to this X-ray procedure is the storage capacity of an associated computer.

The number of pixels has an important influence on the resolution of the final picture. (However, it would be wrong to infer that pixel numbers are the only influence on the production of detail during CT imaging: in order to accentuate the point, we have here disregarded other factors upon which the production and perception of detail are dependent. Within these limits, the next statement in the paragraph is true.) In simple language, the more pixels there are, the more detail will the final picture display.

There is a natural law of gain and payment: we do not get anything for nothing; and images of high detail, with little noise (see p. 478), can be obtained only by increasing the amount of radiation. This is explained as follows.

A pixel is simply a small piece of information and is identified with one element in a matrix. A picture file in the computer, which has many such data in its composition, will have been obtained by the use of a fine matrix; that is, through a proportional number of irradiations of many small anatomical 'chunks' of a subject. So there is a trade-off here between resolution and radiation dose: we may have an image of high resolution, if we are prepared to administer to the patient a relatively high radiation dose. Whether an image of very high resolution is required in all clinical situations is a different point, to which further reference is made on p. 491.

CT numbers

The data gathered by the computer consist of a large number of attenuation coefficients. For many tissues the differences between these coefficients may be quite small and difficult to appreciate in the long range with which we are concerned. A scan of the chest, for instance, may contain all values, from that of air within the lungs to those generated by the thoracic skeleton.

In order more usefully to display such absorption differences, a conversion factor is applied: this factor is called a *CT number*. It is obtained by means of an equation, which takes a relation between the attenuation coefficient (μ) of the tissue in question and that of water and multiplies by a constant (K), known as the magnification (or magnifying) constant. For the mathematically persuaded reader—if any there is—this expression may be written thus:

$$\text{CT (number)} = \frac{K\,(\mu_{\text{tissue-water}})}{\mu_{\text{water}}}$$

The function of K is in establishing a scale. Some systems use a magnifying constant of 500; whilst in others K may have a value of 1000. The choice of scale does not affect the precision of the equipment; although the resolution afforded by the scale (that is, its ability to differentiate between adjacent pieces of information which are close in value) must be at least as great as the accuracy of the calculated attenuation coefficients.

The reader perhaps wonders what this association means in practical terms. Contemporary CT scanners are said to calculate attenuation coefficients to an accuracy of less than ±0.5 per cent. Putting this another way, the equipment is precise to an error of less than 1 in 200 and the magnifying constant should not be less than 200, if the scale's resolution is to be adequate.

However, it is important not to confuse these two aspects of resolution in equipment for computed tomography. A statement of the magnifying constant describes the resolution afforded by the scale of CT numbers: it will mislead us if we believe that it refers to the precision or resolution inherent in parts of the system which acquire the data and make the reconstructions.

Another aspect of CT numbers which may be overlooked is that they are not absolute for any particular tissue but will vary with the kilovoltage applied for the scan. This is bound to be so, since these numbers are derived from absorptive occurrences, which in turn are a function of the applied kilovoltage when a tissue is irradiated: at higher kilovoltage, linear attenuation coefficients become smaller. Thus, CT numbers may vary between different equipments, depending upon the kilovoltage calibration of a particular scanner; and also upon the filtration of the X-ray beam.

The language of computers

Reference to Chapter 6 may remind the reader that computers do not use decimal notation for counting: they employ instead binary numbers. The binary system has a radix of 2: each place to the left of the radical point carries a value which is twice that of its righthand neighbour. (In the decimal system the radix is 10.)

A binary digit (see p. 206) is the fundamental unit of computer storage and is called a *bit*: it occupies one 'space' in the computer's store. Eight bits form a unit called a *byte*. The term K-byte for 1000 bytes is another which is frequently used . (One K-byte = 8000 bits.)

Using one byte, a computer is able to store 256 combinations; whereas, to place a 3-digit number in a decimal counting system would require 30 'spaces' in the store. Computers associated with computed tomography can store or 'memorise' about 66 million bytes (528 million bits of information).

If its ability to compress information is one attractive feature of binary counting, another is its use of only two digits: these are 0 and 1 (see p. 195). Computers store information through electrical circuits called *flip-flops*. These are circuits which have only one function and that is to be either ON or OFF. A flip-flop used in a computer is dignified with the name *logic element* (see p. 194). Each bit in the computer requires one logic element. An activated flip-flop circuit indicates 1 to the computer; an unactivated ('off') circuit indicates o. Combinations of flip-flops can thus be used to feed to the computer vast amounts of numeric information.

The storage capacity of a computer is described as its *core memory*. This is part of the computer itself and essentially is contained in a large number of very small pieces of an easily magnetized metal. Magnetization of an individual among these components indicates 1 to the computer; demagnetization represents o. Typically, the core memory of the host computer in a CT scanner might have a capacity of about 64 K-bytes.

Storage and documenting

Information in the core memory is lost when the power supply to the computer is broken and so is available only for immediate access. On completion of a scan and the departure of the patient, storage in a longer term must be provided. For filing and recall of all CT picture information, two forms of store are available: 1, magnetic discs; 2, magnetic tape.

Magnetic discs

Magnetic discs may be flexible or rigid. The flexible variety is smaller and has a lower storage capacity but is a very convenient—and a usual—form of medium term storage.

A *floppy disc* is about 20 cm in diameter and is made of vinyl. Information can be recorded on the disc magnetically but may deteriorate if it is kept over a lengthy span of years. Floppy discs may appropriately be included in a patient's case notes, for retention during a period of treatment and medical supervision; but these discs are less reliable for the archival storage of CT images.

A *hard disc* is larger and is used for long-term file storage and programme storage. These discs are coated with magnetic oxide and are kept in plastic, dust-free containers when not in use. They rotate continuously at speeds of more than 1500 rev/min. One may remark a tendency for hard discs to be replaced by floppy discs for day-to-day use. As they are cheaper, floppy discs may be preferred despite their lower capacity.

Magnetic tape

Magnetic tape is relatively less expensive than are floppy discs; other virtues relate to its reliability for the retention of information over a long term and its virtually unlimited capacity as a store. The tape is usually about 2·5 cm (1 inch) in width and binary information is put on it in the form of dots.

Whether on a disc or on a tape, information which is to be retrieved and used in calculations has first to be recalled to the computer's core memory: this recall takes a little longer in the case of tape storage.

Hardcopies

The computerized image resulting from a CT scan may be documented by means of a *hardcopy*. This term is descriptive of—and is applied to—the products of two dissimilar processes, which are explained below.

The first employs a high-speed line printer which records the CT numbers put forth by the computer. This is described as a printout and necessarily consists of rows and columns of figures, a form of communication which the majority of clinicians are not trained to appreciate. A further inconvenience arises from the large quantities of paper which may be involved. It is hardly a matter for wonder that printouts are seldom made and computerized images are much more often visualized by means of television monitors.

For documentation purposes a photograph may be obtained of the televised image, by means of a camera associated with a slave monitor. The camera may be of the Polaroid type and produce an almost immediate print, in a manner which must be familiar to any reader possessing such a camera for amateur use. Alternatively, the camera may utilise 100 mm cut film or may operate in conjunction with a multiformat system; this permits several exposures to be made upon one subdivided sheet of film, of a size which is about 20 cm × 28 cm (8 inches × 10 inches), or sometimes about 28 cm × 35 cm (11 inches × 14 inches).

Polaroid material is expensive and perhaps its sole strength is in its self-processing characteristic, when scanning equipment is situated remotely from a film-processing facility. Otherwise, the advantages are with film. It is not only less expensive but better able, than is a paper, to record the long grey scale between black and white.

Recording of a CT image by means of photography of its televised display differs significantly from storing such images on magnetic discs or tape. In the first instance, what the sensitive material records is merely the image which occupies the monitor screen when the camera shutter is operated. The 'picture' which results is a transfer of a particular setting of window width and window level (see p. 475). Furthermore, its characteristics may reflect other processing of the image, made in order to obtain from it a specific category of information. (Some of these evaluation techniques are discussed later in this chapter (see p. 477).) The photograph may be filed and used as documentation of a patient's condition or the effects of treatment, but it cannot provide a record of an entire CT scan. Recall of all picture information is possible only from the magnetic stores associated with computer practice. Redisplay from discs or tape retrieves in full every facility for windowing and other treatment of the computerized image, provided that all 'raw' data has been stored. If it is preferred, the magnetic tape or disc may be used as a store for pictures only.

Viewing the image

Television monitors offer a suitable means of displaying the signals from the voxels. Thus, CT numbers, with their varying values, can be shown as varying shades of grey on a black-and-white monitor (or colour may be used on a colour monitor).

We must recognize, however, that an incompatibility exists between the small number of grey shades recognizable on a television monitor and the very great range of attenuation values acquired by the scanner. We have cited absorption characteristics of air and bone as marking the extremes of this range, which is very much longer than the 15–20 grey steps on a black-and-white monitor screen which the eye may appreciate.

To meet this discrepancy—which is the classic one between the pint pot and the quart—scanners use a 'windowing' system. This refers to the selection at any one time of only a group of CT numbers for display on the monitor. For example, a typical equipment assigns CT numbers as follows:

+ 1000	dense bone
0	water
− 1000	air.

Push button selection allows the operator of this scanner to select one width of *window* among a number of widths, which vary in a binary progression from 32 units of the whole scale of attenuation values, to 1024 units of the scale.

The level of the window—that is, its position on the scale—is under the control of the operator and is continuously variable over the whole range of CT numbers.

It is always necessary to incorporate with the image a superimposed display of alphanumeric data (name of the patient and of the hospital or institute, the date etc). These legends should include the following information about the window:
— the selected width of the window (for instance, it might be 256);
— the window's upper limit (for instance + 146);
— the window's centre (for instance, + 18);
— the window's lower limit (for example, − 118).

Density values (representing attenuation values) reproduce white on the monitor screen when they lie above the window limit and black when they lie below the window limit; giving a continuous grey scale of CT numbers 'enclosed' within the window.

The window setting given above has been quoted only to provide a practical instance (see also Fig. 13.30), which may help a student to recognize indications noted on CT equipment: it would be appropriate during a cranial scan. Some CT systems allow the operator to make a double window display, by which one image includes two attenuation ranges.

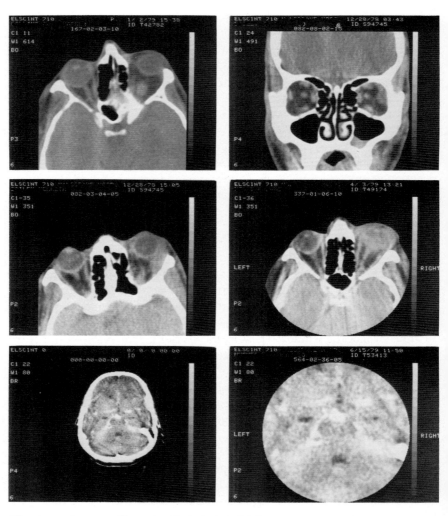

Fig. 13.30 A CT scan, illustrating the inclusion of alpha-numeric data relating to the circumstances of the scan.

Evaluation of the image

The use of a windowing technique during visualization of a CT image—which we have just described—is an instance of an applied process which permits, or may facilitate, the recognition of information contained in such images. Other manipulations for the same purpose are possible: indeed the ability to modify the image at will, in order to obtain specific information, is one of the assets of computed tomography. These manipulations are easy to make, as all the information is stored in the computer in digital form.

For example, the equivalent of subtraction radiography is readily obtained by subtracting values of one CT slice from those of another of the same part of the body, after the administration of a radiological contrast agent. A similar process of subtracting slice values could be applied to the determination of the results of a course of treatment; this is technically difficult to achieve, because it requires re-orientation of the patient, at the second examination, to exactly the position he occupied during the first.

In the present state of computed tomography there are now very sophisticated options for image evaluation, independent of the scanning procedure itself. A region of particular interest may first be defined by means of a circular or rectangular cursor (see Fig. 13.31), or may be outlined with

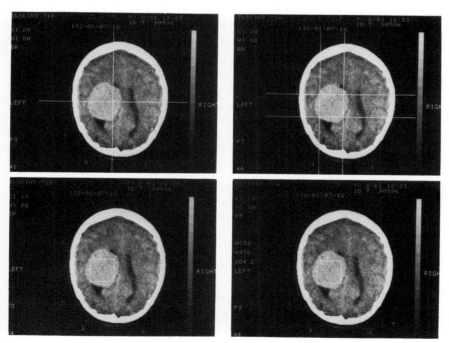

Fig. 13.31 A CT scan, illustrating the use of a cursor.

a light pen if it is irregular in shape. Statistical calculations can then be performed by the computer, showing—for instance—the mean and standard deviation of absorption values within the identified region. Other possibilities, among many, involve the measurement of density or of distances and angles. So rich a mine is image processing that some CT scanning equipment offers a separate evaluation unit, dedicated to the revelation of these seams of knowledge.

However, a fundamental and important process, which is sometimes described as 'optimising' the picture, should be considered more fully here. This process needs the operator to choose between two types of information which he may want from the image: in general terms, does he wish to see the sizes and shapes of structures; or does he wish to differentiate between tissues of similar attenuation values? The first of these is a requirement for good spatial resolution. In the second case, good density discrimination is needed and this will depend on accuracy in the determination of absorption values. It is a disagreeable fact of life that these two functions—good spatial resolution and absorption accuracy—are mutually incompatible in computed tomography. In order to understand why this is so, we must first consider the significance of random variations occurring in CT numbers; or rather, in the attenuation effects from which CT numbers are derived.

When a number of X-ray photons enter an absorber—such as composite tissues in a human subject—three physical effects may be expected to occur:

1 some photons will emerge and be counted by a present detector;
2 some photons will be absorbed by photoelectric inter-reaction;
3 some photons will be scattered by compton inter-reaction.

The second and third of these are random occurrences. This means that if the same number of photons were caused again to be incident upon the same tissues, the number of emergent—and therefore measured—photons would not necessarily be the same as before; indeed it is unlikely that the quantities would exactly match.

This random variation in individual transmission values can appear to increase its effect during the mathematical manoeuvres of image reconstruction; and it necessarily introduces an uncertainty to the computed distribution of attenuation values which are present in a scan. The effect, which becomes increasingly evident, is described as a spatial noise in the CT signal. (In a system which is conveying information—whether visible or audible information—*noise* is any part of the signal or message which does not contribute to the information concerned, from whatever cause.) It should be said that photon flux is not the only agent which introduces noise to a CT system. All electronic operations are associated with noise but we can make a distinction by using the terms electronic noise and quantum noise.

Variations in the data of a scan, arising from random behaviour by photons, impose a limit on an equipment's sensitivity to changes in tissue attenuation: that is, on its ability to discriminate between tissues, which is what we mean by density discrimination. A small change in beam attenuation, within a scanned subject, may not be detected if the change which it produces in the signal is smaller than the noise.

The uncertainty originating from photon flux can be reduced if a larger number of photons is used. This means increasing the radiation dose and the number of rays crossing a voxel at different angles: that is—assuming optimum performance from the detectors—we have improved the equipment's sensitivity to tissue change at the costs of higher radiation dosages.

Photon-counting statistics and the signal-to-noise ratio can be improved alternatively by increasing the size of the aperture through which the X-ray beam is reaching a detector. However, the width of this aperture (usually about 1·5 to 2 mm) fundamentally determines the resolution of a CT system. Increasing the size of the aperture decreases spatial resolution; a system offering high spatial resolution is associated with increased levels of quantum noise.

Coming back to the point of optimizing an image display, a fine picture matrix is needed if the information obtainable from a high resolution system is to be presented without degradation of detail. At the same time it has to be recognized that when the pixel size is small, quantum noise becomes greater; and that when we reduce noise, that is improve absorption accuracy, we introduce a source of blur to the image.

Reference was made on p. 471 to a trade-off between radiation dose and resolution. Now we have seen that—for a given radiation dose—spatial resolution and sensitivity to tissue change similarly may be bartered against each other.

In computed tomography there is an intimate connection between radiation dose, spatial resolution and the accuracy with which absorption differences are detected and displayed. The best equipment for computed tomography should allow the operator to balance these inter-related elements, in consideration of the needs of a particular clinical situation. The questions to be asked are: what radiation dose is justified?; do the structures to be examined possess high contrast?; is the probable lesion within an area of low contrast? In this as in any other radiodiagnostic procedure, the most difficult diagnostic problem is proposed by a small lesion involving organs of low contrast.

Resolution and accuracy (sensitivity to tissue change) are complex subjects in computed tomography. Below is given a list which attempts to summarize the features of scanning equipment which relate to the production of spatial resolution and absorption accuracy.

Resolution depends on:

1   the size of the aperture in front of the detector;
2   the matrix size and the number of pixels;
3   the algorithm used for the reconstruction;
4   the scanning speed (because this influences the period of time during which photons may reach a detector).

Accuracy depends on:

1   inherent quantum noise;
2   introduced electronic noise;
3   the algorithm used for the reconstruction;
4   the quality of the X-ray beam;
5   the geometry of the scanning system.

EQUIPMENT FOR COMPUTED TOMOGRAPHY

All major manufacturers of radiodiagnostic equipment now include a CT scanner in the market. These scanners have been extensively developed within the comparatively few years of their existence, although—like pluridirectional tomographic tables—they are not to be found in every general X-ray department.

Naturally there are some differences in design between different equipments but all can be considered to possess four main functional elements. These are:

1   a scanning gantry or frame which takes the essential numerous readings of radiation intensity;
2   a processing section which converts these numeric data to picture information;
3   a viewing/evaluation unit for the visual presentation of this picture information and for provision of any required manipulation of the image, which may improve diagnostic accuracy;
4   a storage facility so that information may be recalled subsequently.

The equipment embodying these four elements consists of the following essential parts, which in one form or another will be found in every CT scanner. They are:

1   a table, on which a patient may lie and which permits his precise positioning for the purpose of the scan;
2   a scanning gantry which contains (a) the X-ray tube, (b) the radiation detectors and (c) the electronics associated with acquisition of the radiation data;
3   an X-ray generator;
4   a computer;
5   viewing and control consoles.

The patient-positioning table

Fig. 13.32 shows the patient-positioning table and the gantry of a typical scanner for CT examinations of the head and neck. It can be appreciated that the function of the table is both to support the patient and to move him in a controlled manner within and outwards from the gantry, so that any selected transverse section may be scanned; location indicators—usually including a laser beam—are essential.

The equipment shown in Fig. 13.32 is capable of examining only the head and neck but the general principles of design are similar in the case of

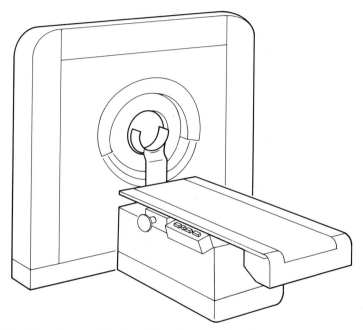

Fig. 13.32 The patient -positioning table and gantry of a typical scanner for computed tomography of the head and neck. *By courtesy of Siemens-Elema AB.*

equipment which can investigate the whole body. Certain obvious physical differences are seen: the table is designed to move much further through the gantry and the gantry's aperture necessarily is larger (for instance, 53 cm in diameter, as distinct from 29 cm) in order to accommodate the patient's trunk. In either case, the table has a motor drive for adjustment of its height. Horizontal transport also is automated and may be provided through a conveyor belt or worm drive. Accurate control of these movements is important since they determine the patient's position relative to the X-ray source and thus influence the topography of the CT slice. Positioning of the patient is controlled close at hand from a console incorporated in the table but there may be the additional facility—available at the scanner's operating console—of moving a patient as little as a millimetre at a time during an examination.

In many equipments the gantry may be tilted cranially/caudally relative to the patient on the table, usually about 20 deg to either aspect of the vertical. A large gantry aperture is necessary to accommodate a patient at an angle. It may be possible, also, to slew the table to a limited extent to either side of the midline, the head-end of the table being towards the centre of the movement. This mobility may facilitate positioning in such instances as a comatose, injured patient who maintains his head in a canted posture; or it can be used to obtain an angled abdominal slice.

The scanning gantry

The X-ray tube

X-ray tubes used in CT scanners are not essentially different from others. The following descriptions refer to typical examples.
1   A fixed anode tube, which is oil-to-water cooled and has a continuous rating of 4 kW, is similar to X-ray tubes used for radiotherapy. It has a focal area of 10 mm × 2 mm and may operate at 80–140 kV and at 38–21 mA.
2   A rotating anode tube which has a heat storage capacity of 1,000,000 H.U. and an effective rating of 10–15 kW. In this example the effective focal area is stated to be 0·5 mm × 0·5 mm.

Rotating anode tubes are usually associated with equipments offering short scanning times (less than 20 seconds). Oil-cooled, fixed anode tubes of a radiotherapy type may be run continuously during a scan; whilst their rotating anode fellows are sometimes pulsed during scan times of a few seconds. Scan times are further considered in the next section of this chapter.

The scanning system

To simplify our account of computed tomography, we began with an assumption of a simple translate-rotate scanning system, which is sketched in Fig. 13.14 and utilizes a pencil X-ray beam and a single detector to measure one radiation profile. Data acquisition by this type of equipment, although simple in procedure, is necessarily slow. The length of time required to complete a scan (about 4 minutes) has confined the equipment's application to the head. Patients may be sedated or otherwise persuaded to keep their heads still for a while but the respiratory and involuntary movements of thoracic and abdominal organs pose another problem. Later scanning systems have been developed which much reduce scanning times but employ a different geometry and more complex detector arrays. These systems are described briefly below.

Modified fan beam (multiple detectors)

The name modified fan beam scanner refers to the collimation of the X-ray beam. In this case, instead of being a 'pencil', the beam may have a width of about 30 deg and is faced by a multiple array of detectors (about 30 for the more common systems of this type).

The X-ray tube and the detectors are coupled as before and the scanning principle of translation and rotation is employed. For example, a 30 deg beam directed at an appropriate array of detectors could take 30 profiles, each at an interval of one degree from its immediate neighbours. If the tube-detector assembly then traversed through say 10 deg before taking another set of radiation profiles, it could complete a scan of 180 degrees (180 radiation profiles) much more quickly than the equipment depicted in Fig. 13.14; in practice, times of about 20 seconds per CT slice are cited.

Whilst this system remains as mechanically complex as the earlier one, the faster scanning times associated with multiple detectors extend its applications from the head to whole body scans.

Wide fan beam (rotate–rotate systems)

In order further to reduce scan times, solely rotational (rotate–rotate) scanning systems have been devised. These use a wide fan beam of 30–50 deg and the movement of the X-ray tube is a simple rotation of 360 deg around the patient (see Fig. 13.33). Some equipments make more than one rotation.

X-ray generation may be pulsed, with one beam to each element of a multiple array of detectors and each acquiring its own radiation data. If each detector is focused on the X-ray source, as are the strips of a focused secondary radiation grid, less scattered radiation is received by the detectors. When detectors are inefficient in rejecting scatter, the sensitivity of the system to contrast is reduced and density discrimination impaired.

It would be a feature of the ideal scanner that the detectors were subject to no scattered radiation: in practice this cannot be realized and scanning systems should be designed to ensure that the acceptance of scatter is as low as possible. This is achieved mainly through beam collimation, but focusing the tungsten plates of a gas ionization detector (see p. 487), in the way described, must increase the effect.

As we have so far explained the operation of rotate–rotate scanning systems, their geometry appears to fix the width of the fan beam (look again at Fig. 13.33). If this width is to be compatible with the largest subject, a

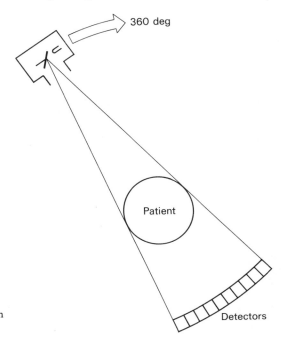

360 deg

Patient

Detectors

Fig. 13.33 A rotate–rotate system for computed tomography.

question arises of the beam's appropriateness to a smaller subject. In this case it must appear that some of the primary X-radiation passing from the tube is not received by the patient and thus cannot contribute to the production of diagnostic information.

All scanners of the rotate–rotate variety make provision for such an occurrence in one or other of two ways:

1 the width of the beam is adjustable by means of entrance (pre-patient) collimation;

2 the distance between the patient and the X-ray tube can be altered.

Either of these arrangements inflicts a larger radiation dose; the first because limitation of the X-ray beam necessitates higher milliampere settings; and the second because the X-ray tube and the patient are brought close together.

Scanners in the rotate–rotate category, using a wide fan beam and multiple detectors, achieve rapid scanning speeds: for instance, a scan of 360 deg can be made in a period varying from 2 to 8 sec. One of the major problems inherent in such fast systems is to obtain an adequate dose (that is, a sufficiency of X-ray photons) during a scan time. As we have seen, when photons are few the image is subject to increased noise (see p. 478). Because of this limitation, these fast scanners may have to run at less than their maximum speeds, if pictures of high diagnostic quality are to be produced.

Stationary detectors

As opposed to translate–rotate and rotate–rotate systems, there is a type of scanner which has a fixed ring of detectors, surrounding a patient, and moves the X-ray tube in a full circle, within the ring (see Fig. 13.34). The

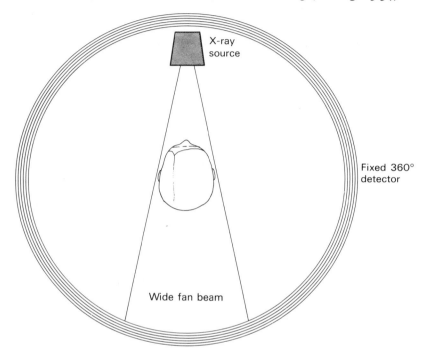

Fig. 13.34 A system for computed tomography using a fixed detector.

beam is described as a fan and scanning times are from 1·5 to 10 seconds. Whilst such a system possesses relative mechanical simplicity, it appears to suffer from a number of drawbacks which are explained below.

1   The large number of detectors which is required add to the costliness of the scanner and may decrease its reliability.

2   At any given moment, only a portion of the detectors are receiving radiation; in this respect, the system is not cost-effective. In translate–rotate and rotate–rotate systems, the detectors are always in the X-ray beam.

3   The geometry of the system is poor. To permit the passage of the X-ray tube, a space is necessary between the patient and the detectors. This allows a spread of penumbra and limits spatial resolution.

4   Geometry requires the detectors to be spaced further apart, with decreased utilization as a result.

5   Rejection of scatter is less efficient and sensitivity to contrast may be lost.

6   The system has inherently high magnification.

$$\left(\text{Magnification} = \frac{\text{source to detector distance}}{\text{source to object distance}}\right)$$

The detectors

Radiation detectors used in CT scanners may be one or the other of two kinds:

1   crystal scintillation detectors, working in conjunction with photomultipliers or photodiodes;
2   gas ionization detectors.

Whichever type is employed, the detector should possess good *detection efficiency*. This term refers to its ability to 'catch' X-ray photons. Photons which are not detected cannot contribute to the diagnostic picture but, of course, are contributors to the dose received by the patient.

The 'detective' ability of the material of the radiation detector is not the only parameter in the design of a detector system, however. Of related importance are the spacing of detectors and the size of a detector's aperture. Aperture is obtained from an exit collimator; that is, a collimator placed in front of the detector and limiting the X-ray beam emergent from the patient.

A close packing together of a relatively large number of detectors in an array is the ideal, if all emergent X-ray photons are to be converted to useful information. A small aperture increases spatial resolution and assists in low acceptance of scatter but also reduces dose efficiency, because some unscattered emergent X rays are prevented from reaching the detector. The ratio of aperture to spacing is a determinant of the system's geometric efficiency. In attempts to assess the overall efficiency of different scanning systems and in their design, none of these factors should be considered in isolation.

Another important characteristic of a detector is its *dynamic range*. This term refers to a detector's ability to receive a wide range of X-ray intensities with proportional output. The dynamic range of a detector determines the range of signals between which it may correctly discriminate. If the signal exceeds the dynamic range, then errors occur in the acquiring of radiation data and streaky artefacts are seen in the image.

Crystal detectors

In the case of crystal detectors, the substance used may be sodium iodide, caesium iodide, or bismuth germinate. It is necessary to associate with the detectors a device which can 'pick up' the scintillations occurring when the crystals are irradiated. Such a device may be a photomultiplier tube (see p. 185) or a photodiode. This is not unlike a photomultiplier but is a simpler and smaller tube which has only two electrodes, a cathode and an anode. The cathode is photo-emissive and will emit electrons when light falls on it. Connected in a suitable circuit, a photodiode is capable of passing a small current in response to a light signal; the strength of the current varies proportionally with the intensity of the light which the photodiode is 'watching'.

Photomultipliers are physically larger than photodiodes and are inconvenient for close packing in a large array of detectors. They are also susceptible to the influence of magnetic fields and may degrade with age.

The main disadvantage of photodiodes is a typical weakness in the produced signal, which consequently requires a high degree of electrical amplification; this amplification introduces additional noise to the system. Photodiodes have other foibles, too, among which are that their gain is temperature dependent and that exposure to X radiation may damage them.

Apart from the characteristics of the pick-up tubes with which they must be associated, the scintillation crystals themselves possess various plus or minus features. The detection efficiency of a 'good' crystal generally is higher than the same property of a detector which depends on the ionization of a gas; but a crystal array may be less stable in the long term, from a number of causes. These include:

1 lack of uniformity in the crystal's response, for several reasons such as quantum noise (see p. 478) and perhaps non-uniformity of the material itself (producing circular artefacts);
2 dependance on temperature;
3 persistence of a light emission after irradiation has ceased (afterglow);
4 current output.for a given X-ray input changes with the age (history of usage) of the crystal.

Frequent calibration of a crystal detector array is necessitated by the last two of these effects. Furthermore, it is difficult and costly to construct a large array of several hundred scintillation-crystal photomultiplier tube (sc-pm) detectors.

Gas ionization detectors

Detectors which depend on ionization effects use an inert gas called xenon. The detection efficiency of xenon is relatively low in comparison with the same feature of a single scintillation crystal. It has been calculated that a single xenon detector requires about 1·7 times the intensity of X rays to reach the same signal-to-noise ratio as the best sc-pm detector.

In detector arrays which use xenon, the gas is maintained at high pressure to increase detection efficiency, but with the effect, too, of inhibiting contamination by impurities and thus heightening the detectors' uniformity of response. Advantageous aspects of a xenon detector system include:

1　constant sensitivity in both short and long terms;
2　indifference to changes in ambient temperature and humidity;
3　wide dynamic range;
4　rapid response, without afterglow;
5　efficient conversion of X rays to current;
6　less frequent calibration;
7　relatively small size favours construction of large detector arrays.

The X-ray generator

To study the technical data which manufacturers provide within pamphlets advertising their CT scanning systems is to find relatively scant mention of the X-ray generator; yet—together with the X-ray tube—it originates the entire process.

However, scanning systems do not require generators to have special characteristics, particular to the function of computed tomography. An earlier part of this book (Chapter 3) was given to the consideration of X-ray generators and now it is necessary to make only a little further comment.

The majority of X-ray generators at present in use in CT scanning systems are identified as providing constant potential. They are 6-pulse or 12-pulse in type; and it is claimed of a typical example that the high voltage ripple is not greater than 0·1 per cent. The stability of the applied kilovoltage is important during a scanning cycle, since any fluctuation causes severe artefacts.

The operating/display console

The control and computer rooms associated with CT scanners are bound to appear to beginners as profoundly recondite. Certainly, they contain advanced equipment, which will include at least the following items:
1　an operator's console, providing push-button control of numerous functions, from the simple (for instance, shifting the patient, starting the scan), to higher orders, such as window manipulation, selection of scan parameters and the initiation of image filing, among others;
2　a computer system, incorporating a control or host computer, a floppy disc drive and a high-speed image-processor controlled by the host computer;
3　a data or dialogue monitor with keyboard, for the input of patient identification, the image number, scan parameters and so on (this monitor may also indicate errors, through an output of suitable messages);
4　a viewing monitor, usually black and white although sometimes a colour monitor may be provided as well, as an 'optional extra'.

Fig. 13.35 suggests a possible plan for a CT suite, showing how the listed—and other—equipment might be disposed. Readers of this book may

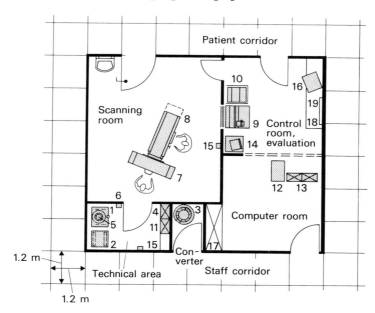

Fig. 13.35 A plan of a suite for computed tomography.

1 High tension generator	11 Power supply for gantry
2 Capacitor assembly	12 Control computer with floppy disc drive
3 Converter	13 Image processor and gantry control unit
4 Generator control unit	14 Black and white monitor
5 Cooling assembly on stand	15 Intercom
6 Water installation	16 Colour monitor
7 Gantry	17 Cabinet for documents and filing of
8 Patient's table	record media
9 Operator's console	18 Worktop
10 Dialogue monitor	19 Film viewing illuminator

By courtesy of Siemens-Elema AB

encounter much more elaborate installations than are here described. These can include additional modules relative to evaluation, storage and documentation of the image. Manufacturer's pamphlets on their CT scanners are recommended reading for students who may wish to expand their knowledge beyond the scope of the art's fundamentals.

However, any suite containing a CT scanning system will be found to have a controlled atmosphere. This is important for the accurate functioning of computers and a manufacturer usually specifies the environmental requirements of his equipment. Typically, a room's temperature should be within the range 15°C to 27°C; and relative humidity should be 55% ± 10%, free of condensation.

CRITERIA OF PERFORMANCE

All systems for computed tomography have the same tasks to perform, through the same stages. We may try to summarize these on the following lines.

1 Information is collected in a raw form, by means of an X-ray source and radiation detectors.

2 Raw information—received from the scanning gantry—is processed. Processing involves analysis by a computer and then conversion to a form which can be displayed as a visual image or picture.

3 Processed information must be viewed by means of a television monitor.

4 Finally, information must be stored. Storage may refer to the immediate use of an image or to its retention for periods considered to be of medium duration (some weeks) or of archival duration (many years). Floppy discs and magnetic tape are such storage systems associated with computers.

If we attempt to specify performance criteria for a CT scanner, we find that it is no simple matter but should embrace several aspects of the scanner's employment. We may, for example, consider the following headings:

1 image quality;

2 dose efficiency;

3 available scanning functions, for instance the ability to perform sagittal and coronal reconstructions, or dynamic scans to analyse blood flow;

4 patient-throughput, which relates to operation time but perhaps is more often influenced by factors which are not connected with the scanner.

In this catalogue, headings 3 and 4 are concerned with a scanner's relevance to particular clinical needs; their importance will vary with the point of view of the assessor. Numbers 1 and 2 are fundamental characteristics and may be said to separate good performers from bad ones. We have tried to sum-up image quality and dose efficiency below.

Image quality

The quality of CT images is derived from many attributes of the scanning system, including the sometimes forgotten parameter of the size of the focal area of the X-ray tube. The following parameters are prominent in determinations of image quality:

1 spatial resolution, giving the ability to see small objects separately defined;

2 density discrimination, giving the ability to see objects of low contrast;

3 scan speed, in reducing motional blur;

4 slice thickness in the discrimination of small objects (thinner slices give more accurate CT numbers and reduce artefacts);

5 the elimination of artefacts.

As we have seen in earlier sections of this chapter, there is not a mutual compatibility between all of these and good equipment allows different modes of operation to be selected. It is usual for an examiner to decide what he will 'go for', in relation to the particular clinical problem to be solved.

For example, we might say that in computed tomography of the spinal column an essential requirement for effective function is the detectability of low contrasts; skeletal examinations of the base of the skull need a thin slice capability; and in dynamic scanning, the use of short scan times of variable periods may be critically important.

Within the scope of this book, we may categorize certain features of CT equipment which participate in the production of image quality and have attempted to show how one may affect another; but how they should be deployed is another matter, which is outside the jurisdiction of this work.

Dose efficiency

Any X-ray examination entails the administration of a radiation dose to a patient. Patient-dose and image quality are two scales in the balance of equipment performance: a true comparison of CT images can be made only in the knowledge of the doses used to obtain them.

We may perhaps broadly define patient-dose as the total quantity of X rays delivered to a patient. During computed tomography, optimal dose efficiency is obtained when all the X rays which pass through a patient are converted to a usable signal. There are several features of CT scanners which may result in photons, emergent from the patient, becoming 'lost', with consequently poor dose efficiency. These 'danger areas' are explained below.

1   If detectors are widely spaced some photons, emergent from the patient, are lost between them.

2   Poor beam collimation may result in the projection of X rays outside the detector area, if the beam width is greater than the extent of the detector array.

3   Information may be lost within a detector because the detector itself is inefficient. (Detector efficiency is a combination of photon collection and photon conversion to electrical current.)

We may link these three areas together in a statement that dose efficiency is the product of detector aperture, beam width and the photon conversion factor.

Dose efficiency is always an important parameter of performance in computed tomography; and during paediatric examinations it might be considered to be the first essential requirement.

Chapter 14
Equipment for Rapid Serial Radiography

Whenever a radiographic record is to be made of some rapid physiological sequence it becomes necessary to take a number of films very quickly; too quickly to permit cassettes to be changed ordinarily by hand even by a practised radiographer. We have already seen (Chapter 12) how the serial changer on the gastrointestinal table makes radiography of the duodenal cap more efficient: this is one example of equipment which has been especially devised to enable dynamic physiological events to be filmed.

However, the filling of the duodenal cap with barium sulphate entering it from the stomach is a slow and prolonged effect compared with the rates at which the major arteries become and remain opacified, following their injection with a radiological contrast agent. At most, the phase of arterial filling persists for only a few seconds. Radiography of the vessels must be completed within this short period. For all arteriography some form of rapid serial changer is necessary if an adequate examination is to be made.

The tasks of any serial changer may be summarized as first to send a film—or enable a film to be sent—from a 'protected' station to a station where it can be exposed to an X-ray beam; and secondly to allow the exposed film to be withdrawn and replaced by another, prior to a succeeding exposure. These tasks can be effectively performed whether the equipment in question moves a film (either a cut sheet or a roll) or whether it moves a cassette which contains a film; but readers of this book should recognize the gulf which separates a film changer and a cassette changer. They are widely dissimilar equipments in detail.

The fundamentally significant difference between the two categories of changer relates to their speeds, that is to the rate at which a film-change can be effected. A film—being lighter than a cassette—can be handled from one place to another more quickly and easily (this is true whether the handler is a human or a machine); so it is not an unexpected finding that cassette changers are slower than film changers and thus have limited applications compared with them.

The title at the head of this chapter could almost have been 'Equipment for Angiography', since angiography is the radiodiagnostic discipline which needs rapid serial changers for its successful performance; the several changers now to be described are designed to this end. Readers of this book, if they inspect the angiographic equipment in use in their various hospitals, are more likely to discover film changers than cassette changers and it is toward these that the balance of this chapter will lean.

Some classification of angiographic equipments can be made in accordance with the work to which a particular equipment is primarily suited. Within the discipline, the following groupings are recognized:

1   general angiography (the appropriate equipment may undertake peripheral, abdominal, thoracic—but not cardiac—and cranial examinations);
2   peripheral and abdominal angiography by themselves (the equipment is planned to undertake only these examinations);
3   specialized cardiac angiography (dedicated equipment);
4   specialized cranial angiography (dedicated equipment).

The equipments applicable to 3 and 4 above are found in regional and subregional centres for cardiac surgery and neurosurgery. Their special features relate less to the film changer itself than to the arrangements made for the support and direction of the X-ray tube and the positioning of the patient. For instance, angiocardiographic equipment includes one form of mounting for the X-ray tube which is described as a variable-geometry U-arm. This feature ensures that the X-ray tube and a linked image intensifier automatically tilt, in order to maintain the heart at the centre of the field of view and the central axis of the X-ray beam at right angles to the input screen of the intensifier. Such equipments are both complex and inapplicable to other than their specialized work. Here we shall consider angiographic equipments in a broader sense.

A RAPID FILM CHANGER

Whilst it is not the only one available, the film changer now to be described is a typical equipment which is in widespread use. It utilizes cut film and can be obtained in two 'sizes', one model being suitable for 24 cm × 30 cm film and the other for 35 cm × 35 cm film. The usefulness of the smaller version is confined to cerebral and selective angiographies; the larger obviously has wider applications.

Any two of these changers may be combined to provide bi-plane operation from two oppositely sited X-ray tubes; this entails positioning one changer beneath the table which supports the patient and the other changer vertically at one side, in the manner sketched in Fig. 14.1.

Such an arrangement as that shown in Fig. 14.1 can be applied not only to the changer with which we are concerned but to another long-established film changer known as the AOT. The AOT rapid film changer is a bigger equipment; it uses either cut or roll film; it is faster and has a greater range

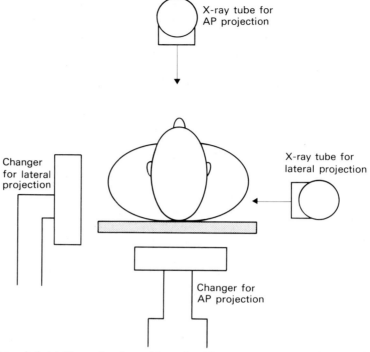

Fig. 14.1. A sketch illustrating the positions of two film changers to provide bi-plane operation.

of exposure rates, which may be significant determinants in its choice for certain angiographies.

Coupling together two changes of the same type permits anteroposterior and lateral radiographs to be obtained following a single injection of a radiological contrast agent. The changers may operate simultaneously or alternately: in the second case each changer makes radiographic exposures during the intervals when the other changer is moving films from a supply magazine to an exposure station.

The rapid film changer to be described is supported on a suitable stand, the characteristics of which affect the usage of the changer and are to be separately discussed. We may consider film-changing equipment to possess three major components, as follows:

1   the film changer itself, which includes a supply or loading magazine, an area for the exposure of a film and a receiving cassette for exposed film;
2   a programme selector and handswitch for the control of the changer;
3   a stand on which the changer is mounted.
It is logical now to describe the equipment under these three headings.

The film changer

Principles of operation

Fig. 14.2 is a simple sketch of the film changer, illustrating its compact design and the relationships of the magazines to the exposure area and to each other.

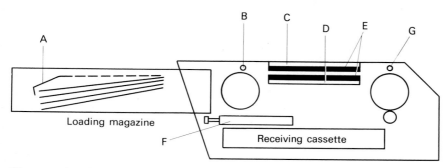

Fig. 14.2   A rapid film changer.

A film puller	E intensifying screens
B feed-in rollers	F marking rod
C upper compression plate	G feed-out rollers
D pressure table	

The supply magazine is detachable for loading purposes: when it is in position, the length of the larger changer is 860 mm (34 inches); it is 173 mm (29 inches) in depth; and its width is 396 mm (15½ inches). The changer for 24 cm × 30 cm film is proportionately less in length and width.

Fig. 14.2 is largely self-explanatory of the principles of the changer's operation. In outline, the sequence of events is:

1   a pick-up arm (A) in the loading magazine collects the topmost film and is pulled towards the changer;

2   the film enters the changer under feed-in rollers (B), which transfer the film to the exposure area (C);

3   the film is held stationary at C by means of a spring-loaded pressure table (D);

4   after exposure, the pressure table is lowered and the film thus is released;

5   feed-out rollers (G) grasp the film and guide it under roller H to the receiving cassette below;

6   if this film is one of a series, simultaneously with the occurrence of 5 above the next unexposed film is introduced to the exposure area.

It should be noted that the overlapping of the feed-in cycle (events 1 and 2 above) with the feed-out cycle (event 5 above) means that two operating cycles are required to transfer one film from the loading magazine, through the changer to the receiving cassette; but the overlap means also that an exposure occurs on every cycle.

The loading magazine

The loading magazine is a large, flat metal box, about 75 mm (3 inches) deep. When it is withdrawn from the changer (a daylight operation at any time), the end further from the changer can be opened. Inside is a film-holder which can be withdrawn from the magazine, after release of two thumb-pressure catches.

A darkroom is necessary for loading the magazine. The magazine is opened and the film-holder removed. Up to 20 sheets of film are then placed in the film-holder, which incorporates 19 small separators on a loose-leaf style of mounting. Care should be observed to make sure that only one sheet of film is inserted between any two separators and—at the end of the task—that the films and separators are secured in the holder by operation of a snap clasp. The holder is then re-inserted in the loading magazine. The magazine is closed and is ready for return to the radiodiagnostic room, where it can be fitted in position on the changer.

To fit the magazine to the changer, it must be introduced at a slight angle over two heavy projecting pins. Raising it to its level working position allows an operating rod to open a feed-slot at the rear of the changer, through which contained films can leave the magazine and enter the changer. At the same time, two locking hooks engage the magazine firmly in position and these must be released by the radiographer—thus also closing the feed-slot—before the magazine can be withdrawn; there is a strong sliding catch beneath the magazine for this purpose.

The exposure area

On the upper surface of the changer, the exposure field is apparent as a rectangular, slightly inset area, which contains a fixed secondary radiation grid. Beneath this is a heavy metal frame on which is mounted, in sequence, a sheet of carbon fibre, a plastic layer and an intensifying screen. This assembly—of which Fig. 14.3 is a cross-sectional sketch—constitutes the front compression plate of the changer.

It is important that the material of this upper pressure plate should not significantly absorb X-rays, though it must be mechanically strong. Carbon fibre is very suitable in both respects and the total absorption of the plate (excluding the intensifying screen) is said to be only 0·4 mm aluminium at 70 kV.

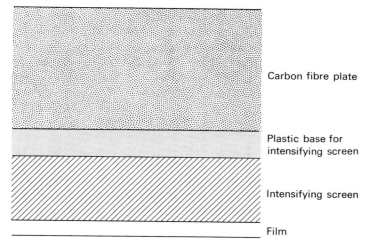

Carbon fibre plate

Plastic base for
intensifying screen

Intensifying screen

Film

Fig. 14.3   The cross section of the upper pressure plate in a film changer.

Opposing the intensifying screen which is on the upper compression plate is another on the pressure table beneath. During the film changer's cycle of operation, this pressure table is raised by cams and compresses the lower intensifying screen upon the upper one; it compresses also the sheet of film which at that stage of the cycle should lie between them. After the X-ray exposure, when the film is to be removed from the exposure area, the pressure table is lowered and this releases the grip on the film.

Whilst each film is in the exposure area of the changer, an automatic identification occurs.

1   Each film is optically marked with a serial number running sequentially from 0 to 9999. This enables every radiograph to be placed in time within a series of exposures.

2   Each film is optically marked with the text on a label which is inserted in the changer by means of a special marking rod (see Fig. 14.1). Before beginning any procedure, the radiographer must complete the necessary label with the patient's name—or number, depending on local practice— and the date. The label is then fitted in the marking rod and the rod inserted in its place on the changer.

The receiving cassette

The receiving cassette is a shallow, steel box which is situated in the lower part of the changer (see Fig. 14.2). When a retaining bolt is lifted, the cassette is removable at any time from the same aspect of the changer as is the loading the magazine. The cassette has a sliding lid which is held closed by a strongly acting spring and is self-opening when the cassette is properly mounted in the changer. This lid has no handle and consequently is rather difficult to open manually. Darkroom procedure for removal of the exposed films is facilitated by the use of an accessory jig. This can be clamped to the darkroom workbench and when the cassette is inserted the jig automatically opens it; films are then easily removed for processing.

The programmer and handswitch

The programmer is a separate wall-mounted unit and—together with the connected handswitch—controls the operation of the changer. Exposures may be made singly—for example, in order to obtain a preliminary scout radiograph—or in a programmed series at a rate of 3 per second or 2 per second. The maximum duration of a programme is 20 seconds and the function of the programmer is to determine the number of films to be exposed (up to the 20 films which the loading magazine can contain) and the intervals at which the exposures will occur. These determinations are made by means of a punched card.

The punched card

Insertion of a punched card in the programmer automatically switches the unit from a single-cycle mode (one film fed through the changer and one exposure made) to a programmed series of continuous exposures. The programme is selected by the operator who must punch a series of holes in a special card and insert the card in the programming unit on the wall.

Punching is done by hand with a stylus and a punchboard: the use of these tools is both a convenience and a precaution, since they enable the card to be accurately punched and avoid any bending of the card or other inadvertent damage to it.

The card contains a number of lines of prepared potential holes. Each line refers to a parameter of the examination, the following being of first importance:

1   the timescale (0–13 sec) for an exposure rate of 3 cycles per second;
2   the time scale (0–19 sec) for an exposure rate of 2 cycles per second;
3   a line which permits a switch-over from one rate to the other;
4   a line which introduces a pause at any stage;
5   the exposure line, from which every hole punched out by the operator results in one film-feeding cycle through the changer.

Other provisions of the card which may be significant refer to the time of release of an automatic injector; the choice of a longer exposure interval; and automatic shift of the table during peripheral angiography (see p. 509).

Duly completed with the patient's name and other identification, the card may be filed with the patient's radiographs and remains a useful record of the procedure employed for the examination. If a number of blank cards is punched in advance with a prescribed programme, this can be a useful aid in establishing routine techniques for the guidance of less experienced staff.

The panel and handswitch

The panel of the programming unit presents several switches which provide for mains supply and manual control of the feed movement. In addition are seen monitor lamps which show the preparedness of the changer for use. These lamps illuminate to give the following indications:

1 Mains ON.
2 Film in the exposure position.
3 Failure of a film to transport.
4 Magazines correctly inserted in the changer.
5 Ready to expose.

The panel incorporates a cardholder and a reader for the punched card, which is seen to advance through the reader as the programme proceeds.

The handswitch is used to initiate a programmed series. This little unit possesses actually two rocker switches. There is one on the top of the handpiece which obtains an emergency stop of the film changer, should such a manœuvre be necessary. The second switch, on the front of the handpiece, is identified with a camera symbol and this is the one which operates the programmer.

The changer is driven by a motor which runs at either 1920 revolutions per minute or 2880 revolutions per minute, depending on the exposure rate (2 exp/sec or 3 exp/sec) which has been determined. Fitted to the motor is a spur gear which—together with another—enables the drive to be taken to a system of shafts, cams and chains responsible for both the mechanical movements and the actuation of microswitches and solenoids which the changer requires if it is to perform its function.

Selection of the changer's velocity is usually derived from clinical consideration relating to the rapidity of the blood flow to be filmed; but the exposure rate chosen influences the maximum exposure interval which may be obtained and thus has radiographic as well as clinical importance.

It is evident that exposures should be made only during that part of the cycle when the film is held stationary by the pressure table; this is approximately 30% of the duration of the full cycle. Sometimes an angular description is given to this period when the film is compressed between the intensifying screens: it is called the *exposure angle* of the changer and in the changer under discussion is specified as 140 deg. This is merely another way of describing intervals of time in terms of a revolution (360 deg) of a rotating part. (That rotating parts *are* involved is evident even if we think only of the cams which—rotating with revolving shafts—create the up and down movement of the pressure table.)

The changer with which we are concerned cannot utilise an exposure interval longer than 0·1 sec when the rate is 3 exposures/second; or longer than 0·16 sec when the rate is 2 exposures/second or less. (When two changers alternate exposures, the highest permissible frequency of exposure is 1·5 per second). In practice the maximum exposure time allowed must be a little less than the actual duration of the period when the film is compressed on the pressure table. This provides for the inevitable delay in the equipment (about 10 to 20 milliseconds) whilst electrical 'messages' are passed; the term interrogation time is usually applied to this brief 'dead' period.

Stands

Several varieties of stand are available for the film changers of which some account has just been given. The basic stand is a mobile unit on universal wheels, which either may be employed as castors or may run on a floor-track. The base of the stand has plunger-type foot-operated floor locks which fix the position of the stand at the chosen location.

The base supports a short vertical column which carries the film changer itself. Some vertical movement of the changer, to the extent of 400 mm (about 15 inches), upwards and downwards on this column, is possible. This capability of movement gives several advantages:

1 it permits a magnification technique (macroradiography) to be used;
2 it makes the changer adaptable to different heights of table;
3 it facilitates positioning a patient's head directly upon the changer during cerebral angiography.

Support of the changer includes a turn plate, allowing the changer to be turned at increments of 90 deg to obtain three different positions of the magazine in each of the horizontal and vertical planes.

Apart from its use on the basic stand, this changer may be attached to other forms of support—for instance a C-arm—which increase the flexibility of its applications: it may be used even upside-down. If it is fitted to a stand affording a spherical movement (for a comparable example see p. 553), the changer may operate in the hemisphere above the patient, as well as in the hemisphere below him; these positions are shown in Fig. 14.4. However, the changer should not be put in a stance which directs the magazine upwards. In this circumstance, the transfer of a film through the changer would be affected by the forces of gravity.

(a)

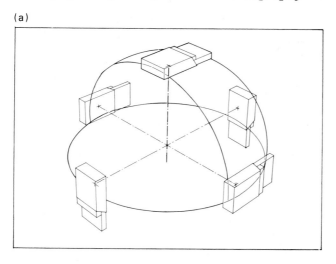

(b)

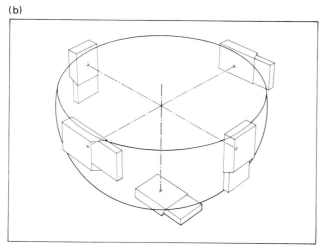

Fig. 14.4 Spherical positions for a film changer; (a) in the hemisphere above the patient, (b) in the hemisphere below the patient. *By courtesy of Siemens-Elema AB.*

RAPID CASSETTE CHANGERS

A variety of apparatus is available for the rapid change of cassettes. Different kinds of this equipment are applicable to cerebral angiography and to arteriography of the lower limbs from the abdominal aorta. Removal of the cassettes from the exposure area may depend upon withdrawal by hand: rates of change faster than 1 film per second are not likely to be attained.

Cerebral angiography

General structure of the changer

Figure 14.5 shows a typical rapid cassette changer for cerebral angiography. It consists of two boxes which hold a number of cassettes and are attached to each other at right-angles in the form of an L. The complete device is suitably mounted, usually on a specialized unit for skull radiography such as those made by Barazetti or Schonander (see Chapter 15). A patient supine on the couch can be placed so that his head lies on the foot of the L, while the vertical arm of the letter is against the left side of his head and face (Fig. 14.6).

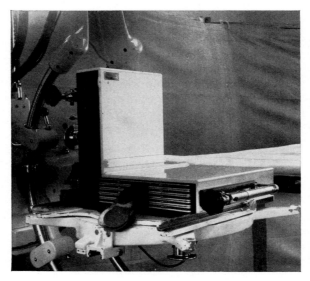

Fig. 14.5   A cassette changer for cerebral angiography. *By courtesy of Barr and Stroud Ltd.*

In the changer illustrated, each box can hold four cassettes. At the back of each pile of cassettes in the box a spring-loaded disc pushes the cassettes against the surface nearest to the patient. Removal of the proximal cassette results in the one below or behind it being thrust into the space so provided and this will continue to occur until the box is emptied. A mechanism of this kind is necessary if the anode-film and object-film distances are to remain constant.

Withdrawal of the cassettes is by hand and for this purpose each is equipped with a leather tongue or handle. The position of this is slightly staggered through the series to diminish the chances of the operator attempting to seize two at once. The cassettes used may be 18 × 24 cm or 24 × 30 cm (or their equivalent in inches) or a combination of these, depending upon the size of the changer. They are light in weight and of conventional design except for the insertion of a lead sheet in the back of each. This sheet should be at least 1 mm thick since its function is to protect the film in the cassette behind it from the primary beam.

An alternative arrangement to modifying cassettes in this way is to use a standard cassette fitted into a lead-lined tray. In this case the tray—and not the cassette—will carry the withdrawing-handle and again this can be staggered—usually in respect of its length—relative to the one above and below it, so that two cannot easily be grasped at the same time. This arrangement means that the changer can utilize cassettes generally available in the department but it may be thought a more clumsy system than the other and more likely to be subject to vibration: certainly a cassette and its tray are heavier to move than a cassette alone. Furthermore the changer may accommodate fewer films, perhaps only three or four in each box, as opposed to five.

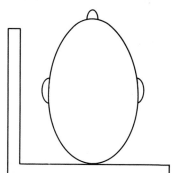

Fig. 14.6

The fronts of the boxes are made from a light metal alloy similar in density to aluminium and therefore radioparent. These surfaces are faced with white perspex and incorporated in each is a secondary radiation grid with a lattice of 75 lines to the inch. Sometimes the grid itself forms the front of the box. These grids are unfocused (see Chapter 8).

Anatomical identification is provided by R and L lead letters in both sections of the changer. The position of each radiograph in the series can be established by opaque numerals marked on the back screen of each cassette and corresponding to a similar number on the handle.

The design of the changer illustrated in Fig. 14.5 is such that in each section the cassettes in position for exposure project slightly into the companion section. This greatly facilitates radiographic positioning. Without this provision, it is necessary before taking the lateral view to raise the patient's head on a suitable support—for example, radioparent foam blocks—in order to ensure that the back of the head is included on the films. Similarly, with reference to the frontal view, without this feature of the changer the patient must often be shifted to his right to maintain alignment of the median plane with the midline of the cassette. Neither manœuvre is desirable during angiography, quite apart from the time saved if the patient's position can be established at the beginning of the procedure and not subsequently altered to any extent.

Immobilization of the patient

The changer includes accessories to be used to immobilize the patient's head. One of these is a linen, cotton or nylon band of which the ends interlace. It is put round the cranium, crossing on the forehead when the patient is supine. Each end is then attached to a ratchet device at the side of the changer which will apply tension to the band or release it, as the need may be. The band can be used not only to prevent movement but also to rotate the head to obtain oblique projections.

The alternative device—or it can be employed additionally—is a clear perspex plate with a quick release adjustment. This is possibly more unpleasant for a conscious patient than the head bandage.

Using the changer

The changer is normally operated in conjunction with a generator of high output and preferably an X-ray tube capable of sustaining repeated loads at short intervals; however, these loads are cumulatively not so great as those implicit in the use of the film changers described in the earlier sections of this chapter.

Two accessory features are necessary to the generator.
(a) It must have a switch which will maintain rotation of the tube anode independently of the radiographic exposure switch. In the absence of this feature, the anode will lose speed on release of the exposure switch and a 'prepare' interval of about 0·8 second must occur before the next exposure can be made. This delays the sequence of exposures too much. When a switch of this nature is fitted it is preferably operated by means of a key, similar to that used for the ignition of a car. This can be removed from the control desk on completion of the special X-ray examination and there is then no danger of its being accidentally left 'on' during ordinary use of the unit. Such a mishap would certainly result in serious overheating of the X-ray tube, because when the stator coils are energized during a long period of time they become very hot.

(b) The generator should have an additional radiographic exposure switch on a long lead to allow the X-ray exposures to be made by a radiographer standing remote from the control desk; that is, close to the cassette changer. This switch and lead should be connected in the exposure circuit by means of a plug so that they may be removed altogether when not required: furthermore, the switch should be not hand-operated but a footswitch.

As the cassette changer is not automated, its successful operation depends upon a practised radiographer. The following would be an appropriate method of procedure. When the patient and the X-ray tube are correctly positioned relative to the changer and the radiologist has indicated that he is ready to begin injection of the contrast agent, the radiographer then should:

1 check that all lead protection is in position;

2 check exposure factors;

3 operate the special switch which initiates continuous rotation of the anode;

4 inform the radiologist of this;

5 on receipt of the radiologist's agreed signal, make the first exposure, using the footswitch;

6 as soon as the exposure is terminated withdraw the top cassette by hand, placing it upon some suitable adjacent surface—for example a padded trolley top or even upon pillows laid on the floor which will diminish noise and preserve the life of the cassette;

7 immediately make the next exposure;

6 and 7 are repeated until the supply of cassettes is exhausted.

The anode rotor is then switched off and the cassettes are taken for processing.

This sequence of events can be more quickly performed than described and the rate of change is of the order of 1 film per second.

Peripheral angiography

The equipment previously described enables a number of exposures to be made in quick succession at one site in the body. However, in some circumstances this is not enough.

Patients suffering from peripheral vascular disease often do not have a sufficient blood supply to their feet and lower legs, because of an obstruction of the arteries of the thigh or pelvis. Injection of a suitable contrast agent into the abdominal aorta, at a point above where it divides into the right and left common iliac arteries, will result in a flow of opacified blood down the vessels of both legs simultaneously. Films must be obtained successively between the regions of the pelvis and the ankles which will record the arteries as they opacify and thus reveal the sites and degree of obstruction.

The time taken for the opacified blood to pass from the lower abdomen to the feet will vary with individual patients but it is of the order of a few seconds only. Consequently equipment for aortography is required to:

1   obtain a number of exposures quickly;

2   provide for either (a) coverage of the whole lower limb at each exposure, or (b) movement of the patient relative to the positions of the X-ray tube and a film, so that different sites may be successively recorded. We shall consider (a) first, as it involves a cassette-changer. The specialized tables necessary for (b) are the subject of this chapter's next section.

Large field serial radiography

The problems in obtaining complete radiographic coverage of the lower limbs at each exposure are real but they are not insuperable and apparatus has been devised which makes this a feasible procedure. Implicit in the construction and operation of such equipment are the following points.

1   The use of a long cassette, for example one of dimensions 35 cm × 1·3 m (14 × 51 inches). This holds three 35 × 43 cm (14 × 17 inch) films placed lengthwise.

2   The use of a long film-focus distance (of the order of 2 metres or 72 inches or more) to obtain a sufficiently extensive film-coverage. This means that the X-ray tube must have a special mounting close to the ceiling. Consequently the room height must not be less than about 3 metres (10 feet).

3   The use of a special cone or diaphragm limiting the beam to a narrow—although long—rectangular field. This collimator may feature a double slot and thus provide a discrete field of irradiation of each leg.

4   The use of measures giving correct exposure of all three films in the cassette, despite that each records a body part of different thickness. This might be done, for example, by means of different speeds in the film/intensifying screens combination, such as those stated below:

abdominal area; high- or medium-speed film with a pair of high-speed intensifying screens;

thigh; medium-speed film with one medium-speed intensifying screen;

lower leg; direct-exposure film without intensifying screens. This and the thigh parts of the cassette should have black cards placed where the screens would otherwise be, with the double object of maintaining screen-film contact and absorbing any light spread from adjacent fluorescing areas.

Grids are often used in relation to the abdominal and thigh parts of the cassette.

Another method of balancing an exposure technique against diminishing thickness of the part X-rayed is to fit a graduated filter to the tubehead. This can be composed of three different wedges of aluminium and obviously must be placed in its slide so that the thickest section is toward the patient's feet. Such a filter might be used instead of or as well as the film/screen manipulations just described.

Several tables have been designed which can handle cassettes of these large formats and can change a cassette in slightly less than one second. Fig. 14.7 is a sketch of such a table, which features a revolving hexagonal drum

Sliding table top

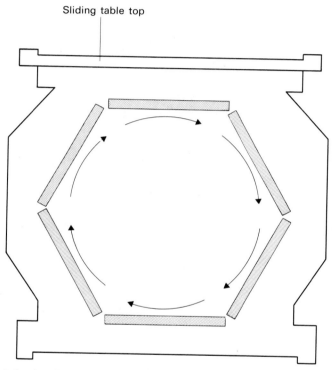

Fig. 14.7   A sketch to illustrate the principle of operation of a large-cassette changer suitable for single-exposure representation of blood vessels in the pelvis and leg.

beneath a floating table-top. The drum is loaded from one side of the changer; opening the door brings an automatic rotation of the drum to the loading position and the cassettes are inserted one after another. Each cassette in this case is 30 cm × 120 cm (12 inches × 47 inches approximately) and a special trolley, which can transport up to 12 cassettes, is a helpful accessory; a number of them together is not easy to handle.

Like the film changers previously described, this cassette changer is fully automated and is controlled from a programming unit. This gives preselection of the pauses—in a range from zero to 12 seconds—between the six exposures of a single series. The maximum exposure rate is 1 frame per second; this is derived from an exposure time of 0·1 second and a period of 0·9 second for the further transport of a cassette.

The programmer also provides a 'free' mode of operation in which radiographs can be exposed and the cassettes transported at any time.

TABLES FOR ABDOMINAL AND PERIPHERAL ANGIOGRAPHY

At present, the majority of equipments for abdominal and peripheral angiography achieve their purpose by methods which permit one or more radiographs to be taken at each of several anatomical sites (usually between the lower abdomen and the ankle). These equipments as a rule pose less difficult technical problems than are entailed in the rapid change of large cassettes. They often have the further advantage of versatility, being as suitable for angiography at one anatomical site as at several.

Rapid radiography at each of a number of preselected sites is made possible if the equipment moves the patient in relation to the X-ray tube; or alternatively moves the X-ray tube and the film together as one entity in respect of the patient. Apparatus in each of these categories has been employed for a number of years. However, the specialized tables presently available from the major manufacturers of X-ray equipment operate on the first principle: the patient is moved, while the X-ray tube and the film—usually in an automatic changer—remain stationary.

Some of these tables are specifically catheterization tables. They are designed for several angiological applications and are appropriate to a suite planned for a full programme of these examinations. However, simpler equipment is also available. It is likely to be chosen for a department where a limited number of patients are referred for angiography, which is then a minor part of the total workload. In such circumstances the purchase of highly refined X-ray equipment for these procedures represents uneconomic expenditure of both money and space. A typical, relatively simple arrangement for abdominal and peripheral angiography is described below.

Sliding table-top with film-changer

Figure 14.8 illustrates the significant parts of a simple installation for aortography which would not preclude the performance of other X-ray examinations at other times. It consists of:
1 a sliding table-top;
2 a rapid film-changer (the one shown is an AOT);
3 a motor unit and roller mechanism.

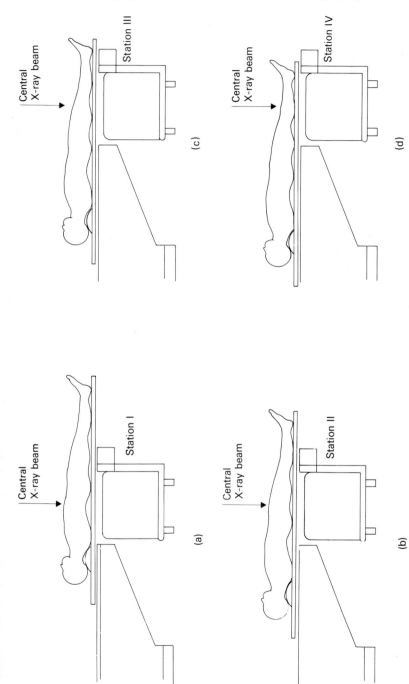

Fig. 14.8 A simple system for peripheral angiography of the pelvis and lower limbs. A sliding table top is driven over an AOT rapid film changer, being halted at each of certain stations, where a preselected number of exposures is made. Four stations are shown in drawings (a) to (d).

The sliding table top fits—and will move within—a standard type of groove on each side of a general-purpose fluoroscopic table with an image intensifier. This would be used as an aid to placing the intra-arterial catheter at the start of the investigation. The sliding top, on which the patient is able to remain during the entire procedure (including any fluoroscopy), is driven over the AOT film-changer, towards and along the X-ray table, by means of a roller mechanism and motor unit. This assembly is mounted on a vertical column on the stand supporting the AOT changer.

Figure 14.8 makes these features clear and illustrates how a patient, who is lying on the sliding table-top, may be moved through an X-ray beam centred on the film-changer.

Movement control

Control of the movement of the table-top is provided by a special series selector which is additional to the standard programme selector of the film changer. This special unit has four selector switches—one for each of the four sites indicated in Fig. 14.8—and permits up to 10 films to be exposed at each site.

Two press buttons marked *Start position* and *Test* respectively:

1   bring the table-top to the starting position;
2   allow a trial to be made of the table-top's excursion.

When the motor unit is in the starting position a green pilot lamp is illuminated on the series control.

Figure 14.9 illustrates how the four positions of the table-top produce some overlap of the irradiated areas and can result in a complete examination of the vessels of the lower limb. The total length of the patient recorded by the excursion is 105 cm, constituted as follows:

Station I covers 25 cm;
Step I–II   25 cm;
Step II–III   27 cm;
Step III–IV   27 cm.

The time required for the movement of the table-top is about 2 seconds for each step.

Exposure control

Measures for obtaining radiographs of the correct density at all four anatomical sites (that is, allowance for the decreasing thickness of tissues between hip and ankle) depend on reductions in kilovoltage at stations II, III and IV. The kilovoltage across the X-ray tube is automatically decreased by means of a number of variable resistors connected in series with each

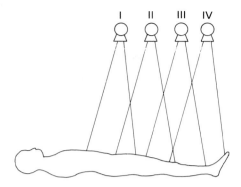

Fig. 14.9

phase (three) of the *primary* leads of the high tension transformer. The kilovoltage selected for the exposure at station I is progressively reduced at steps II, III and IV by the inclusion of resistors of successively higher values. This is a straightforward application of Ohm's Law: the voltage drop is proportional to the resistance present in a circuit.

Patients, of course, are not standard subjects for radiography; X-ray departments use different radiographic materials; nor are the observers of the resultant radiographs more predictable. All these introduce variables which cannot be predetermined and require the equipment to provide flexibility of the selected exposure factors. This flexibility is achieved in two ways.

1   To obtain appropriate kilovoltage reductions for an 'average' subject in the specific conditions (for example, type of film, processing factors and others), the values of the series resistors can—and will—be adjusted during installation.

2   Some available variation in the kilovoltage-reduction occurring at each step will enable the radiographer to cater for a different 'size' of subject at any time. This variation is found by varying the milliampere factor in the exposure (while keeping the milliampereseconds value constant).

To understand (2) above, the student should refer to earlier discussions in this book which explained the proportional relationship between the magnitudes of the voltage-loss on-load and the load current (see page 17, for instance). Thus we can change the voltage drop at the steps of the series by altering our choice of tube current (milliamperes). A higher value of milliamperes results in a greater reduction in kilovoltage at every step of the programme.

The programme

Depending on the patient's condition, the velocity of the blood stream is another variable. We do not know precisely when the opacified blood will reach the ankle from the site of injection in the groin, or whether this interval of time is the same for both legs. Knowledge of these factors greatly influences the conduct of the examination, which will need to vary for differing individuals. The following programme is suggested as a suitable mean.

Loading the magazine

Sixteen (35 cm × 35 cm) films are loaded in the supply magazine of the AOT changer in the following spaces:
1 and 2 (these are for test purposes);
3 to 10 inclusive;
12, 14, 15, 17, 19, 21.

Rate of change

The programme selector of the AOT is set to change films at the rates given below:
3 films/second for 2 seconds;
1 film/second during the remainder of the series.

The exposure series

The series selector for the sliding table top is set as follows:

Station I	3 films;
Station II	4 films;
Station III	3 films;
Station IV	4 films.

The first exposure should be automatically initiated to occur 0·4 second after the beginning of the injection, thus ensuring exposure of the second film at 0·7 second and the third film at one second after injection. After this the stepped movements of the table top will begin. Since each step needs an interval of two seconds and the remaining films are exposed at the rate of one every second, the last radiograph in the series is taken 20 seconds after the beginning of the injection.

Specialized angiographic tables

Several varieties of table particular to angiography are made to meet the needs of departments where the workload and number of available X-ray rooms justify such an installation. The performance required of these catheterization tables is not in essence different from what has just been described for a simple version of similar equipment, but they present greater refinements of operation.

For instance, one apparatus offers four steps, giving five exposure fields and recording a total length of 125 cm. The length of each step may be varied as required. A punched card inserted in a sensor is used to control the kilovoltage reductions and to pre-determine the automatic injection of the contrast agent, the exposure timing and the finish of the programme.

Another catheterization table is variable in height, making macro-radiography possible (it would be applicable to the renal arteries, for example). This table further offers a number of interchangeable tops, one of which is a rotary patient-cradle to facilitate oblique projections.

In conjunction with the account just given of a simple angiographic table, students should study the equipment at hand in their own departments and notice its particular and significant features, including the type of rapid-film changer with which the table is associated.

Chapter 15
Equipment for Cranial and Dental Radiography

For radiography of any part of the skull and of the teeth specialized equipment is by no means essential. These examinations can be—and often are—made to high technical standards on any general purpose medical X-ray equipment. Nevertheless, both cranial radiography and dental radiography are easier, faster and generally more accurate procedures when equipment is used which is designed specifically for each kind of work.

Whenever the X-ray department is large enough it is often planned so that certain rooms undertake certain categories of examinations: thus we have the 'barium room', the 'chest room', the 'IVP room' and the 'skull room'. It is in the last, or in suites intended for cerebral angiography and similar procedures, that we find the highly organized skull table and its accessories.

Equipment suitable solely for dental radiography may be provided in the main X-ray department but perhaps is more likely to appear in the dental clinical rooms or in X-ray departments serving dental hospitals, particularly when we consider the more sophisticated and exclusive versions of this equipment.

THE SKULL TABLE

General features

A skull table is much more readily appreciated from practical observation than from written descriptions. For a start, the word *table* can be misleading to a reader who is not aware that the area so described has nothing to do with the 'dining table' proportions of general X-ray equipment.

A typical skull table is depicted in Fig. 15.1, and there is one to be seen also in Fig. 4.12. The table is characterized by a number of distinct parts.

1 A fixed column which supports the object table and X-ray tube together; this is either on a T-shaped base or designed for floor-ceiling or floor-wall mounting.

2 An object table which essentially is a bucky tray; this is counterbalanced in its movement up and down the column. The distance between it and the

X-ray tube is not variable and results in an anode-film distance of 90 cm (36 inches).

3 Double semi-circular arches at either end of which are (a) the X-ray tube, (b) a counterweight for the tube. The object table and these arches are mounted on the column by means of a single carriage.

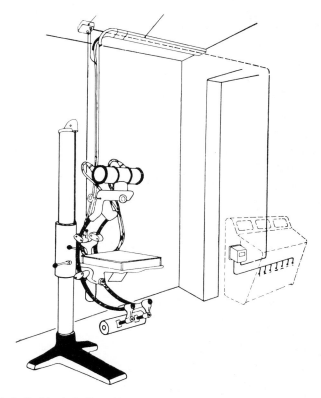

Fig. 15.1 A skull table. A similar table is seen in Fig. 4.12 on p. 151. *By courtesy of Elema-Schonander.*

The patient's couch

Associated with the skull table is a trolley or couch on which the patient can lie, positioned so that his head is over the skull table itself. This couch is neither an integral part of the equipment nor as a rule in a fixed relationship to it.

Sometimes the couch is of a specially constructed type and in this case its heavy pedestal base may mean that it virtually *is* immobile in the room, or at least that it will be moved very little; alternatively it may be designed to run on a carriage and floor rails.

A couch of this kind can be raised and lowered hydraulically and is usually built in three hinged sections. By tilting one-third at a reclining angle (the end third nearest the skull table), this can make a back-rest; the middle third remains horizontal to form a seat; the remaining third is dropped vertically downwards to support the knees and calves. Thus the couch converts to a chair and can be used for the examination of patients in the sitting position, particularly during cerebral air studies. Arm, head and shoulder rests and a sling for the chin provide the means adequately to immobilize the patient or to support one who is incapable of maintaining himself erect.

Movements of the table and X-ray tube

The principal conceptions behind the design of the skull table are:

1 to provide apparatus which is capable of moving about the patient with great flexibility in preference to changing the patient's position to suit certain angulations of the X-ray beam;

2 to provide apparatus in which the X-ray beam—whatever its inclination—is normally constantly centred upon the secondary radiation grid and film. Both principles are bound to result in increased accuracy of projection.

In achieving these aims the apparatus is notable for its capacity to be adjusted in the following ways, which are illustrated in Fig. 15.2. All moving

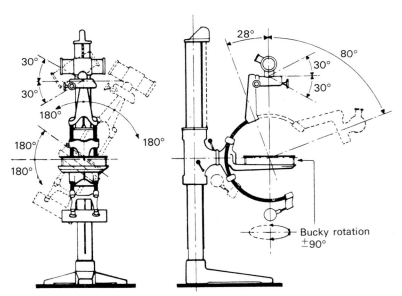

Fig. 15.2 Diagram illustrating the various angular movements of the Schonander skull table. *By courtesy of Elema-Schonander.*

parts of the equipment are graduated in degrees to facilitate setting up and reproducing specific positioning techniques.

1   The whole device of the object table and the arches containing the X-ray tube and its counterweight can be moved *en bloc* up and down the supporting column. This adjusts the height of the table to that of any stretcher or couch or of any patient who is examined erect.

2   The whole device again can be rotated through 360 degrees. This permits the object table to be employed in the vertical and associated positions.

3   The X-ray tube and object table can be moved independently. While the table remains stationary the tube and its arcs can be rotated round it.

This permits angulations of the X-ray beam in the sagittal line of the patient; for example, to obtain a Towne's projection. The full 30 degrees of beam inclination needed in this case may be obtained by any of the following approaches:

(a) angulation of the X-ray tube only;

(b) tilting the object table only;

(c) a combination of putting some of the tilt on the table and some on the X-ray tube.

4   The X-ray tube can be swung on its arcs in a direction along the arcs. The total range of movement is about 120 degrees; this comprises 30 degrees towards the column and 90 degrees away from it. In the latter position of the tube a lateral projection of the skull may be taken with the patient lying either face upwards or face downwards; the cassette in this case is held vertically on the far edge of the table by means of a special attachment. Fig 15.2 shows how at all other angles the X-ray tube remains centred upon the table.

5   The X-ray tube can be tilted independently on its own axis ± 30 degrees, as shown in Fig. 15.2.

6   The bucky is on a pivot and can be rotated through 360 degrees so that beam inclinations obtained under (4) and (5) do not involve slants across the grid elements (see Chapter 8).

The object table

In addition to turn-table support for the grid and its mechanism the object table has other unusual characteristics. The action by which in a normal X-ray table the bucky tray is removed results in this case in the withdrawal of the complete structure of film holder and grid movement; these hinge and either hang vertically downwards or by engagement of a support hook can be held in a vertical position to permit the cassette to be loaded into clamps from beneath.

The upper and lower sections of the table are made of transparent

Plexiglas (see Fig. 15.3). On the upper surface are etched a pair of cross-lines intersecting at the centre of the field and a large circular protractor, scaled in four quadrants of 90 degrees each or two semi-circles marked from zero to 180 degrees.

Underneath the table are a pair of lighted mirrors. So long as the bucky mechanism is withdrawn from its radiographic position, these mirrors reflect towards the radiographer a view of that aspect of the patient which is in contact with the inscribed transparent surface. This facility permits the X-ray beam to be centred accurately on surface anatomical landmarks which are near to the film and ordinarily lost to sight because of this.

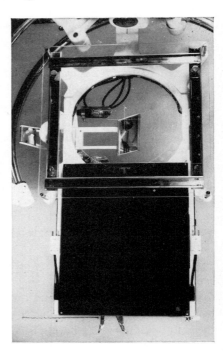

Fig. 15.3 A skull table with the bucky withdrawn. *By courtesy of Elema-Schonander.*

Accessories

A skull table is likely to have some or all of the following accessories not already mentioned.

Immobilizing devices

The best form of immobilizing device is a band on double ratchets of the kind described in Chapter 14 (p. 504). Alternatively head clamps may be used which fix to the sides of the table.

Beam limiting and beam centring devices

Usually limitation of the X-ray beam is obtained by removable diaphragms which are slotted into the tubehead, rather than by cones. A number of diaphragms of different sized apertures are supplied, some giving a circular field and others a rectangle; for example the areas covered by a series of seven might be circles 9 cm, 13 cm, 18 cm, 24 cm and 30 cm in diameter, and rectangles 11 cm by 3·5 cm and 11 cm by 2·9 cm.

Visual indication of the direction of the primary beam is provided either by a centre-finding pointer or by Varay lamps (see Chapter 8, p. 303).

Spring-loaded cassette changers

Spring-loaded cassette boxes for cerebral angiography of the kind described in Chapter 14 are usually combined with a skull table. The bucky mechanism is removed and replaced with the box which will be employed for the anteroposterior (Towne's) projection; the box for the lateral projection is fitted to the edge of the table in the same position as the cassette holder described earlier (p. 517).

Special techniques

The skull table which has been depicted and described here is a classic type. In fact a number of skull tables are available which differ from this in certain constructional aspects while operating on the same general principles. These may include facilities for tomography, macroradiography (enlargement of the radiographic image) and even television fluoroscopy of the skull.

GENERAL DENTAL X-RAY EQUIPMENT

Much less dental radiography is undertaken in hospital than in places elsewhere, for now almost every dentist's surgery possesses equipment which enables him to take radiographs on the spot. Even in hospital it is quite likely that most of the dental radiography will be done similarly at the chairside in the dental consulting rooms in preference to the main X-ray department. There is clearly a place for apparatus which is designed for use in these specific conditions and is intended to undertake only dental and facio-maxillary examinations.

We can list the main requirements of chairside dental X-ray apparatus as follows.

1 It should not occupy much space.

2 It should be simple, light, easy to manœuvre and capable of maintaining a position without brakes.

3 Precise angulations of the X-ray beam must be readily obtainable.

4 The radiographic output must be sufficient for all dental and some facio-maxillary examinations. However, the output need not—and therefore should not—be greater than these purposes suggest since many dentists will require the set to operate from their domestic supply.

5 The set must afford the operator and the patient certain standards of radiation protection; it must also be electrically safe.

Most of the above observations apply also to portable X-ray equipment (see Chapter 9) and consequently it is no surprise to find that chairside dental X-ray units employ a similar tank construction for the tubehead (see page 333), with all its attendant advantages. These units have even simpler controls and seldom possess measuring instruments, other than a mains volts meter; sometimes not even this is present.

There are three significant parts of such dental equipment to consider:

1 the tubehead;

2 the tubestand;

3 the timer.

The tubehead

In Fig. 15.4 is seen the tubehead of a modern unit for dental radiography. The head is oil-filled and vacuum-sealed. In it are the high tension transformer; the filament transformer; the X-ray tube; an oil-expansion diaphragm. Each of these features is discussed fully in Chapter 9 and need not be explained again here.

The tubehead is mounted in a contrivance known as a gimbal in which it is free to rotate in two planes. A scale at the side indicates angles of rotation round the axis of the tube. The head is light and easy to adjust with finger-tip pressure; it remains steady in whatever position it is put and consequently requires no locks or brakes.

A localizing cone is provided for the tubehead giving an anode-skin distance of 18–23 cm (7–9 inches). The inherent filtration of the tube is 0·5 mm Al and it has an effective focal spot size of 0·8 mm. Additional aluminium filtration should be added. (Total filtration should be 1–2 mm Al in the United Kingdom).

The generator can have a fixed output of 12 mA at 55 kVp. In this instance the tube current and the kilovoltage are each rather higher than those offered by many dental X-ray units; for example 7 mA and 50 kVp are quite usual values.

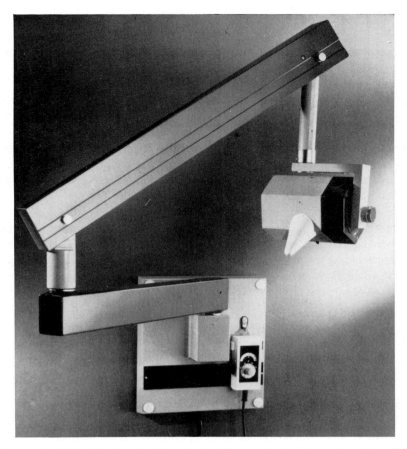

Fig. 15.4   A tubehead for dental radiography. In this example the tubestand is of the wall-mounted variety. The handswitch and timer unit is seen on a hook nearby. *By courtesy of Picker International Ltd.*

The tubestand

The tubehead is mounted on a tubestand. This is seen in Fig. 15.4 and comprises essentially a horizontal bar to one end of which is fitted another. The second can rotate upon the first and also hinges in the vertical plane; this enables the height of the tubehead—which is attached at the other end of the bar—to be altered freely.

The tubestand itself is mounted in one of the following ways:

1   on the wall by means of a bracket;
2   on a mobile pedestal which moves on four large castors;
3   on the dentist's pedestal control.

While slightly different features of design characterize the tubestands of various examples of chairside dental X-ray equipment, the choice of a bracket or mobile pedestal mounting is frequently found. The first and third have the advantage that the equipment occupies less space but the disadvantage that its use is restricted to one room.

The timer

The hand timeswitch should be on a flexible lead which permits the operator to stand at a distance from the X-ray tube when an exposure is made. In appearance the timeswitch is similar to those found on portable X-ray sets for general work.

In the case of the unit depicted in Fig. 15.4, the timer is of the electronic type (see Chapter 5). It provides a maximum exposure interval of 5 seconds. Between 1 and 5 seconds the calibrations are in steps of 0·25 seconds; between 0 and 1 second there are ten divisions of 0·1 second each. A red pilot lamp indicates when X rays are 'on' and the exposure push-button is designed to prevent any operation as the result of accidental pressure.

SPECIALIZED DENTAL X-RAY EQUIPMENT

Cephalostats (craniostats)

A cephalostat or craniostat is an apparatus which permits a precise correlation of position to be established between an X-ray film, the head of the patient and the anode of the X-ray tube. This correlation can be reproduced exactly for the purpose of later examinations during orthodontic treatment, strict radiographic comparisons being necessary for the assessment of progress. The process may be described as a teleradiographic dental examination.

Figure 15.5 is a photograph of a cephalostat and Fig. 15.6 is a diagram in which the main parts of the apparatus have been numbered and are described in the key below. The cephalostat is wall-mounted and of a strong rigid structure. In essence the patient is literally pinned by the ears by means of ear plugs in a fixed relationship to a cassette-holder; the X-ray tube, which is shown in neither illustration, is at another fixed point. The orbital indicator, nasal positioner and scales showing certain distances all play a necessary part in the indication, recording and subsequent reproduction of a particular radiographic situation.

Some cephalostats incorporate a metal—for example duralumin—filter which can be adjusted in position relative to the patient when lateral

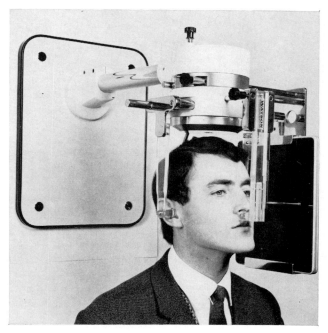

Fig. 15.5   A craniostat. *By courtesy of Picker International Ltd.*

projections of the face and jaws are made. The purpose of the filter is to prevent over-penetration on the radiograph of the nasal bones and soft tissue profile, since the relationships between these and the teeth are significant for the orthodontist.

A further accessory which should be employed with the apparatus whenever possible is a secondary radiation grid (see Chapter 8). This is placed in the cephalostat's cassette-holder or alternatively a gridded cassette may be used. The recommended grid is of the Lysholm type: it has 100 lines to the inch (45/cm) and a ratio of 12 to 1 and is focused at 140 cm.

The X-ray generator

Othodontic radiography entails serial examinations of the teeth, facial bones and soft tissue structures in relation to each other and from an X-ray point of view it is radiography of the skull. A small dental unit of fixed output—such as was described in the previous section—can be used in association with a cephalostat but it is not the most satisfactory type of generator.

A more acceptable—although necessarily more expensive—source of X-rays is a tubehead unit of similar tank construction which includes solid

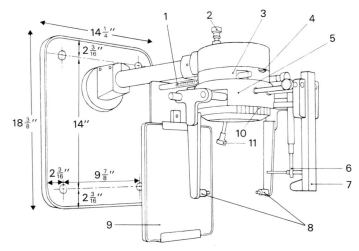

Fig. 15.6 A craniostat.

1 Scale to indicate the distance between the median plane–or the midcoronal plane–of the head and cassette
2 lock for rotating head
3 cassette support which can be rotated through 360 deg. Its position in this drawing may be compared with Fig. 15.5
4 lock for cassette support
5 head rotates through 360 deg. with four stop positions
6 orbital indicator
7 nasal positioner
8 ear locators
9 cassette
10 scale indicating the distance between the ear locators
11 control for adjusting the ear locators

By courtesy of Picker International Ltd.

state rectifiers and can be combined with a comprehensive control. Such an outfit can be expected to offer tube currents up to 150 mA and kilovoltages up to 125 kVp, provided the mains supply is adequate (see Chapter 9). The X-ray tube could be of the rotating anode type with a single focus of perhaps 0·8 mm.

Whatever form of generator is employed, installation of the cephalostat requires the tubehead to be mounted in a permanent position at some fixed distance relative to the cassette-holder. It is an advantage of the more powerful generators that they enable a longer anode-film distance to be successfully employed, with obvious improvement in radiographic definition. When the X-ray generator can provide a maximum of only 7–12 mA and kilovoltages no greater than 50–55 kVp, then the anode-film distance must be severely reduced if adequate exposure of faciocranial radiographs is to be obtained. The cephalostat illustrated provides a correction scale to indicate on the radiograph the degree of image enlargement which occurs at short anode-film distances.

Pantomography

Pantomographic equipment provides the means to obtain panoramic tomographs of the jaws and face; that is, all the teeth, together with the mandibles and maxillae, are seen on a single 15 cm × 30 cm film. The technique is simpler to perform than standard peri-apical radiography of the teeth and entails a smaller radiation dose than would a full-mouth survey of 10 to 14 intraoral films; it is admirable, too, for the demonstration of the temporomandibular joints, fractures of the facial bones, developmental annormalities and large dental cysts.

Readers of this book, familiar with X-ray requisition forms from the dental departments of their hospitals, may find that often the letters OPG are used to denote this form of pantomographic investigation. Strictly speaking, OPG is a reference to a trade name and applicable only to a particular equipment, the Othopantomograph of Siemens Ltd; but—like *wellingtons* and *cardigan*—in English usage OPG seems to have become a widely understandable term for a genre.

The tubehead, cassette-carriage and patient-support

A general view of a unit for panoramic tomography of the face and jaws is shown in Fig. 15.7. Its planigraphic principle of operation requires the X-ray tube and the film to circle a stationary patient during the course of the X-ray exposure. The duration of the exposure may vary between different examples of the equipment: in the model illustrated it is 15 seconds.

As Fig. 15.7 shows, the X-ray tube is contained in a tank-construction (see page 333). The tube has an effective focal area of 0·6 mm × 0·6 mm and the total filtration is equivalent to 3 mm Al. By means of an overhead horizontal support the X-ray tube is connected to a carriage and holder for a curved cassette, of which the convex surface is facing the tube.

A radiographic cone is provided but effectively the beam is collimated by means of (a) a primary diaphragm in a choice of widths for adults and children and (b) a secondary slit panel which is adjustable and situated immediately in front of the film. A plan view of this means of collimation is shown in Fig. 15.8.

The tubehead and the cassette-carriage oppose each other and are able

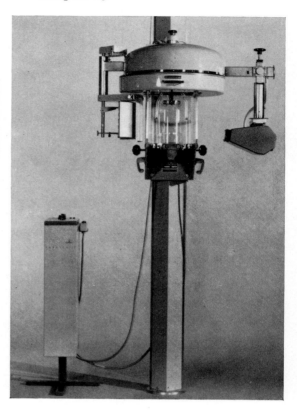

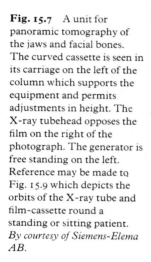

Fig. 15.7 A unit for panoramic tomography of the jaws and facial bones. The curved cassette is seen in its carriage on the left of the column which supports the equipment and permits adjustments in height. The X-ray tubehead opposes the film on the right of the photograph. The generator is free standing on the left. Reference may be made to Fig. 15.9 which depicts the orbits of the X-ray tube and film-cassette round a standing or sitting patient. *By courtesy of Siemens-Elema AB.*

to rotate round a refined system for accurately positioning and immobilizing a standing patient. The system incorporates:

a bite block;

a chin support;

a forehead support;

right and left temporal supports;

right and left perspex face-plates;

a handle on either side of the unit which the patient may grip.

The total assembly of tubehead, cassette-carriage and patient-support is counterweighted and can be moved as one structure vertically on a wall-fixed pillar. An electromagnetic brake controls this movement, the range of which is such that the equipment may be used to examine subjects ranging in height from young children to adults up to 6 feet 5 inches tall. As with this particular unit the patient normally stands during the examination, no chair and therefore less space are required. However, a sitting patient is equally acceptable to the equipment. Another variety of such a panoramic

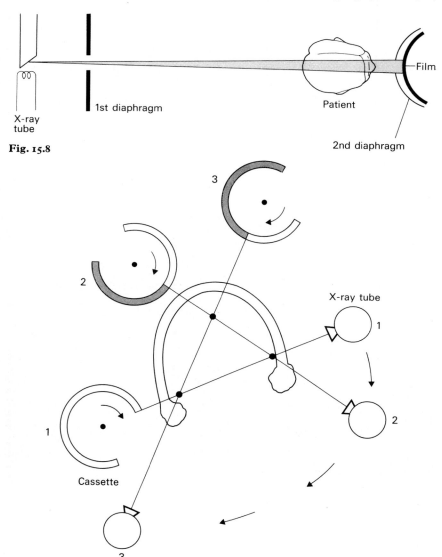

1st diaphragm

Patient

Film

X-ray tube

2nd diaphragm

Fig. 15.8

3

2

1

X-ray tube

1

2

Cassette

3

Fig. 15.9 A plan view of orbits of rotation during pantomography.

radiographic system includes a chair but, even so, a floor area of approximately 4 feet by 4 feet ($1 \cdot 2$ m × $1 \cdot 2$ m) is adequate to contain the total arrangement.

The cassette

The film format and the design of the cassette vary in some respects in different models. 15 cm × 30 cm or 5 inches by 12 inches are the usual sizes of film.

For the purpose of the technique the film must be supported in a curved plane. This requires the cassette either to be of a conventional rigid type but curved along its major axis; or to have the form of a flexible vinyl—or similar—envelope, closing with press studs and adaptable to the curvature imposed on it by the cassette holder. Whichever type of cassette is in use, it contains a pair of intensifying screens.

Having been loaded in the darkroom, the cassette is fitted in its curved holder and secured behind a similarly curved aluminium filter and mounted appropriately on the carriage.

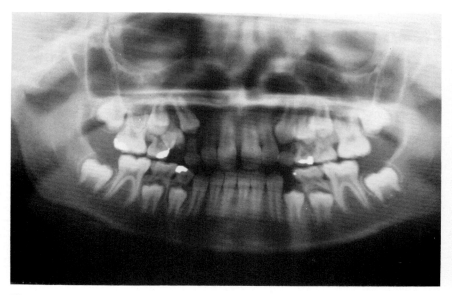

Fig. 15.10   A typical pantomograph of the teeth and jaws.

The generator

A single-pulse generator (self-rectified operation of the X-ray tube) provides a sufficient output. The equipment depicted in Fig. 15.7 functions from a generator which offers a radiographic kilovoltage from 55–85 kVp in nine steps, a fixed milliamperage (15 mA) and a constant exposure time of 15 seconds.

In another example, the kilovoltage range is from 40 to 100 kVp and the tube-current variable between four settings which give respectively 8 mA, 10 mA, 12 mA and 15 mA. As this particular generator can serve a total of three X-ray tubes, it provides exposure timing which is variable from 1/60–15 seconds; however, during panoramic tomography a fixed exposure interval of 20 seconds must be selected.

Mode of operation

Fig. 15.9 is a plan view of the lower jaw, showing the points of rotation of the X-ray tube and film-cassette, their circling of each other during an examination of the teeth and jaws and the turning of the cassette on its own axis of curvature past the second beam-collimator.

Fig. 15.10 (page 528) is a copy of a panoramic tomograph which has been obtained as a result of a similar procedure. It will be noticed that the subject is recorded larger than life on these radiographs. In respect of the unit shown in Fig. 15.7 the magnification is actually 1·4. The relatively short anode-film distance and the greater-than-usual separation of the film from the part X-rayed contribute to this magnification. The use of an X-ray tube with a small effective focal area is essential.

Chapter 16
Specialized Radiographic Systems

CASSETTELESS SYSTEMS

Modern X-ray departments are using what have become known as daylight systems for the production of radiographs. A daylight system is one in which the film is so handled that it goes from its exposure to radiation in the X-ray room to its viewing as a finished radiograph without at any stage progressing through a darkroom with safelight illumination. The advantages of such systems which allow the whole progression of the film to proceed in actinic light may be enumerated as below.

1   Radiographers spend more time with their patients, not being required to go away to darkrooms to process films.

2   Time is saved and departmental capacity is increased: that is, the department can handle a greater workload in a given time or a given workload in a shorter time.

3   Skilled staff are more effectively used.

4   Working conditions are improved.

5   Automated handling reduces the risk of damage to films and the production of artefacts in radiographs.

6   An X-ray room equipped with a suitable daylight system need not be close to a darkroom and so there is widened scope in departmental planning.

There are no serious disadvantages to offset the gains but there are certain questions to be answered when planning the installation of a daylight system. These are as follows.

1   How much space is needed?

2   What arrangements must be made to cover breakdown?

3   Can the costs of purchase and installation be met?

4   What arrangements are to be made for films which are not handled through the daylight system?

The daylight systems which are currently available come in two categories:

1   systems which provide automatic unloading and reloading of cassettes in ordinary room-lighting, linked to automatic processing;

2   systems which have been described as cassetteless radiography, linked to automatic processing.

The first type implies the use of special cassettes and special devices for their loading and unloading but does not entail modifications to the bucky table or X-ray vertical stand. The second type certainly does entail special tables and stands. Because of these facts, we describe here only cassetteless systems as a part of equipment for radiography and consider that the first category (which has been elsewhere described) is away from the planned scope of this book.

Cassetteless systems can be considered in three separate categories which are as follows:

1 cassetteless systems which are part of automatic bucky tables for general radiography;
2 cassetteless systems which are embodied in erect stands for chest radiography;
3 cassetteless systems which are the spot-film devices in diagnostic tables designed for fluoroscopy.

Cassetteless bucky tables

Features of a cassetteless bucky table are as follows.

1 A floating table-top.
2 A system of magazines which are protected from radiation and from light. These magazines store the films in readiness for their automatic transport into the position which they must occupy during the exposure.
3 A film-transport system. This automatically takes a film from one of the supply magazines and conveys it to the exposure position, which is located between a pair of intensifying screens.
4 A means to record on the radiographic film the required identifying data. These are, for example, the patient's name, the date, the hospital, the radiographic projection and any anatomical identification and technical information which may be needed.
5 A continuance of the film-transport system after the radiographic exposure has been made. This part of the system takes the film to its processing in an automatic processor which is directly coupled to the bucky table.

The X-ray tubes which may be used in connection with automatic bucky tables may be:

1 mounted on a stand which is integral to the table as indicated in the sketch in Fig. 16.2 so that the tube is centred to the film and has a constant tube-film distance which is 102 cm (40 inches);
2 ceiling-mounted on an overhead support as indicated in the sketch in Fig. 16.1;
3 carried on a floor-mounted or ceiling-to-floor stand. The last two

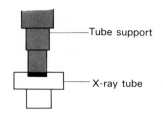

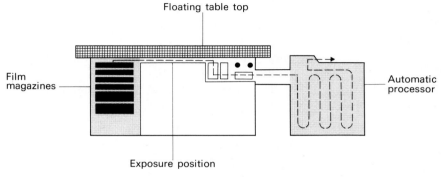

Fig. 16.1

arrangements allow the X-ray tube to be used for other equipment in the X-ray room.

Magazine systems

The supply magazines of automatic bucky tables have various formats. Fig. 16.1 is a sketch of a table which carries 6 supply magazines. For these, the following formats are available:

    18 cm × 24 cm vertical
    24 cm × 30 cm vertical
    20 cm × 40 cm or 18 cm × 43 cm vertical
    35 cm × 35 cm or 30 cm × 35 cm vertical
    35 cm × 43 cm vertical
    35 cm × 43 cm horizontal

Each supply magazine here holds 60 films without interleaved separating sheets of paper and a warning lamp lights when any magazine holds less than 10 films.

Fig. 16.2 is a sketch of a table which has 4 magazines, each of which stores 100 films of the size appropriate to the magazine. The supply magazines must be loaded in a darkroom under safelights and then placed in their protected situations in the bucky table. Making the X-ray

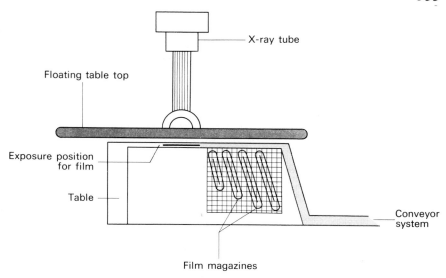

X-ray tube

Floating table top

Exposure position for film

Table

Conveyor system

Film magazines

Fig. 16.2

examination, the radiographer selects the required film format by pressing a push-button. This selection also gives automatic collimation of the beam to cover the film-size which is being used. A closer collimation can be carried out as usual by hand if it is wanted.

Film transport

In the operation of an automatic bucky table, a film from the selected supply magazine is automatically brought into the exposure position beneath the table (indicated in the sketches in Fig. 16.1 and Fig. 16.2). Here the film is held between a pair of intensifying screens which may be selectable: for example, there may be push-buttons to allow choice between a pair of fast screens and a pair of high-resolution screens. Very good contact between the film and the screens is mechanically achieved, usually enhanced by the use of air-evacuation.

After the exposure, each film is automatically removed from the exposure position and conveyed to a coupled automatic processor. This can be closely adjacent to the table as sketched in Fig. 16.1 or it may be remote if the conveyor system is extended. Such extension allows flexible planning to meet the needs of particular installations. For example, one processor can serve two automatic tables or stands (as sketched in Fig. 16.3) by a suitable module for the conveyor system. In such a case, the automation must

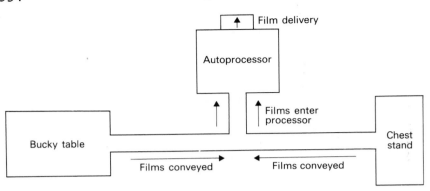

Fig. 16.3

obviously include circuitry and a storage region so that films can take their place in a queue and enter the processor singly.

Identification

The data which must be put on the radiograph in order to identify it are placed there at the time of the exposure. There is a slot or opening to take the card which contains the information. An automatic bucky table may include, among the controls of its operation, suitable sliders on the console which can be set to record on the film the letters AP or PA and the words Left or Right.

The table

The requirements of the floating table-top are that it should have an adequate range of easy movement, effective locks and a short table-top-to-film distance. Typical are an excursion range for the table-top which is plus/minus 70 cm lengthwise and plus/minus 12 cm crosswise and a table-top-to-film distance which is 4 cm. A bucky grid is of course incorporated over the exposure-position of the film and in some tables this grid may be easily interchangeable. In that case, the radiographer may vary the grid so that it is appropriate to the technique which is to be used.

It is possible to link the bucky table to an automatic exposure-timing device. This is done by the provision of a detector-chamber which can be placed in position over the film through the use of actuating push-buttons.

Cassetteless chest stands

Essential features of a chest stand which is to function without cassettes are as follows.

1 A magazine to hold the films protected from radiation and light prior to the X-ray exposure.

2 An exposure area in which each film in turn is held with good contact between intensifying screens for the period of the exposure. The front of this exposure area constitutes a support against which the patient places his chest as indicated in the sketch in Fig. 16.4.

3 A film-transport system to take each film in turn from the holding magazine to the exposure area.

4 A means to record on the radiograph the data of identification such as the patient's name and the date.

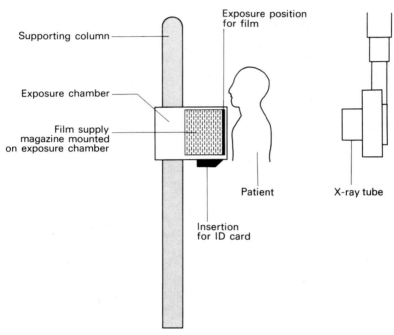

Fig. 16.4

5 An extension of the transport system so that the film may be conveyed to an automatic processor.

An X-ray tube which is to be used in conjunction with a cassetteless chest stand may be:

1 directly coupled to the stand with the X-ray beam centred to the exposure chamber, operating at a fixed tube-film distance of, say, two metres;

2 ceiling-mounted on an overhead support as indicated in the sketch in Fig. 16.4;

3   carried on a floor-mounted or floor-to-ceiling stand. An X-ray tube directly coupled to the exposure chamber can be used only with the chest stand of course. The other arrangements allow the tube to be used with other equipment in the room.

Magazine systems

In a cassetteless chest stand, the magazine which holds the films in a protected position before exposure is required to hold films of one size only.

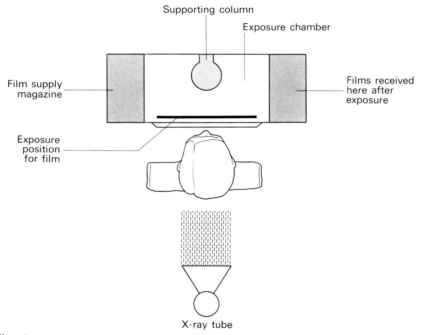

Fig. 16.5

Typical examples are magazines to hold 100 or 125 films of size 35 cm by 43 cm (14 inches by 17 inches). In some equipment the magazine must be removed from the unit and taken to a darkroom for loading under safelights. In some equipment the magazine is designed to be charged in the X-ray room by loading with a special pack which eliminates the necessity for safelights.

Figures 16.4 and 16.5 are sketches of a chest unit in which the film-supply magazine is mounted on one side of the exposure chamber, which is adjustable in height up and down a supporting vertical column. A container which receives the films from the exposure position is mounted on the other side of the exposure chamber. Fig. 16.6 is a sketch of a different arrangement in which the film-supply magazine is at the top above the exposure chamber, while the container which receives films as they pass on from the exposure point is beneath it. So the three essential sections (a supply section, an exposure section and a receiving section) can be brought together in more than one way.

Film transport

Each film must be automatically placed into the exposure position from the supply magazine before the exposure can be made: in some units the initiation of this movement is coupled to the insertion of the card carrying

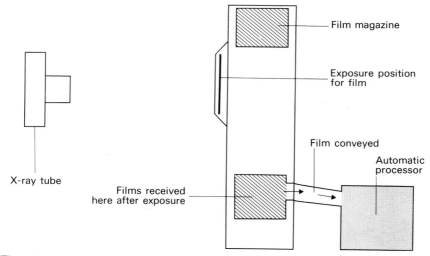

Fig. 16.6

the identifying data. In the exposure position the film is compressed between intensifying screens, the essential close contact often being assured by means of a vacuum. Immediately following the exposure, the film is automatically moved from its position to a containing section so that it may go onward for processing. The conveyance for processing may be achieved in various ways according to the type of cassetteless equipment in use. The possibilities are as follows.

1   The film may pass from the exposure position to the container section where it is automatically taken into a conveyor system that forms a direct link with the input point of an automatic processor. This processor may be

adjacent to the chest stand as shown in the sketch of Fig. 16.6 or it may be remote from the stand as indicated in the diagram of Fig. 16.3. A remote processor may serve more than one X-ray unit by appropriate arrangements for the film conveyor.

2   In the container section the films may be lodged in a case which can hold about 50 films and is a combined transporter and feeder. This means that the case can be removed in daylight from the stand and can be carried by hand to an automatic processor (that is its transporting function). At the processor, still in daylight, the transporter can be attached to the processor and it then automatically inserts the films singly for processing (that is its feeding function).

3   The case in the containing section may be simply a transporter to hold about 50 films. This transporter is removed from the chest stand in daylight and carried to the darkroom. Under safelights it is opened and the films are removed by hand and fed into the processor.

Identification

Incorporated into a cassetteless chest stand is a location for a card to carry the identifying data which are required. This information is recorded on the film at the time when it is in the exposure position. It is usual to make the movement of the film to the exposure position and the initiation of the exposure depend upon there being a card in place in its locating slot. The purpose of such an arrangement is to reduce the chance of a film's being exposed without any record upon it of data by which to identify it.

Cassetteless Spot-film Devices

Equipment for fluoroscopy is available in which systems of magazines provide a cassetteless method for spot-filming to record fluoroscopic appearances. Such a method replaces the conventional serial changer for which films in cassettes are changed by hand. An important advantage of a cassetteless method is speed in making the record since films can be changed automatically at much faster rates than can be achieved by even the most dextrous operators who are changing cassettes by hand.

The table

The diagnostic tables in which cassetteless systems are embodied may be (a) of the type which uses an under-table X-ray tube, the image-intensifier and TV pick-up tube being mounted over the table as sketched in Fig. 16.7, or (b) of the type in which the image intensifier and TV pick-up tube are held

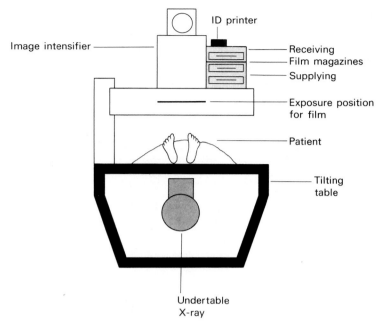

Fig. 16.7

underneath the table as sketched in Fig. 16.8 and an overtable X-ray tube is on a tubestand which forms an integral part of the table.

Whichever of these arrangements is used, the fluoroscopic table is, as usual, a tilting one with sliding table-top. The reader is referred to Chapter 12 for features of tables designed for fluoroscopy, since fluoroscopic examinations are still the prime purposes of this equipment. What has been altered is only the method to make spot-film records on standard full-size X-ray film so that the use of cassettes is eliminated.

Film magazines and transport

Essential to the cassetteless systems are the following.

1 Supply magazines to hold the film prior to exposure. These are loaded under safelights in the darkroom.

2 An exposure position where each film in turn can record fluoroscopic appearances in accordance with a selected exposure programme and with variable film formats. At the exposure position each film is compressed between intensifying screens for the duration of the exposure, with a secondary radiation grid between the patient and the film.

3 A receiving magazine into which the films are passed after exposure.

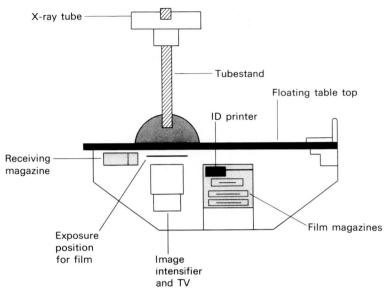

X-ray tube

Tubestand

Floating table top

ID printer

Receiving magazine

Film magazines

Exposure position for film

Image intensifier and TV

Fig. 16.8

When it is full, this is taken out of the equipment and is unloaded under safelights in the darkroom.

4   A transport system to move the films from supply to receiving magazines through the exposure position.

The equipment sketched in Fig. 16.7 has two supply magazines mounted to one side of the image intensifier. These supply magazines are the lower two in the tier of three which is shown. The third and uppermost magazine in the tier is the receiving magazine. The supply magazines are for two different sizes of film (10 inches by 12 inches and 14 inches by 14 inches or metric equivalent), the controls giving selection between the two sizes and choice among programmes for formats chosen for the exposures. The capacity of all three magazines is in this case about 50 films each. On the control console there are warning indications when the numbers of films in the supply magazines have fallen below a certain value (say 9 or less) and when the numbers of films in the receiving magazine are near to an overloading amount (say 40 or more).

The equipment sketched in Fig. 16.8 has the image intensifier underneath the table and the supply magazines as illustrated to one side of it. In this case two supply magazines (14×14 and 10×12 films or metric equivalent) are standard to the equipment. A third supply magazine (for 11×14 films) is available as an extra accessory. These magazines each hold 50 films of the appropriate size. The receiving magazine is indicated in Fig. 16.8 to the viewer's left beneath the table-top and in this case it has the capacity for 100 sheets of film. For each of the magazines there is a separate display of the number of films which it holds and warning lamps show when each supply magazine has 9 films or fewer still within it and when the receiving magazine has gathered 90 films or more. The controls include selection switches for film-sizes and for programmes of exposure-formats.

As can be seen in both Figs. 16.7 and 16.8 the exposure position for the film is central to the image intensifier whether that is above or below the table. The sketches do not indicate any secondary radiation grid: such a grid would of course be in a position between the patient and the film when it is placed for exposure. Typical of such grids are the following examples:

1   fixed grid, 10:1 ratio, 40 lines per cm;
2   reciprocating grid, 10:1 ratio, 34 lines per cm;

Important points on the transport of the film from its supply magazine to the exposure position are as follows:

1   it should arrive there as quickly as possible so that transient appearances may be recorded without needless delay and to this end the film should travel fast;
2   when the exposure begins the film must be motionless or its movement will add to the unsharpness of the image and to this end the film must come to a sharp stop;
3   the faster the film travels the longer is the time required to halt it.

There are thus two conflictions to be reconciled in the practical arrangements. In some of the available equipment, the compromise used is to make the film travel very fast at the beginning of its journey and then become slower in its rate as the exposure-position is neared so that it may be the more certainly stopped within a short time.

Identification

Figures 16.7 and 16.8 both indicate a placing for a card which carries identifying information about the patient and the examination which is being undertaken. When the card is properly placed the information from it is recorded on the film at the time of the exposure. This is on a part of the film (for example, the lower left or the upper right hand corner) which is away from the area of diagnostic interest. In addition to the printer there may be a number marker which operates through a switch on the control panel. This number marker (with a range 00 to 99) is used to print a serial number in addition to the other data in one corner of the film.

SYSTEMS AND EQUIPMENT FOR TRAUMA

From the time of the occurrence of an accident, experiences within an X-ray room constitute only one phase of the total care of an injured person. Radiographic equipment which is orientated to the investigation of injury—if it is to be appropriate in every respect—should refer to the needs of a patient before he arrives in the X-ray department and after he has left it; and it should be useful not only to radiographers but to others to whom the patient may transiently be committed, from abulancemen to surgeons.

It is this thinking which has led to the development of complete systems for use in accident and emergency departments. These systems are centred upon facility of the X-ray examinations concerned, but their overall aim is a minimum amount of movement from—and disturbance of—the injured subject. They provide for:

1 transport of the patient;
2 any required immediate measures of intensive care;
3 X-ray examination;
4 minor surgery, such as the toilet of wounds.

In the radiodiagnostic room itself, such a system for trauma may include other X-ray equipment which is designed particularly for cranial and skeletal examinations. In this chapter both are to be considered.

Patient-transfer systems

Total systems for accident and emergency procedures are often described as being patient-transfer systems; but this should not blind us to the first purpose of these equipments, which is to allow radiographic—and indeed also fluoroscopically controlled—examinations to be made with the least physical disturbance of a subject. The essentials of any such system may be stated as follows:

1 a trolley, upon which a patient will remain from the time of his arrival by ambulance at the hospital until he is either sent away again or is admitted to a bed;
2 equipment available in the radiodiagnostic room which endows the trolley with the salient characteristics of an X-ray table and permits accurate radiography to be quickly—and from the patient's point of view, easily—performed.

The transfer trolley

In various respects, the design of a particular patient-transfer trolley is governed by the nature of the X-ray equipment which is at the centre of the system. It is not practicable to combine the trolleys of one system with the radiodiagnostic concomitants of another. This aside, we may notice a number of features which a patient-transfer trolley should—and often will be found to—possess. These include:

1   a top which does not significantly absorb X rays (for instance, an aluminium equivalent of 1·3 mm at 70 kVp would be appropriate), together with a similarly radioparent mattress;

2   a means to tilt both head and foot ends of the trolley (particularly important for resuscitative purposes is a downwards head tilt of about 15 deg);

3   a means to adjust the height of the trolley surface (to enable the trolley more readily to adapt to the functions of a treatment table and to match the various heights of hospital beds);

4   a back rest which may be inclined at various angles or may lie flat;

5   side supports (cot sides) which may be fitted for the safety of an unconscious or restless patient;

6   an arm support which can be fitted to maintain the position of the limb for a patient who is receiving an intravenous drip;

7   a drip-bottle holder, which has telescopic adjustment of its vertical height and is capable of occupying any of a number of positions on the trolley (this may be at each of the four corners or alternatively the drip-stand may be locked anywhere along side rails on the trolley top);

8   a large wire basket for the patient's possessions, preferably readily accessible for cleaning and other purposes;

9   a holder or rack for an oxygen cylinder (again easily accessible, to allow the cylinder to be changed);

10   a holder for a suction bottle;

11   a means to attach a cassette holder to either side of the trolley, in order to have support for a film during radiography with a horizontal X-ray beam;

12   wheel brakes.

The X-ray equipment

Student readers of this book are likely to encounter one or the other—or perhaps even both—of two available systems which are purpose designed for accident and emergency radiography, but are different from each other in significant respects. One of these systems depends on trolleys which have removable tops and the other uses trolleys which have a fixed top. The first is the more complex system of the two and potentially has the greater scope; indeed its makers say that the system is inappropriate only to gastrointestinal radiology. This is because the associated X-ray table may be adapted to angiographic investigations and overtable or undertable fluoroscopy. It should be said, however, that within the health service of the United Kingdom, these procedures are not a usual part of the initial examination of injured people. Both accident and emergency systems are now to be described.

The system using trolleys with a removable top (A)

For the sake of convenience and brevity, we shall designate as A the system which employs trolleys having a removable top. These trolleys consist primarily of a wheeled base-frame which has a cantilever at either end (see Fig. 16.9). Foot-operated hydraulic pumps raise and lower these cantilevers; they may be put into action either simultaneously or separately. Mounted on the cantilevers are locking devices which will secure a table top and when this is fitted the combination becomes a patient-transfer trolley. As part of system A, a radiolucent mattress is available, which—carried in ambul-

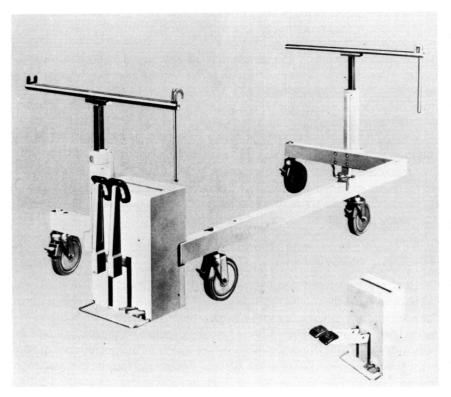

Fig. 16.9   The wheeled base-frame of the trolley which is used by system A for accident and emergency radiography. *By courtesy of Siemens-Elema AB.*

ances—can be used as a stretcher at the scene of an accident and is placed on the transfer trolley upon arrival at the hospital, obviating any need to move the patient again.

In the X-ray room, a basic unit (see Fig. 16.10) takes the place of a conventional radiographic table. The basic unit is constructed of two pillars which stand—on a floor-inlaid base—about 115 cm (40 inches) apart and are approximately 80 cm (30 inches) in height. The pillars support a carriage

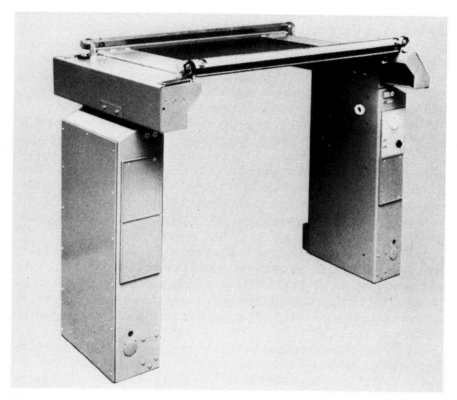

Fig. 16.10 The basic unit with which the trolley of Fig. 16.9 is associated. *By courtesy of Siemens-Elema AB.*

which is able to accept the table top (that is, the trolley's top) and allow it to 'float' in two directions. The crossways excursion permitted by the carriage is 15 cm (6 inches) to either side of the midline; the lengthwise movement is about 100 cm (40 inches), although this measurement is influenced by the length of the table top, of which more than one variety can be supplied for different purposes.

On the pillars of the basic table, four blind panels are to be noticed: these can be exchanged for connection panels for auxiliary equipment—such as a rapid film changer—when a more sophisticated version of the table is to be used. As our present concern is with initial accident and emergency radiography, it is upon this table that we shall now concentrate.

The basic unit for accident and emergency examinations includes a permanently mounted bucky, having the usual features which permit a cassette to be loaded in a tray and locked in a position central to the bucky top. In radiographic practice, a ceiling-suspended X-ray tubehead includes a cross-brake which automatically locates the central X-ray beam to the bucky grid, in the transverse line. Once the radiographer has performed the preliminary centering manoeuvres and the table top—with its load—is in position beneath the X-ray beam, the patient can be 'floated' to orientate with the central beam, through the means of the moving table top and the use of a footswitch to release and apply the table brakes, as required. This of course is an easy manoeuvre for both people involved.

On the patient's arrival in the X-ray room, it is necessary to transfer the trolley top from the wheeled base to the bucky unit, the patient meanwhile remaining recumbent where he is. The design of the base frame is such as to allow the trolley top to surmount the bucky unit, assuming that the height of the trolley has been adjusted for the purpose by means of the hydraulic system. A magnetic aligning guide at the back of the table carriage (that is, on the side of the table opposite the radiographer's working station) assists correct positioning of the top.

When the table top is above and in proper alignment with the bucky unit, it can be lowered, by operation of the appropriate foot pedals, until it beds on the carriage and engages with two heavy side rails; the top is now locked to the carriage and will float with it. The trolley base frame may be taken away and the radiographer has unencumbered access to the patient on the table.

At the end of the examination, it is necessary to reverse the manoeuvres just described. When the trolley base frame is repositioned at the table, the top can be locked to the cantilevers. If these are then raised by the hydraulic system, the resultant upwards thrust tilts the carriage rails inwards and releases the top; the trolley is once more a secure independent unit on which the patient may be moved from the examination room to his next destination.

To use the basic bucky unit to examine other than stretcher cases, between times as a conventional X-ray table, requires the provision of a spare table/trolley top. This can remain on the basic unit until the arrival of a stretchered patient. A set of special brackets is available which can be mounted on the wall of an X-ray room, about 70 cm (28 inches) from the floor and on which the spare table top may be parked as required. To move it, however, two people are needed, one person lifting from either end. (The table top's weight is about 40 kilograms.)

The next system to be described, which we shall denote as system B, does not possess the same range of applications as A; but it is simpler to operate and has concentrated on the needs of a radiographer working virtually alone in an emergency situation, as may be often the case.

To operate either system effectively, the hospital receiving accident cases needs more than one trolley, obviously. The number required depends upon estimated work loads and available funds. It is to be remarked that the choice of a particular system must be influenced by its acceptability to medical, nursing and portering as well as radiodiagnostic staff. However popular a system may be in the X-ray room, if it is not liked elsewhere in the accident department the appropriate trolleys will not be used.

The system using trolleys with a fixed top (B)

The accident and emergency system which uses a trolley having a fixed top is less elaborate than system A; it is particularly orientated to a radiographer working apart from readily available assistance; and it is independent of an X-ray table.

The crucial feature of B's trolley is that it includes a slot, which runs the length and breadth of the trolley and is about 50 mm wide: this slot accepts a tray which may contain a cassette (Fig. 16.11a).

Apart from the trolley, the other essential components of system B are (1) a mobile cassette carrier and (2) an optical light-beam positioning unit which is fitted to the light beam diaphragm of a ceiling supported X-ray tube for preference, although the tube of a high-output mobile generator could be used.

The mobile cassette carrier is seen in Fig. 16.11 (b) and (c). It is an ingenious cabinet on wheels which combines several purposes. These are explained below.

1   The base of the cabinet is lead-protected and is designed for the temporary storage of several exposed and unexposed cassettes.

2   On the top of the cabinet, a cassette holder is supported on slides and incorporates a secondary radiation grid having a ratio 8:1 and 40 lines/cm (85 lines/inch).

3   The cabinet top can dispense a cassette, in its holder, to the cassette-tray slot of the trolley; or alternatively the top of the cabinet may be raised, like the hinged lid of a box, to a vertical position and thus support the contained cassette upright, alongside the trolley, for radiography with a horizontal X-ray beam.

The dispensing process is easily performed. The radiographer begins this by wheeling the cabinet to the side of the braked trolley and then slides the cassette holder from the cabinet to enter its shelf (slot) on the trolley, their two levels being matched in height from the floor. The cabinet can be wheeled to one side, to any convenient parking site in the room, and the trolley effectively has become a simple radiographic table. The cassette holder accomodates a 35 cm × 43 cm cassette, either way round, and an adaptor is available which allows smaller cassettes to be used.

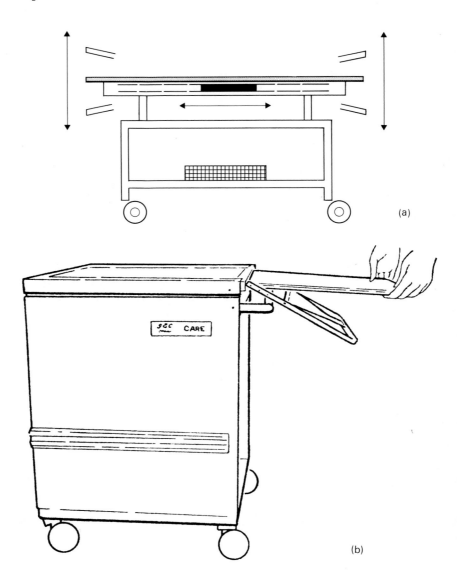

(a)

(b)

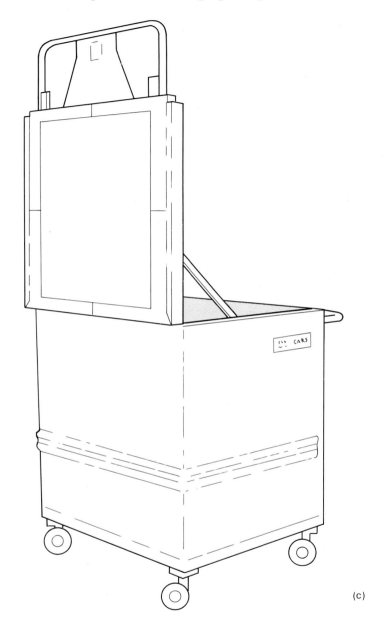

(c)

Fig. 16.11 (a) A trolley for accident and emergency radiography which features a slot for the acceptance of a cassette tray as used in system B. (b), (c) a mobile cassette carrier which is associated with the trolley sketched in (a).

(b) and (c) are reproduced by courtesy of Picker International Ltd.

We may note at this point that the carrier/cabinet has latches which ensure ease and safety in its operation. These are:

1 two thumb latches on either side of the handle of the cassette tray, to allow the tray to be pulled to an open-drawer position so that a cassette may be inserted;

2 a bar-activated latch beneath the cassette tray which releases the tray for its slide towards the trolley and can be operated only when the carrier top is horizontal;

3 a latch which prevents the top of the carrier from being raised to a vertical position, unless the cassette holder is drawn fully within its slides and thus held by the previous latch. The interlocking of (2) and (3) above is to preserve the cassette holder from an injurious descent to the floor if the equipment were to be carelessly or ignorantly operated.

The light beam positioning unit is brought into use when the trolley has received the cassette tray and a cassette is in the tray, positioned for the required examination. As it is connected in parallel with the light source of the beam delineator, the beam positioning unit does not require separate switch control. It projects twin beams of light to a target point near the handle of the cassette holder. With adjustments of the position of the ceiling supported X-ray tube, these lights superimpose in the form of a cross on the target area when:

1 the central X-ray beam is currently meeting the centre of the cassette and the overlying secondary radiation grid;

2 the focus of the X-ray tube is at the correct distance from the film, that is when the anode-film distance equals the radius of the grid (100 cm or 40 inches).

On completion of the X-ray procedure, the cassette holder may be returned to the cassette carrier, if the carrier is wheeled again to the side of the braked trolley. The carrier remains as before in the radiodiagnostic room and the patient continues his travels on the trolley.

What has been described are the essential components of system B for accident and emergency radiography. Additional fitments for the trolley are available, which include the items given below.

1 A slotted mattress. This has cut-outs in a number of places (for instance there is a long slot between the legs of a recumbent patient) which give support to a cassette placed vertically for radiography with a horizontal beam.

2 A cassette holder styled like a small backrest. This fits in slots in the mattress and can be used to support a gridded cassette directly beneath a patient's head. It may be angled up to 30 deg above the horizontal.

3 A triple jointed device which can be fitted to the side rail of the trolley. It will grasp a cassette and maintain it in positions suitable for a

lateral projection of the femoral neck and infero-superior views of the shoulder.

Equipment for cranial and skeletal radiography

In Chapter 15 a table has been described which is purpose built for the performance of cranial radiography to a high degree of accuracy. In principle, there is no reason not to employ this table for cranial surveys in accident and emergency situations. The table can be operated in conjunction with its own couch (to which it would be necessary to move the patient) or one of the patient-transfer systems already described (p. 542). However, the dedication of these skull tables to the precise execution of complex cranial projections must reduce the equipment's relevance to a wider radiographic scope. Radiographers working in the accident and emergency rooms of a busy general radiodiagnostic department will find more useful some equipment which has a wider range of purposes and has been planned in relation to both cranial and skeletal X-ray examinations. This type of system is now to be described.

A unit for cranio-skeletal radiography may be generally described as tube-linked. This means that the X-ray tube and a cassette-holder (which might be a bucky but often is not) are linked together by the placement of each at either end of a vertical straight arm. This arm is mounted on a support, upon which it can rotate in the vertical plane, in the fashion of a centre sweep second hand moving over the face of a wall clock (see Fig. 16.12).

The link-arm's support may be floor mounted or may be suspended from the ceiling, as in Fig. 16.12. In this case, rotation (360 deg) about the point of ceiling attachment gives, to the X-ray tube and its linked cassette, movement which is spherical about a fixed centre. On this fixed centre the central X-ray beam is continuously directed (see Fig. 16.13).

The vertical arm, which is constructed telescopically, can be motored upwards and downwards in a total excursion of about 600 mm (24 inches). The cassette carrier independently may be moved upwards and downwards, over a distance of about 350 mm (14 inches), in order to obtain different anode-film distances and different degrees of magnification. All these movements are recorded on appropriately placed scales and thus may be visually controlled.

Tube-linked equipment of the kind just described effectively brings the mountain to Mahomet: it allows radiographic positionings for various examinations of the skeletal system to be achieved through manipulations of the X-ray tube and the film, relative to a recumbent or seated patient, who is not required himself to adapt his position to the equipment. The unit

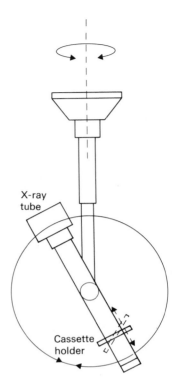

X-ray
tube

Cassette
holder

Fig. 16.12   Essential construction of a tube-linked
unit for cranio-skeletal radiography.

associates particularly well with a narrow, skull positioning board which can
be fitted to the patient-transfer table tops described on p. 544; but, with a
patient brought to the tube-linked unit and his head supported on any
radioparent surface which is free of obstruction, all cranial and facial X-ray
examinations can be performed whilst he remains in a supine position. Many
other skeletal projections are similarly facilitated; and the horizontal-beam
view, which is so often a significant radiograph in the accident and
emergency department, should be readily and accurately obtained.

EQUIPMENT FOR MAMMOGRAPHY

In order to produce satisfactory mammograms it is necessary to meet the
stringent requirements of a successful technique. The difficulties present
can be seen on considering the following facts about radiographic
examinations of the breast.

1   The part concerned is soft tissue.

2   The tissues of normal structures in the breast and of lesions in the breast
are very nearly the same in the extent to which they absorb X rays; that is,
they have nearly the same degree of radiolucency.

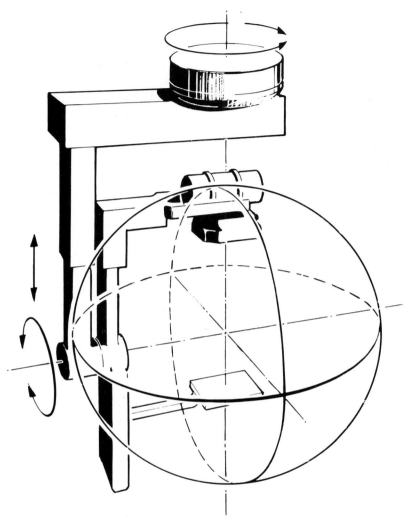

Fig. 16.13 The spherical movement of the X-ray tube and the linked cassette in a tube-linked equipment for skeletal radiography. *By courtesy of Siemens-Elema AB.*

3 Because of this, an X-ray beam of soft radiation is required and hence a low kilovoltage must be used. High kilovoltages and penetrating beams diminish differences in radiolucency between the parts of any subject. In a subject where differences are small anyway nothing must be done to diminish them.

4 The method used to record the image must be capable of resolving fine detail. That is, it must be able to record very small structures (eg

calcifications of pin-head size) so that they are visible. This need for high resolution means that the film emulsions must be relatively small in grain size and they should be used without intensifying screens or with those of high resolution. Such film materials so used are inevitably a slow imaging system.

5   The necessary low kilovoltages result in beams of low intensity. This low intensity combined with a dismayingly slow imaging system make it necessary to use a high milliampereseconds value in the exposure technique in order to obtain satisfactory density in the image.

6   High milliampereseconds are achieved by the use of relatively long exposure times (in some cases as long as up to 10 seconds).

7   There is considerable risk of movement during these long exposure intervals so careful immobilization is needed.

8   Compression of the breast reduces the thickness of tissue. This compression helps to diminish the problem of being forced to combine a low-intensity beam with a slow imaging system. Compression also aids immobilization. It is not within the scope of this book to consider fully how all the difficulties are overcome for we cannot here explore avenues leading to imaging systems and radiographic positioning techniques. It is, however, appropriate for us to describe equipment used for mammography and our readers will see how this equipment is designed to solve at least some of the problems implicit in radiographic examinations of the breast.

There are two lines of approach towards obtaining suitable equipment:

1   to modify conventional X-ray equipment so that it may be used successfully to do mammography as well as other radiography;

2   to use a unit specifically designed for mammography.

Features of an X-ray unit making it suitable for mammography tend to make it unsuited to all other examinations. Because of this, a special mammographic unit cannot be used to do general radiography. So an X-ray department embarking on the cost in terms of space and money for such a highly specialized unit should be planning to undertake many mammograms.

MAMMOGRAPHY WITH GENERAL EQUIPMENT

The X-ray tube unit

In Chapter 7 we described features of X-ray tubes to be used for mammography. Such tubes are not suitable for general radiography. So, if a general X-ray unit is to be modified so that mammography in addition to other examinations may be done, a conventional X-ray tube insert must be used. There are, however, certain changes which can be made to the tube unit as a whole. The aim of such changes is to maintain in the X-ray beam as it leaves the tube much radiation of long wavelength. The beam will then diminish less the small differences in radiolucency between the several tissues of the breast.

When an X-ray beam passes through filtering material the effect is to remove from the beam the components of longer wavelength. The beam is then effectively more penetrating than one which is generated at the same kilovoltage but is totally unfiltered. In order to make a conventional tube unit more suitable for mammography, filtering material is removed from the path of the beam so that the longer wavelengths may be retained in its composition. The modifications required for such a tube are therefore that it must be possible to remove (a) the additional aluminium filter which is a feature of conventional tube units, (b) the light-beam diaphragm.

The X-ray beam then leaves the tube without passing through any filtering material other than the inherent filtration made up by the glass of the tube insert, the oil in the shield and the portal of the housing; the impossibility of eliminating these in a conventional tube will be understood!

When the filter has been removed for mammography there is a risk that its absence will be overlooked when the unit is next used for some other examination. In order to circumvent the human element in failure to restore the filter, modifications to the unit may include providing an interlock which renders it impossible to make an exposure without the filter if the technique is not a mammographic one. The interlock system may operate a warning signal such as a light when the filtration is inappropriate to the examination for which the controls are set; inappropriate filtration would be the absence of the additional filter for general radiography and the presence of the additional filter in a mammographic technique.

The light-beam diaphragm is replaced for mammography by a long cone which is used to limit the field size just to cover the area of diagnostic interest; this is the full extent of the breast from the nipple to the deep surface attached to the anterior chest wall. This long cone may or may not be used to serve as a compressor for the breast.

The support for the patient and the film

In the absence of a specialized mammographic unit, various supports for the patient and the film have been used. A conventional X-ray table can be made to serve. A universal bucky is more versatile and easier to use with satisfaction. Variable height is required in the table which supports the film and in the seat which supports the patient so that when the patient sits beside the table her breast can be placed in contact with the film whatever her height. Another helpful feature is to have a semi-circular cut-out in the edge of the table against which the anterior chest wall is applied, thus adapting the profile of the table to anatomical contours. This makes it easier to record on the film the full extent of the breast.

The generator

The generator has to be considered in relation to two questions as follows.
1   What kilovoltages can it provide in the lower part of its range?
2   Has its voltage the pulsating waveform of a 2-pulse generator or the continuous rippling waveform provided by 6-pulse and 12-pulse generators or the continuous form of truly constant potential?

In regard to the available kilovoltages it will be understood that an important requirement for successful mammography is the use of low values of kilovoltage. So the modification required for a conventional generator is that it should be able to provide a selection of kilovoltages in the range 20 kV to 40 kV.

As to the waveform, that must be a feature that is established for any given generator, inherent in its operation and to be altered only by choosing a different type of generator. However, let us at least consider which of the voltage waveforms—the pulsating or the rippling and continuous—might be seen as the better choice for mammographic examinations.

The ideal quality of radiation applied to mammography is that of homogeneity: that is, the photons in the beam all have the same energy. This ideal energy is such that photoelectric absorption is a predominant effect in the tissues of the breast and radiation contrasts between the different structures are as great as possible. In practice it is impossible to achieve a truly homogeneous beam with the equipment we use in diagnostic X-ray departments. What we must ask about the various voltage waveforms mentioned here is which of them is most likely to provide an X-ray beam with a range of photon energies which is a closer approach to homogeneity? The answer must be that the rippling and the continuous constant potential waveforms are a better choice than the pulsating one. Generators with a rippling or a constant potential waveform provide for the X-ray tube a voltage which does not fall much below its value at the peak of the ripple or does not change at all throughout the cycle of mains alternation.

The resultant X-ray beam therefore has a range of photon energies from which are absent those photons of low energy which are produced by the low voltages in a pulsating cycle of change. In 2-pulse generators the tube voltage goes down to zero three times in one cycle and as a result the X-ray beam must have in it a number of photons with energies determined by low kilovoltages in the cycle of change. This beam must be of greater heterogeneity (and so further from homogeneity) than is the other. Most manufacturers recommend for mammography a generator which is 6 pulse or 12 pulse or of constant potential and do not recommend 2-pulse generators for this application.

SPECIALIZED MAMMOGRAPHIC EQUIPMENT

Specialized mammographic equipment may be considered in two categories. These are:

1 mammographic stands;
2 complete mammographic units.

These two categories are considered separately in more detail later on (pages 559–561). At present we are concerning ourselves with the sort of X-ray tube to be used in this equipment. The mammographic stands and the complete mammographic units have in common that their X-ray tubes are specifically designed for mammography.

The X-ray tube (insert and tube unit)

Features of an X-ray tube designed for mammography have already been mentioned in Chapter 7. We list them again below.

1 There is closer electrode spacing. This allows the tube to be used with lower filament heat for a given milliamperage.
2 The anode is made of molybdenum. This results in an X-ray beam which has in it a narrow band of long wavelengths which are intense.
3 The window of the X-ray tube through which the beam emerges is made of thinned glass or of beryllium. The thinned glass or the beryllium has less filtering effect than the thickness of borosilicate glass which is used for the rest of the tube envelope and for the windows and envelopes of conventional X-ray tubes. Thus the inherent filtration of the mammographic tube is reduced.
4 The tube has a molybdenum filter. This filter, by its selective absorption, removes from the beam certain wavelengths which are not the ones intended to be used for mammography.

One of the effects of the lower filament temperatures referred to above is that there is less deposition of evaporated tungsten on the tube wall, so the inherent filtration may be further reduced by the absence of this thin metallic layer. In other radiographic examinations the radiation used is sufficiently penetrating for this deposited tungsten to make little difference to the X-ray beam; but in a tube to be used for mammography (when it is so important not to remove long wavelengths from the beam) the elimination of even a thin layer of tungsten may be significant.

Focal spot sizes in mammographic tubes may vary from 0·6 mm to 1·0 mm and in some cases a 2·0 mm focus may be used. The broader focus increases penumbra in the image but to offset this it helps to reduce the risk of movement unsharpness because the higher milliamperes rating of the broad focus allows shorter periods of exposure to be used.

The tube unit is fitted with a long cone which is D shaped; that is, the cone is contoured so that it is better adapted to the necessary close positioning of the tube unit against the patient. For example, when the craniocaudad projection is done, the flat side of the cone is towards the anterior chest wall and the face.

Fig. 16.14 shows a sketch of the tube insert from a mammographic unit. It can be seen that this rotating anode tube has the features mentioned

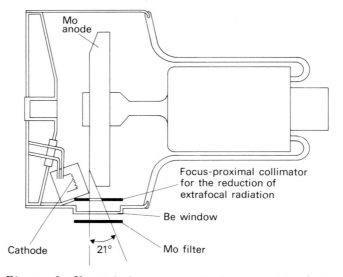

Fig. 16.14 Diagram of an X-ray tube for mammography. *By courtesy of Siemens-Elema AB.*

earlier: close electrode spacing, a molybdenum anode, a beryllium window and a molybdenum filter. Within the glass window there is a collimator close to the focus of the X-ray tube which is intended to cut off radiation arising from parts of the anode other than the focus.

One of the difficulties to be encountered in mammography is that of recording in the radiograph those parts of the breast which are closest to the chest wall. A beam of radiation which can be made tangential to the chest wall is a means to achieving this record. In the equipment of which the X-ray tube in Fig. 16.14 is a part, the patient when positioned as shown in Fig. 16.15 has the flat cathode end of the X-ray tube towards her face. This places

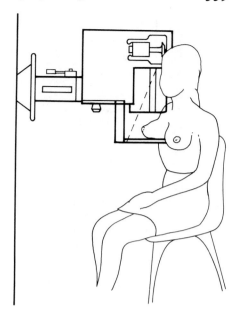

Fig. 16.15 Diagram to show the beam of radiation from a mammographic unit emerging with one edge tangential to the chest wall. *By courtesy of Siemens-Elema AB.*

in one line the focal spot of the tube, one side of the compression cone and one side of the film. The beam of radiation then has one edge tangential to the chest wall.

Mammographic stands

The mammographic stand has its special X-ray tube mounted on a tube carriage. This tube carriage holds the X-ray tube rigidly coupled and aligned to a little table which serves as a holder for the film and support for the breast under examination. Some stands have mounted above the table a radiolucent compressing plate which can be lowered to compress the breast between the table and the plate. In other stands there is no breast compressor as such and compression is achieved by the use of a long beam-limiting cone on the tube unit, the cone having a radiolucent plastic cover over its wide lower aperture. The tube unit and the cone are brought down so that the cone compresses the breast against the film. The carriage which holds the tube unit and the film-holder/breast-support is mounted on a cross-arm, which itself is carried on a tubestand. This may be a heavy steel vertical column which moves on a floor track such as is described on page 286 of this book. An example of a mammographic stand is illustrated in Fig. 16.16.

Mammographic stands are designed to be flexible in operation and easily manœuvrable so that patients may be examined standing, seated or lying down and the required projections can be conveniently and reproducibly obtained. The movements of the tube unit and the film-holder/breast-

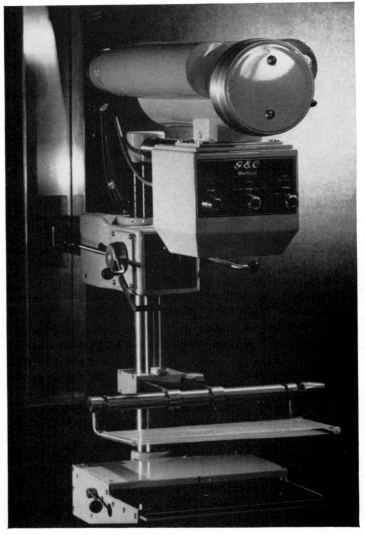

Fig. 16.16 A mammographic stand. The X-ray tube can be seen mounted on its carriage above the film-holder. Between the film-holder and the X-ray tube above is a device for compressing the breast against the film-holder. *By courtesy of Picker International Ltd.*

support are controlled by electromagnetic brakes which hold them firmly when applied.

The generator

These mammographic stands are intended to be used with their X-ray tubes connected to an ordinary high-tension generator which has within its range kilovoltages which are low enough for mammography. The generator might be already supplying other X-ray tubes in the department, the mammographic tube being connected to an unused tube outlet from the generator. Or the mammographic stand might be installed in an X-ray room with its own separate generator as a self-contained unit in an X-ray room.

Complete mammographic units

A complete mammographic unit is a self-contained piece of equipment designed for mammography and for no other procedure. Such units are often made mobile so that they can be wheeled into position for use. Mobility makes them capable of being used to examine a patient lying down on an

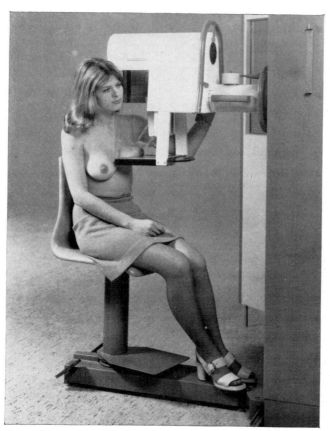

Fig. 16.17   A complete mammographic unit showing the breast support, the breast compressor, the X-ray tube unit and the seat for the patient. *By courtesy of Siemens-Elema AB.*

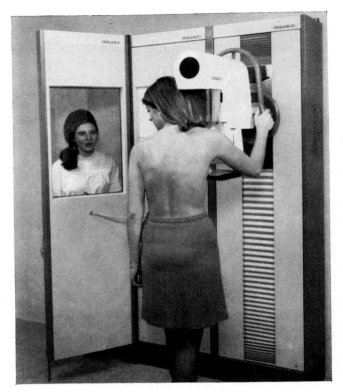

Fig. 16.18   The same unit as in Fig. 16.17 is seen here with the patient positioned erect. The protective screen for the radiographer is shown. *By courtesy of Siemens-Elema AB.*

ordinary X-ray table. However, a mammographic unit is not bound to be like this and may be a fixed installation. The equipment comprises the following features:

1   a breast-support/film-holder which may be designed so that a special cassette for xeroradiography may be put into the film holder as alternative to a conventional cassette or film pack;

2   a breast compressor either as a separate compression plate or integral in the beam-limiting cone by virtue of a radiolucent plate covering its open end;

3   some breast cones;

4   a special X-ray tube;

5   a tube support by means of which the tube unit is rigidly coupled and aligned to the breast-support/film-holder;

6   a full range of movements for the tube assembly and the breast-support/film-holder so that the required projections may be conveniently obtained

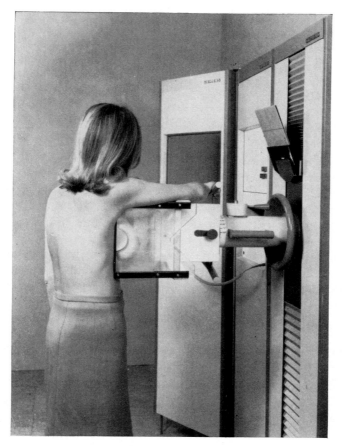

Fig. 16.19 The same unit as in Figs. 16.17 and 16.18 is shown here with the patient erect and the beam directed horizontally. The control panel can be seen to the viewer's right of the lead glass window in the protective screen. *By courtesy of Siemens-Elema AB.*

and the patient may be examined easily seated or lying down;

7 a special high-tension generator for the unit which will provide a range of low kilovoltages (for example, 20 to 40 kVp);

8 an automatic timer to control the exposure.

A mammographic unit is seen in Figs. 16.17, 16.18 and 16.19. It is a complete unit with a three-phase high tension generator and the X-ray tube which is illustrated in Fig. 16.14. A radiographic stand, a seat for the patient, a control panel and a protective screen for the radiographer are all parts of the one complete unit. The timer is an automatic one controlled through an ionization chamber (half-moon shaped) which is behind the film. Details of the patient's identity are recorded on the film by the radiographic exposure.

Chapter 17
Care, Maintenance and Tests

In any hospital the X-ray department is one of the most expensive to equip and maintain. The purchase of major apparatus involves very large expenditures and of this probably most student radiographers are at least vaguely aware. We may, however, be less conscious of the relatively high costs of what seem to us simple articles—cones, centre-finders, ratchets for compression bands—and in our frequent use of them may give to these much less respect than is accorded to more obviously intricate and precious equipment. Yet, indeed there is very little in any radiological department which is not surprisingly expensive. We have a responsibility for the careful treatment of *all* apparatus.

When equipment is used frequently by a large number of people who do not own it, it is necessarily subjected to more than its fair share of wear and tear. Any radiographer who has not a natural respect for expensive and generally well-designed machinery should endeavour to cultivate the trait; for to work long in an X-ray department, especially a busy one, without such a habit of mind, is sometimes to lay a trail of disaster equivalent to the activity of a purposeful saboteur.

In this chapter will be considered certain simple principles of general mechanical care and maintenance, of which faithful observation by everyone can greatly help the department's work. In the second part of the chapter tests will be described which permit a radiographer to know whether apparatus is working correctly or is faulty in a given respect. Some of these may be practised by the student radiographer as helpful experiments during training.

GENERAL CARE

Cleanliness

The cleanliness of apparatus is highly significant to departmental hygiene and this aspect has received emphasis in other contexts. However, it may be important as well to the functioning of the equipment concerned.

If the X-ray tube is not ceiling mounted, a common cause of trouble is accumulated dust and grit particles in the floor-track of the tubestand. These are not readily removed by the procedures usually applied to sweeping or cleaning the floor. They can build up insidiously to a level at which it becomes difficult to move the tube column when the radiographer is standing in the customary position at the other side of the X-ray table—a point which affords poor leverage at best. Fatigue is much increased by the recurrent necessity to walk round the table in order to push the X-ray tube by means of its vertical column and the situation is potentially dangerous, since the tube stand may jump the track if thrust past an obstruction; under a mechanical drive the tube may fail to move at all at the required time, for example during tomography.

A little attention regularly given to floor-tracks is well worth while. It is a simple enough matter, though it may require patience and the readiness to proceed along the track on all fours using a screwdriver or equivalent tool as a probe and removing the larger accumulations of fluff and similar debris. A stiff narrow brush is perhaps the most practical instrument for cleaning away fine grit, although a vacuum cleaner—if available—is obviously better. A few drops of machine oil on the runners of the tube-stand provide helpful lubrication which is of first importance to smooth movement of the apparatus.

Liquids are a potential hazard to X-ray equipment. Tables and film changers do not ordinarily have water-tight covers and liquids used in their vicinity should be handled carefully. A spill can readily provide a short circuit between two electrically live points.

The writers have seen a rapid film changer made inoperative on the occasion of its next use, because a saline infusion set up during arteriography was allowed to drip through a faulty connection alongside the unit. Little importance was attached to this at the time by the 'scrubbed' radiographer assisting at the procedure. Only after the subsequent breakdown of the equipment was the trouble traced to an extensive deposit of dried salt on moving parts of the changer. These had to be renewed at some expense.

While radiographers may fairly be expected to act carefully in X-ray rooms, patients are less likely to be able to do so. In the course of a barium session it is not unknown for drinks to be spilled and enemas to go out of control. The radiographer should 'mop up' at once if possible and in any case, at the end of the list, should go throroughly over the equipment to make sure that the table and its accessories are clean. Once barium sulphate has dried and hardened, its removal becomes a disproportionately difficult matter.

If the gastrointestinal table is unfortunately often to be identified by its crusts of barium, the unit in the IVU room may display characteristic barnacles of its own. These occur from the practice of ensuring that air is not present in a syringe by holding it in a vertical position with the needle upwards and pushing the plunger until the contents appear at the needle tip. This can result in a jet of contrast agent falling anywhere in the vicinity of the operator. The walls of the room are outside the scope of the present discussion but the X-ray table is at even greater risk, and unless a regular cleansing drill is followed it will almost certainly show unattractive signs of its association with urography before very long.

In a busy department it may often seem difficult to give time to the small domestic rituals; in an over-crowded, badly planned one, there may be little pride in their performance. Their real importance to the apparatus—as well as to patients—is sometimes overlooked.

Daily damp dusting of each X-ray room and its equipment is a minimum requirement and whenever possible a regular session should be allotted for more thorough cleaning with polishes and methylated spirit. During this, any obviously loose screws or bolts can be tightened: it is wise to have the unit switched off when this is done. Those discovered to be missing, and likewise homeless screws, should be reported to the superintendent radiographer, together with any other minor faults, such as broken meter glasses, cracked plastic components, or worn cable coverings.

In these performances the needs of portable and mobile units are sometimes forgotten. Ideally, all such equipment should be brought back every night to a parking bay in the main X-ray department or to some other recognized site. Here, there should be arrangements to keep it protected from dust—for example, the provision of a large polythene cover. Apparatus regularly within sight in the department is not so likely to be neglected.

Log book

The keeping of a log book or case record for each X-ray unit is an important part of satisfactory maintenance. In such a book, faults should be recorded by the radiographer as they occur and are reported to the superintendent radiographer; subsequently the visiting engineer should include a brief report of what he has found and the action taken.

Such a record has several advantages.

1 Apart from being a useful catalogue of emergency failures, it ensures that minor faults and suggestive 'symptoms' are brought to the attention of an engineer when the next routine service is due. (For example: 'Note cracked glass in kilovolt meter'; or 'Overtable tube rotor is noisy'.)

2 It provides firm evidence that a particular fault has received attention and makes obvious the painful history of any for which repeated visits by an engineer have been necessary over a period of time. Such a record may be very helpful during any subsequent enquiry.

3 Like a patient's case-record, it provides information about an X-ray unit to someone (a new superintendent radiographer perhaps, or a relief engineer from another area) who has not seen this particular 'patient' before. This will be especially important if there is some unusual feature of the equipment. For example, an engineer may solve a difficulty at some time by means of an alteration to the circuitry. If he remains the only source of information that this change has been made, there may be needless problems and loss of time ahead for anyone else who has to attend to the equipment.

Practical precautions

It is an odd fact that in using X-ray equipment many radiographers have a few bad habits in common. As a single episode perhaps none matters very much but a minor mistreatment of some piece of apparatus, if it is sufficiently often repeated, can lead to eventual breakdown, with implications not only of expense but of disrupted work and lost time for patients awaiting examination.

Brakes and locks

One character to be recognized in our rogues' gallery is a strange tendency to try to move equipment against a brake which is firm. Bucky trays are manœuvred in this way and even more often is the X-ray tube raised or lowered on the vertical column, rotated or pushed along the floor. Locks of the electromagnetic variety are usually able to resist such assaults but a friction-type lock is never intended to be super tight and its opposition can be overcome with moderate impulsion; female radiographers may deny that they can be strong enough to do this but they commonly are! Eventually a situation is reached in which the brake does not hold at all and will have to be repaired.

Properly used, a friction-type lock should not be over-tightened but turned just enough to keep the equipment under control in its desired place. A half-turn is then sufficient to release it, and this simple action should not be beyond anyone. The habit of avoiding loosening a brake perhaps arises from a compulsion among busy radiographers to save time.

High tension cables

High tension cables are often unwittingly victimized in X-ray departments. On many mobile units the horizontal tube-arm can be rotated 360 degrees round the vertical support. However, to go twice in the same direction is not to the benefit of the cables, which inevitably become wound round the tube column. A similar mechanism of ill-treatment can occur when any X-ray tube on either a mobile or a static unit is tilted from the position of a vertical beam to that of a horizontal one. Anyone altering the aim of the tube in one of these ways should take time to study the lie of the cables before actually rotating the tube. It has been known for an engineer to have to dismantle an X-ray tube from its supports in order to disentangle a pair of HT cables which owed their condition to nothing more unusual than 'ordinary' ward radiography.

When high tension cables become progressively 'wound up' two things at least happen: (a) the mobility of the tube becomes increasingly restricted; (b) sooner or later the cables will fracture. Because of the possibility of fracture, a high tension cable should not be acutely curved. If undue stress is not to occur a diameter of curvature of 30 cm (12 inches) is the minimum.

There *is* undue stress if electrical equipment is pulled towards the operator by its cable: a common sufferer from such treatment is the fluoroscopic footswitch. It is a careless practice to which no one should resort, no matter what is the electrical apparatus or the category of cable concerned. Points of electrical connection are intended for that, and not to withstand hauling strains of whatever degree.

Meters and controls

The functions of meters and controls are sometimes confusedly put together in the student's mind. Candidates in examinations who are asked to state the controls present on an X-ray unit often include meters in the list. However, a meter is *not* a control: it cannot effect any alteration in a situation. A meter is merely an indicator: it makes a statement about certain existing conditions but it cannot be used to change them in any way.

Meters usually receive from radiographers less attention than they deserve. Most neglected are the milliampere and milliampereseconds meters which tell the radiographer both that the exposure has occurred and furthermore that it has occurred normally. Yet often, when a film is found after processing to be seriously under-exposed or even totally blank, a question about the behaviour of the milliampere meter fails to have any satisfactory answer. Radiographers are wont to say that they were watching the patient during the exposure (it is seldom necessary to do this *all* the time), or that the exposure was too small to be read (yet manufacturers take care to provide meters with shunts for this specific purpose of allowing radiographers to know accurately the value of the current obtained).

A radiographer who discovers operational faults in an X-ray unit only when the radiograph involved has been processed is—in most cases—not using the unit at all thoughtfully. In some circumstances, it is true, a radiographer may have to expose films while actually at a distance from the control stand and consequently does not have the meters within sight. This should always be a matter of slight uneasiness, since to operate the unit in this way is to be deprived of any real knowledge that the exposure in fact has been successfully made. Students should develop the habit of looking at meters and noticing what they record. It is never useless information.

Generally speaking, no control on an X-ray set should be moved during the course of an exposure. An exception to this principle is the 'stepless' Variac control available for the alteration of kilovoltage actually during fluoroscopy. In this case the current involved is very much smaller than it would be for any radiographic exposure.

Tubestands and tracks

In their installations the manufacturers of X-ray equipment are always concerned to provide easy movement of the X-ray tube, whether this is ceiling-mounted or runs on a floor-track. In moving the tube any distance it is important not to allow it to gallop along and hit the end-stops of the track at full speed. This can be harmful in two ways. The tube column may 'jump' the rails. There is also the possibility of fracturing a filament in the insert, particularly if this is hot, or even of shattering the insert.

Much the same risks of filament or insert damage are present if a tube is thrown up the vertical column unnecessarily briskly and comes to an enforced halt at the top. Furthermore, it is usual to fit a 'fail safe' mechanism to such tubestands which operates to prevent the tube falling, should the suspension cable snap (see Chapter 7). A tube travelling smartly upwards simulates the conditions of failure at the cable-end and it is quite probable that the 'fail safe' lock may come 'on'. The tube will then be immovable until such time as it can have an engineer's attention.

When a mobile unit is to travel about the hospital it is the responsibility of the radiographer who last used it to ensure that all the locks on the tube-column remain firm. Those who may be required to move mobile and portable X-ray equipment are not obliged to have any knowledge of its operation and a tube which is capable of sliding or swinging upon its supports as the unit is pushed along is a danger both to anyone in its vicinity and to itself. Its weight will give it considerable impetus and if it strikes, say, a wall or door with sufficient force it is possible for the insert to be thrown out of place in its shield, the glass fractured or—most probably—the stressed glass/metal seal at the anode broken.

Mobile units which have electrically controlled tube-brakes require particular attention. When such a unit is disconnected from a source of electric power the brakes become inoperative, together with the other components, and are—for practical purposes—'off'. Units of this kind invariably are fitted with secondary mechanical locks and any radiographer using the equipment should know their function, where they are and how to operate them.

On completion of any bedside or similar examination there should be a firm drill to ensure that the radiographer leaves the unit tidy, its cable neatly coiled, the tube in a normal position on the column—for example, above the control desk so that its weight is neatly distributed—and all brakes tight. It may then—and only then—be considered fit to travel.

Accessory equipment

Things which have to be often carried from one place to another are sometimes dropped. In the X-ray department, cones, secondary radiation grids and cassettes are all potential sufferers. They are expensive items and care should be taken of them.

If accessory equipment of this kind is found to be damaged in any way its condition should be reported at once. To continue to use it is to invite worse trouble in most cases. For example, a cassette which is only slightly distorted or of which a fastening is loose may become jammed in the serial changer of a fluoroscopic table, resulting in the immobilization of the cassette—usually in some inaccessible position behind the screen.

It is a mistake to enter into a battle of wills with apparatus which is not behaving satisfactorily. No piece of equipment should ever be subjected to force. You may believe that your opponent has submitted but you will undoubtedly lose the contest in the end. For example, a localizing cone, of which the attachment plate had been only slightly distorted as the result of a fall, was once rammed into place by a radiographer anxious to use it. All was well until the X-ray tube was moved from the horizontal to the vertical position, at which time the cone immediately fell off, scoring a near miss on the head of the patient prone on the table.

In a busy department secondary-radiation grids lead difficult lives. A grid survives best when it is enclosed in a cassette and the combination employed as a single entity. This is bound to be more expensive initially : the number of grids required in a given department will inevitably be greater in order to avoid delay between several radiographic exposures. However, there is no doubt that the policy is worthwhile in the much longer grid-life obtained.

A grid which does not have the protection of enclosure in a cassette or other casing is readily damaged during both use and storage, unless care is taken. No secondary radiation grid should ever be employed with a cassette of lesser dimensions than itself. A grid placed between a heavy patient and a small cassette is subject to undue strain along its unsupported margins and sooner or later will crack. Even when it is not actually working, a grid can be damaged while lying on a shelf or trolley in the X-ray room, if heavy objects—such as cones, lead gloves and cassettes—are put down on top of it. The safest place to keep a grid is probably in some form of wall mounting; the radiographer using it is responsible for its return to port on each occasion.

Grids are inherently delicate and complex in structure despite their simplicity of appearance. Anyone carrying one about the hospital to use with mobile equipment should take care not to allow it to fall or become bent or knocked by other articles. We have probably all of us seen grids with damaged corners, of which the expression *frayed at the edges* is truly descriptive. Like this, they may be good teaching aids—since their detailed construction is easily seen—but they are inefficient radiographically and even dangerous, for cracks in a grid can simulate fracture lines in bone or intestinal fluid levels in the abdomen. A damaged grid cannot be repaired. If edges and corners alone are involved, the grid may sometimes be successfully cut down to one of smaller size but those whose responsibility it is to administer X-ray departments have usually to think in terms of its total replacement.

FUNCTIONAL TESTS

Testing the performance of exposure timers

Among tests to be made on functioning X-ray equipment are those for exposure timers. The questions asked about timers are as follows.

1 Is the timer accurate, timing without error?
2 Is the timer consistent in its settings, timing without variation?

Following from the first question is another: what magnitude of error would be considered unacceptable? There is no fixed answer to that since tolerance is related to the length of the time-interval which is tested. A slight error (for example of 0·005 second) will be a large proportion of a very short exposure time (it is obviously an error of 100 per cent if the exposure time is 0·005 second). The same error is an insignificant proportion of a longer exposure time: 0·005 second is only 5 per cent of 0·1 second.

Consistency in timing is considered to be of greater importance than is absolutely accurate performance by an exposure timer. If when a timer is set for 0·1 second the exposure lasts for 0·12 second, the inaccuracy does not matter very much provided that on the 0·1 second setting the timer *always* gives 0·12 second and is not variable in its error. So tests to be carried out on timers seek to examine not the accuracy alone but also the consistency of their actions.

A device which has been used for many years to test the performances of X-ray timers is called a spinning top. It is still a satisfactory test tool when the high tension generator of the X-ray set being tested is of the single phase type with its pulsating tube voltage related to the mains frequency. The conventional spinning top cannot be used to test the timers of generators where the tube voltage is not in the form of discrete pulsations: another tool, which is described later in this chapter, is to be used for three phase generators (which have a continuous rippling voltage waveform) and capacitor discharge generators (which have maintained continuous voltage output).

A sketch of the top is shown in Fig. 17.1. It consists of a metal—usually steel or brass—disc which is a few millimetres in thickness and designed to

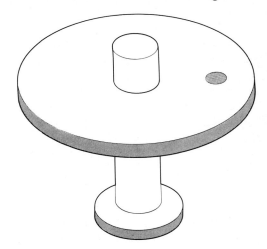

Fig. 17.1   A spinning top.

revolve easily upon a central peg. The peg has a flattened base, so that the whole mechanism can be stood on a cassette or direct-exposure film placed on the X-ray table. At a point near the periphery of the disc is drilled a small hole. This sometimes is circular in outline and sometimes rectangular; the shape is not significant.

The use of the spinning top to test the accuracy of operation of the X-ray exposure timer is described below. The experiment can easily be performed by student radiographers.

Testing a timer's accuracy

The steps of the procedure to test a timer's accuracy by means of a spinning top are as follows.

1 The timer to be tested is set for 0·1 seconds and other exposure factors are also selected; for example, 200 mA, and 75 kVp. (Note that the tube tension should not be too low.)

2 A film (for example 24 × 30 cm) is placed on the X-ray table and the X-ray tube positioned over it. This film can be either in a cassette or of the direct-exposure type. The former of course provides an image of higher contrast and this is generally advantageous in estimations of the timer's accuracy. However, as will be seen, there is other information which can be obtained for which the recording of small tonal gradations is significant; the direct-exposure film may be better in this respect.

3 The film is divided off by means of lead strips, or simply by adjustment of the beam collimator, into six separate sections, only one of which is exposed at a time. The tube is centred to each section in turn.

4 The spinning top is placed in the first section and spun with the fingers. Its actual speed is immaterial but it should be given sufficient impetus to keep it moving for some seconds.

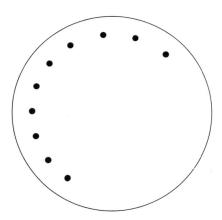

Fig. 17.2

5 The radiographer returns to the controls of the unit and makes the X-ray exposure.

6 A further five exposures are made in this way, each in a different section of the prepared film.

7 The film is processed as usual and viewed.

When the radiograph is examined it will be seen to contain six images, each similar to the one depicted in Fig. 17.2. In this, each dark spot is the image of the hole as it rotates in the spinning disc. If the 'spots' are close together the disc has been revolving more slowly than if they are far apart; their spacing is immaterial to the interpretation of the experiment. What *is* important is their number, since each has been produced by a single electrical impulse through the X-ray tube; that is, each represents a peak in the sine wave or one half-cycle of the supply (Chapter 1). Fig. 17.4 shows three radiographs of a spinning top which has one rectangular hole.

In the United Kingdom, the mains operate at 50 cycles a second and therefore in 0·1 seconds we would expect to see recorded on the film five whole electrical cycles. Remembering that each 'dot' is a half-cycle, there will be ten of them if the unit has full-wave rectification, five if the X-ray set is of the half-wave kind and therefore operates only during half of each complete cycle. Fig. 17.3 will remind the student of these two forms of rectification and illustrate the relationship of the densities on the film to the time interval in each case.

The radiographs in Fig. 17.4 were made with an exposure of 0·05 seconds on a single-phase full-wave rectified unit operating on 50 Hrz supply. There should be 5 rectangular spots on each of the three radiographs but in fact there are six. Any lesser number than the expected one indicates that the

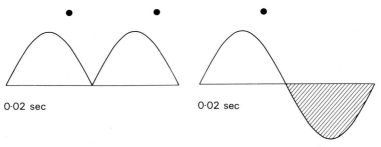

0·02 sec   0·02 sec

Fig. 17.3

timer is giving us an exposure interval which in fact is shorter than the setting on the timer and any greater number means an interval which is longer. Bearing in mind that each single 'spot' represents 0·01 seconds in time, we can discover both the existence and the extent of the timer's fault. The radiographs shown in Fig. 17.4 indicate that on a setting of 0·05 second the tested timer has a consistent inaccuracy and gives a time-interval of 0.06 second.

Unless we are considering very short exposures, a slight inaccuracy in the timer—let us say, of the order of one extra 'spot' or 0·01 seconds—in practice probably will not matter much, providing that it invariably occurs. An inconsistent fault is a much more troublesome matter and this is the reason for making a test always of six similar exposures. The radiograph which we obtain gives us, as we have seen, three pieces of information:

1   whether the timer is accurate;
2   the extent of the inaccuracy, if present;
3   whether the fault is consistent.

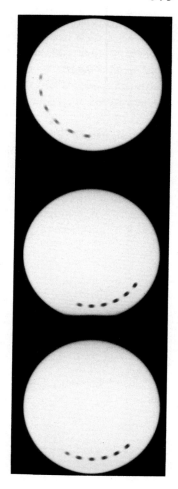

Fig. 17.4

Following a consistency test of this kind, the next procedure should be to make a run down. For this a single exposure of the spinning top is obtained for all settings of the timer between 0·1 seconds and zero. In the case of the two-pulse generator which we are discussing this is likely to be at the following intervals: 0·1, 0·08, 0·06, 0·05 and so on—usually at stages of 0·01 seconds—down to the minimum period obtainable which is 0·01 seconds. In the numerical instances given the number of 'spots' seen on the film would be respectively 10, 8, 6 and 5.

Timing and switching systems used in conjunction with high-powered apparatus may be phased (Chapter 5). A test with the spinning top can be made to determine whether the system is initiating the exposure at the correct phase of the cycle, that is at zero volts.

To do this successfully the spinning top must be made to revolve very fast so that each area of exposure becomes sufficiently extended for the observer to appreciate within it any changes in radiographic density. The timer is set for 0·01 seconds and the exposure made while the top spins at maximum speed. When the film is processed it should be apparent that the exposed area is not a single, even density but contains a relatively dark patch flanked by lighter tones. The point of maximum blackness indicates the instant at which the voltage reached its peak value. If the switching is correctly phased, this obviously should occur in the exact centre of the area concerned. Any deviation from the central position must be evidence that the exposure begins and ends at some other points on the voltage waveform than zero.

Fig. 17.5 is a sketch of a routine timer test which has revealed incorrect phasing in another way. This was a 2-pulse unit and the timer had been

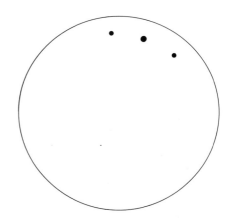

Fig. 17.5   Incorrect phasing.

set for 0·02 seconds. Instead of the expected two, we have on the film a trio of 'spots'. However, the first and the third are noticeably smaller than the second and their combined area is suggestively similar to that of the middle one alone. This led to the conclusion that the exposure had been initiated towards the end of a waveform, had continued through the next complete half-cycle and had ceased at a comparable point towards the end of the third waveform. Fig. 17.6 depicts the situation graphically and we can appreciate from the sketch that the system was accurate enough in giving 0·02 seconds exposure, but was not doing so between zero values of voltage—as it should be if the phasing circuit is correct in operation.

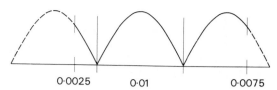

Fig. 17.6   0·0025   0·01   0·0075

Another test tool for timers

The generators found in modern X-ray departments are often not of the 2-pulse type with single phase supply. There are (a) three phase generators which provide 6 or 12 pulses for each complete cycle of mains alternation, with a voltage waveform which is a slight ripple; (b) constant potential generators with such stabilization of the tube voltage that the graphical depiction is not a pulsating nor a rippling waveform but a steady straight line; (c) capacitor discharge units with maintained continuous voltage outputs that similarly are not waves nor ripples but lines.

The spinning top test so far described is based upon the provision of well separated images of black spots. In the case of three phase generators with rippling waveforms, the pattern that results from an exposure when the top is set spinning by hand is not one of discrete spots: it is a continuous band of density with darker striations where the peaks of the voltage waveform occur at regular intervals related to the mains frequency. These striations (shown in Fig. 17.7) may be difficult to count as the discrete spots are counted. They are not easily counted because (a) they are dauntingly many in number (for 0·1 second 6 pulse equipment gives 30 and 12 pulse equipment gives 60 on a 50 Hrz supply); (b) they are very close together (in 6 pulse equipment these peaks of voltage occur at intervals of 0·003 second and in 12 pulse equipment at intervals of 0·001 second on 50 Hrz supply) unless the top is spinning at a much higher speed than can be achieved by hand. In the cases of generators with continuous lines as their voltage waveforms when they are correctly operating, the spinning top tests give images of unbroken lines with neither spots nor striations available for counting. So if timers are to be tested for accuracy and consistency a test tool other than this simple spinning top must be used.

There are available timer test tools for X-ray sets which can be used both on single phase and on three phase generators and on capacitor discharge and other generators with continuous voltage waveforms. These tools can test time-intervals from a few milliseconds up to 1 second.

The Wisconsin Timing and mAs Test Tool is one such in a range of test tools known as the Wisconsin Radiologic Test Tools. These have been developed by individuals in the Medical Physics and Engineering Center of the University of Wisconsin Department of Radiology.

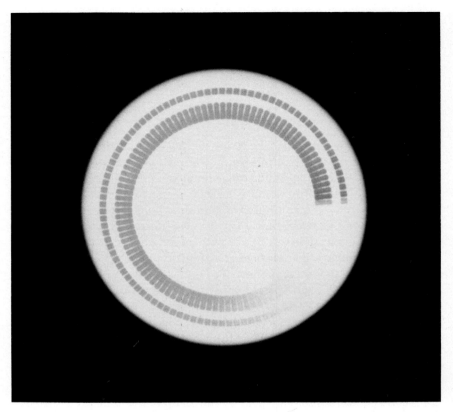

Fig. 17.7

The Wisconsin Test Tool for an X-ray timer (seen in Fig. 17.8) is a plastic box which contains a brass disc 8 cm in diameter. The disc has two slits spaced 180 degrees apart as indicated in the diagram in Fig. 17.9. When the tool is used, this disc is kept spinning by a motor which rotates it at a constant speed such that it makes one complete revolution in 1 second: that is, each slit moves through 360 degrees in 1 second. (Some tools have 3 or 4 slits at 90 degrees spacing.)

If a radiographic exposure is made while the disc rotates, the moving slits each describe an arc which shows as an area of density on the processed radiograph. Such arcs of density are shown in Fig. 17.10 which shows three arcs each of about 30 degrees. Since the disc makes one complete revolution in 1 second, the extent of each arc appearing on the radiograph is related to the period of time occupied by the exposure. Thus, for example, in 0·1 second we could expect an arc of 36 degrees to be described and the 30

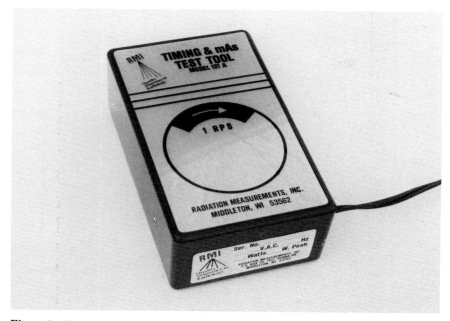

Fig. 17.8 A test tool for the timer and the milliamperes settings. *By courtesy of Radiation Measurements Inc.*

degree arcs shown in Fig. 17.10 could be the result of an exposure of 0·08 second.

A hole may be drilled close to one of the slits just inside its end which is nearer to the centre of the disc. This hole allows the tool to function exactly as the conventional spinning top if the generator under test is a single phase one with discrete pulsations of voltage which provide for counting the black

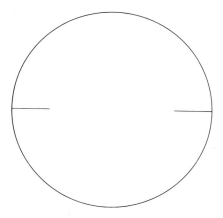

Fig. 17.9

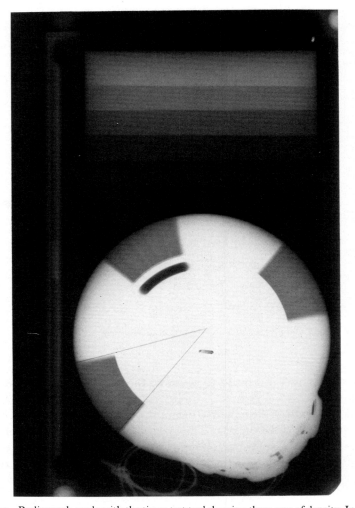

Fig. 17.10 Radiograph made with the timer test tool showing three arcs of density. In this case there are three slits separated by 90 degrees and one of the slits has a small hole near its inner end. The voltage waveform for the X-ray tube is not a pulsating one so the hole has produced an image which is a band of density and not discrete spots.

dots of separate impulses. Inside the box which contains the spinning disc there is also a copper stepwedge. Its images can be seen in the radiographs in Fig. 17.11 and its purpose is to test the relative constancy of output at different milliampere settings: this is explained on page 584. The steps of the procedure for using this tool to test timer accuracy are set out below.

1   The timer to be tested is set for 0·1 second and other factors of exposure are selected. These might be 70 kV, 100 mA and one metre anode-film

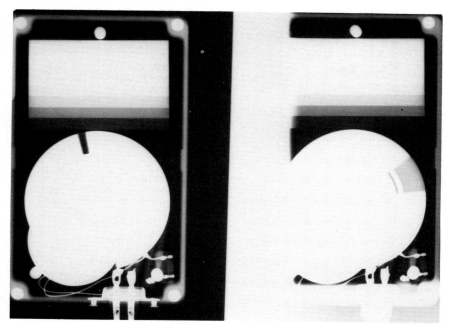

Fig. 17.11

distance: the suggestion from Wisconsin is 70 kV for three phase and 80 kV for single phase equipment.

2 A cassette loaded with film (for example 24 cm by 30 cm) is placed on the X-ray table and the tool is placed on one section of it. The rest of the cassette's surface is screened off with lead so that it may be used for further exposures in the series of the test.

3 The X-ray tube is centred to the test tool and the beam is collimated just to cover the tool.

4 The tool is set running under the power of its motor so that the disc is rotating at one revolution per second.

5 The radiographic exposure is made.

6 This should be followed with a further two exposures. Each is made with the tool positioned on a different area on the cassette and the other areas screened with lead. The time-interval and the other settings of the controls should remain unchanged.

7 The film is processed and viewed.

Interpretation of the results is made by:

1 counting the number of 'spots' produced by the images of the moving hole on the disc if the generator is single phase two-pulse equipment;

2   using a protractor to measure the angles of the arcs of density produced
by the moving slits for other generators. A special protractor may be
provided which is calibrated in exposure times as is indicated in the diagram
in Fig. 17.12.

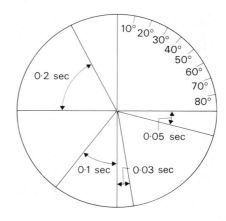

Fig. 17.12

At 0·1 second:
• the correct angle is 37 degrees, allowing 1 degree for the width of the slit;
• the allowed angle is 34·5 degrees to 41·5 degrees;
• the number of single phase pulses on a 50 Hrz supply is 10;
• the allowed number of pulses is 9 to 11.

Since three exposures have been made with the timer setting unchanged
from 0·1 second, the consistency of the timer's action can be assessed by
checking that in all three images the angles of the arcs are the same.

Further time intervals may now be tested. For example, by making three
exposures at 0·2 second with 50 mA; three exposures at 0·05 second with
200 mA; three exposures at 0·03 second with 300 mA. Table 17.1 gives
guidance on the interpretation of the results from these settings.

Of course, any particular setting of the timer which is suspect can be
tested for accuracy and consistency. The milliamperes setting should be

Table 17.1

Time interval in seconds	Correct angle (allowing 1 deg. for slit)	Tolerance limits for angle	No. of single phase pulses	Tolerance limits in pulses
0·2	73	67–81	20	±2
0·05	19	19·5–21·5	5	None
0·03	13	13–15	3	None

adjusted to give an exposure that is as nearly as possible the same as the rest of the series. For the settings described here, the milliampereseconds value is 10 mAs, except for 0·03 second with 300 mA.

For any setting, the correct angle of arc can be calculated by dividing 360 (the number of degrees in one revolution of the disc) by the denominator of the fraction of a second which is the tested time-interval; and then adding to the answer one degree for the width of the slit. For example, 0·25 second is $\frac{1}{4}$ second: $360/4 = 90$: 90 plus 1 = 91.

For any angle of arc measured on the radiograph, the time of exposure can be derived by subtracting one degree from the measured degrees to allow for the width of the slit and then dividing the measured degrees minus one by 360 degrees. So for example: measured degrees are 18: 18 minus 1 = 17: 17/360 = 0·047. So 0·047 second is the actual time for which the exposure lasted.

If the specially calibrated protractor that is available is used to measure the arcs, the time-intervals can be read directly from it. This saves the tester's time whether it is to be spent on mental arithmetic or the use of a calculator.

Towards greater accuracy in the results, Wisconsin make the following recommendations:

1 for times up to 0·5 second, use the special protractor to measure the angles of the dark areas produced by the moving slits;

2 for times between 0·5 and 1·0 second, use the special protractor to measure the curved line of arc produced by the hole drilled close to the inner end of one of the slits;

3 for single phase generators (2-pulse equipment) count the impulses or black spots produced by the moving hole and the pulsations of the voltage;

4 if it proves not possible to make measurements because the arcs start or stop behind the shadow of the motor (seen in the lower left quadrants in the radiographs in Fig. 17.11) carry out a repeat exposure. This coincidence of the arcs with the motor may sometimes happen at exposure times 0·5 and 1·0 second.

Assessing the milliamperes settings

The controls of modern X-ray sets usually provide selections through a range of milliamperes. For example, a typical selector provides the following settings: 100 mA; 300 mA; 400 mA; 600 mA; 800 mA; 1000 mA. The exposure dose given to the film is proportional to the product of the milliamperage and the exposure time: that is, it is proportional to the milliampereseconds. Any given milliampereseconds value may be expected to give a reasonably constant exposure dose of X rays and result in a reasonably constant radiographic density whatever the individual values of milliamperes and seconds. Thus, for example, 10 mAs can be expected to have the same radiographic effects when it is given as any of the following: 100 mA for 0·1 second; 200 mA for 0·05 second; 400 mA for 0·025 second; 800 mA for 0·0125 second; 1000 mA for 0·01 second.

This expectation of equivalence is valid when:

1 the timer is accurate and is consistent in its performance;

2 the milliamperage selector functions precisely to give at each of its settings a consistent milliampere value and output of X rays. When the selector is consistent, the radiographer may expect the 200 mA setting to give twice the output of the 100 mA setting, the 400 mA setting to give twice the output of the 200 mA setting and so on in proportion to the change in milliamperes which is made;

3 the kilovoltage is maintained at a given value despite the rise in milliamperes (of which there is more on p. 602);

4 the processing conditions are standardized.

We have seen in the previous section how the performance of the timer may be tested. Now we are concerned with how the consistency of the milliampere settings may be assessed. The tests described in the following paragraphs do *not* involve the direct measurement of the milliamperes through the X-ray tube. They are rather tests which a radiographer might make with the aid of available special devices. Two of the three methods described entail the use of films for radiographic exposures.

Using the Wisconsin test tool

The Wisconsin Timing and mAs Test Tool described in the previous section provides a means to check the constancy of output at various settings of the milliamperes selector. Within the box which encloses the spinning disc to be used for time tests there is also a copper stepwedge with five steps. It is seen above the spinning disc in the radiographs in Fig. 17.11. The procedure for using this stepwedge to test the consistency of the milliamperes settings is as follows.

1 A cassette loaded with film (for example 24 cm by 30 cm) is placed on the X-ray table and the tool is put on one section of it. The rest of the cassette's surface is screened with lead so that it may be used for further exposures in the series of the test.

2 The X-ray tube is centred to the tool and the beam is collimated just to cover the tool.

3 A radiographic exposure is made with one of the sets of factors in the series given below:

0·1 second	100 mA = 10 mAs
0·05 second	200 mA = 10 mAs
0·025 second	400 mA = 10 mAs
0·02 second	500 mA = 10 mAs
0·016 second	600 mA = 10 mAs
0·0125 second	800 mA = 10 mAs
0·01 second	1000 mA = 10 mAs

For all the exposures in the series the kilovoltage is kept constant at 70–80 kV and the tube-film distance is one metre. The milliampereseconds are kept constant and the milliamperes are varied through the series using whatever settings of the selector it is wished to test. If the disc is kept spinning for the exposures, the performance of the timer is shown in the radiographs.

4   After the first exposure is made, another set of factors in the series is used to make a second exposure with the tool positioned on a different area of the cassette, all other areas being screened with lead.

5   For each setting to be tested an exposure is made, using as many different areas of a film or separate films as required.

6   The exposed radiographs are processed and the results are viewed.

To interpret, you compare all the images of the stepwedge and assess whether they match in density for corresponding steps in all the radiographs. Thus, do all the images of the first step which is nearest to the disc have the same density? Do all the other steps similarly correspond in all their images?

The questions may be adequately answered by a visual assessment carefully made in optimum viewing conditions, for that is the way in which radiographs are generally judged and interpreted. If it is wished to eliminate the uncertainties of subjective judgment and to reduce the amounts of time and energy that the decisions may consume, then the densities must be measured with a densitometer.

In practice it is not necessary in fact to measure or to assess by eye *all* the steps in *all* the images. In practice the visual assessment of very low and very high densities is of no value since the eye cannot detect very small density-differences at such extremes of a range. So you can select for estimation or measurement just one step of each wedge-pattern. Choose a step which has a density about the middle of the range shown and then compare the densities of the *same step* in all the wedge-images.

If step-for-step correspondence is found in all the patterns and the timer is accurate, the milliampere settings are consistent throughout the range tested. It is unacceptable if the densities in any of the images are out of correspondence by more than one step: this situation is shown in the radiograph in Fig. 17.13. In such a case the settings of the selector should be checked and adjusted by a service engineer.

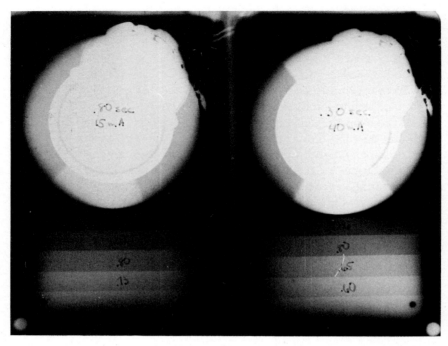

Fig. 17.13 A radiograph which reveals inconstancy between two milliamperes settings. In the radiograph on the left the density measured on the third step of the wedge (counting from the foot upwards) is 0·80. In the right-hand radiograph the density 0·80 is measured on the fourth step of the wedge, so this mA setting is out of correspondence by 'one step of the wedge'. (Other radiographs at other settings in this series have not been included in the illustration.)

Using an aluminium stepwedge

As we have seen, the Wisconsin Timer and mAs Test Tool contains a copper stepwedge with 5 steps. This is a very limited number to use to test the constancy of output at different milliampere settings, especially if the resultant test radiographs are to be assessed by eye. Five steps provide only four density-differences and it could turn out that the exposure conditions which were used gave images which lacked, within this short range, a useful density for estimation by eye. All the densities might be either too high or too low in value. The test must then be repeated with altered exposure conditions and a waste of time and material.

It may be more satisfactory to use a stepwedge such as is shown in Fig. 17.14. As can be seen, it is a little flight of steps made of metal. The one shown is aluminium and has 14 steps each of which is 3·0 mm thick: it is suitable for use up to about 130 kV. Fourteen steps are 13 differences and

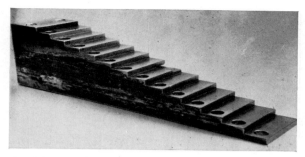

Fig. 17.14 An aluminium stepwedge.

the selection of exposure factors becomes less critical to obtaining some useful densities in the range. If a stepwedge such as this is used in place of the Wisconsin tool as previously described, the performance of the timer must first be separately tested since the radiographs obtained of the stepwedge hold no evidence of the timer's functioning.

The procedure to be carried out in using this aluminium stepwedge is the same as that described on pages 584–586, with the aluminium stepwedge replacing the Wisconsin tool. The method of interpretation is the same: that is, the patterns are compared by eye or densitometer for equivalencies in density.

Fig. 17.15 shows just two radiographs of this aluminium stepwedge made at 80 kV and 120 mAs; in one 300 mA was used for 0·4 second to test the 300 mA setting and the other 100 mA was used for 1·2 seconds to test the 100 mA setting. It can be seen by eye that there is step-for-step matching of densities in the two images if you consider the five steps of the wedge between which density-differences can be readily perceived. In Fig. 17.15 these are on the left side of an imaginary centre line in the illustration moving towards greater density.

So Fig. 17.15 shows constancy of output at the 300 mA and the 100 mA settings of the milliamperes selector. It can be seen that in the stepwedge illustrated a hole been drilled through each step to the depth of the step. This results in each recording two densities, one due to itself and another due to its predecessor. This is not an essential feature: it simply makes the comparison of adjacent densities easier. As we have seen, the images should not be more than one step out of correspondence.

Using ionization dosimetry

A non-radiographic test for the consistency of the milliampere settings can be made by means of ionization dosimetry. This method uses an ionization

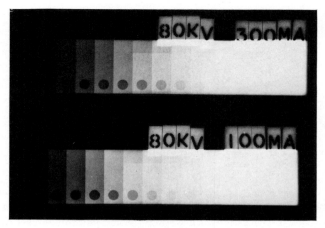

Fig. 17.15   Radiographs of a stepwedge which show that the kilovoltage is maintained for two values of tube current.

chamber in place of a film as the 'detector' of the radiation from the X-ray tube and it could be argued that ionization dosimetry is preferable on the following grounds:

1   there are fewer variables to be taken into account (for example, response of the film to the exposures, processing conditions, characteristics of intensifying screens);
2   there are savings in time and materials (films and chemicals);

The practice of this method does of course imply the purchase of or the availability of a special piece of equipment: that is, an ionization dosimeter. The method rests on the basis of fact that if all other conditions of output of an X-ray tube stay the same, then dose is proportional to milliamperage. Irregularity in the milliampere settings is revealed by irregularity in the expected linear relationship of dose to milliamperes.

Testing available kilovoltages

The control consoles of X-ray sets allow the radiographer to select appropriate values from a useful range of kilovoltages. Settings are provided in steps of about 2 kV from 40 kV up to perhaps 130 kV.

Careful selection of the kilovoltage across the X-ray tube is a most important factor altered by the radiographer to determine contrast in the resultant image. Variations in the effective penetrating power of the X-ray beam change significantly the differential absorptions by the tissues to be traversed. Yet direct knowledge of the kilovoltage applied for any given setting of the selector is not available to radiographers through conventional control consoles.

It may be considered to be unimportant that kilovoltage settings should provide exactly the value which is stated. In choosing kilovoltage, the radiographer makes a subjective judgment which is empirically based, although modified by knowledge of the principles which are involved. More important perhaps than the accuracy of the settings is their consistency: any given setting should provide a value of kilovoltage which is repeatable and for that setting remains the same whenever the setting is used.

In assuring the quality of the radiographic result it is necessary to check the kilovoltage applied from the control-settings of the X-ray sets which are in use. If all the X-ray sets consistently provide kilovoltages close to the stated values, the radiographers are much more likely to achieve a high standard of work that is reproducible and is maintained. It may be possible for one radiographer working with one X-ray unit to make adjustments through familiarity with the inexactness of the settings (so long as the settings are consistent in their erroneousness) and so to achieve a satisfactory radiographic result on every film which is exposed. But in a department with several X-ray sets and many radiographers if the kilovoltages actually available differ widely from the values stated by the settings, then these variations are a plentiful source of repeated radiographs. With so much present emphasis on the conservation of materials and energy and on limits to expenditure, such repeats are intolerably wasteful.

Several methods are available for estimating the kilovoltage applied to the X-ray tube. Some of them are not such as would be used readily by a radiographer making a check on the X-ray sets of the department: so there seems little point in describing them here. Instead we concern ourselves with a technique that can be applied easily and quickly by radiographers. This technique uses an X-ray film to detect the radiation emerging from the tube and it is based upon the use of a special cassette.

The Wisconsin test cassette

The Wisconsin test cassette is a special cassette which can be used to determine by a radiographic method the effective kilovoltage across the X-ray tube when the test was made. The accuracy of the result is assessed as generally within plus/minus 2 per cent and certainly within plus/minus 5 per cent. At 100 kV, 2 per cent is a 2 kV variation and 5 per cent is a 5 kV variation. While some people might say that a 5 kV change makes to the radiograph a difference which is perceptible to the viewer's eye, most would doubtless agree that in the general run of radiographs a 2 kV change does not appreciably alter the image.

The cassette (see Fig. 17.16) allows the kilovoltage to be assessed in four regions: 60 kVp region; 80 kVp region; 100 kVp region; 120 kVp region. It is said to be most accurate in the first two regions and least accurate in the highest one. It has higher accuracy when it is used on three-phase generators as compared with single-phase ones.

The cassette further enables its user to estimate the half-value thickness (half-value layer) of the X-ray beam which comes out of the tube when it is energized at the 60 kVp setting. Students may recall from their study of physics that the half-value thickness of an X-ray beam is a statement about

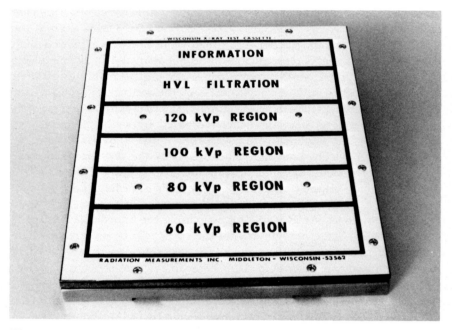

Fig. 17.16

its penetrating power. The half-value thickness is defined as being the thickness of a stated material which is required to reduce the intensity of an X-ray beam to half its original value: the Wisconsin cassette gives an expression of the half-value thickness (half-value layer) in equivalent millimetres of aluminium.

As an indication of the penetrating power of an X-ray beam, the peak kilovoltage at which it is generated makes an incomplete statement. To know the peak kilovoltage is to know of a heterogeneous beam only its minimum wavelength and the related maximum energy for a photon. Radiographers could well question the usefulness of knowing only *that* when they must concern themselves with the ability of a beam to penetrate the tissue of the human body and to have an effect on a film and produce a radiograph. At least the half-value layer gives an indication of the effective penetrating power of a heterogeneous beam since to specify the half-value layer is to indicate the beam's attenuation by the material which is used to state the half-value layer.

When the Wisconsin test cassette is used to determine the half-value layer of the beam produced at 60 kVp, the radiographer gains knowledge of what thickness of aluminium will reduce this beam to one half of its original intensity. This begins to seem a potentially useful piece of information when it is remembered that for the photon energies which are commonly used in diagnostic radiography the half-value layers expressed in aluminium and in calcium would be nearly the same, since aluminium and calcium have linear attenuation coefficients which are nearly the same at photon energies about the middle of the diagnostic range.

Radiographers can approximately equate the absorptive abilities of calcium with those of bone and from this derive the knowledge that the attenuation achieved by, say, 10 mm of aluminium would also be achieved (nearly enough) by 10 mm of bone. A further useful piece of information is that at a photon energy commonly used in diagnostic radiography bone removes about 5 times more radiation than does the same mass of soft tissue. So we could estimate, with some approximation, that the attenuation achieved by, say, 10 mm of aluminium and of bone would also be achieved by 50 mm of soft tissue. So knowledge of the half-value layer of a beam of X rays when it is expressed in millimetres of aluminium is a piece of information which can be of some use to the radiographer who is selecting exposure factors.

A further important point is that a beam generated at 60 kVp which has a very low half-value layer (say less than 1·5 mm of aluminium in contrast to around 1·8 to 2·0 mm of aluminium) must be a beam with a long range of photon energies. This suggests that there is insufficient equivalent aluminium filtration in the tube to remove the low photon energies which will be absorbed in the patient's skin: so this X-ray tube is giving the patient a dose of needless radiation which is not contributing to the radiographic result at all.

On the other hand, if a beam of X rays generated at 60 kVp shows a half-value layer which is thicker than the expected figure of around 1·8 to 2·0 mm of aluminium, then the implication is that the effective filtration in this X-ray tube has *increased*. Such could be the case in a long-used X-ray tube, subjected to heavy loading, where there has been considerable deposition of hot tungsten on the glass envelope of the tube. The layer of metal over the window through which the X rays emerge from the glass insert acts as a filter if it is thick enough and removes some of the photons in the beam which have lower energies. Thus the beam becomes effectively more penetrating and the half-value layer increases in thickness. So this finding may give warning of the state of an ageing X-ray tube and predict its failure.

The construction of the Wisconsin cassette

Figure 17.16 shows the external appearance of the Wisconsin test cassette. The four regions of kilovoltage from 60 kVp to 120 kVp are seen marked on the outside of the cassette, as are the panels for half-value layer and what is described as *Information*: this last one is intended to bear lead legends or other markers which may identify the particular X-ray set which is being tested and the date of the test.

Figure 17.17 shows an exploded view of the Wisconsin test cassette so that the different constituent parts can be seen. Working inwards from the front of the cassette the various elements are as follows.

1   A sheet of copper which is $\frac{1}{16}$ inch thick and is large enough to cover the four regions where the kilovoltages are to be assessed but does not extend over the region where the half-value layer is to be measured. This sheet of copper is intended to act as a filter and remove some longer wavelengths from the heterogeneous beam which comes out of the X-ray tube. With the photons of lower energy thus removed, the energy-range of the remainder in the beam is narrower and the attenuation by the copper wedges which are the next elements in the cassette becomes almost a linear function of photon-energy.

2   Underneath the copper sheet are four copper stepwedges, one for each of the four kilovoltage regions: 60 kVp, 80 kVp, 100 kVp and 120 kVp. They each have a different range of thickness as appropriate to the kilovoltage to be measured. Thus, for example, the copper stepwedge for the 60 kVp measurement has a different thickness-range from its thin to its thick end than does the wedge for the determination of tube-voltage in the 120 kVp region. These stepwedges are used in the measurement of kilovoltage as will be seen. Alongside these stepwedges is a fifth copper stepwedge which is used for the measurement of half-value layer: it is *not* covered by the copper sheet as are the other four for that does not extend into the half-value layer region of the cassette. The important point is that the measurement of kilovoltage is to be done *after* the beam has had the photons of low energy removed from it: a filtered beam is used. The measurement of half-value layer uses an unfiltered beam because the half-value layer depends upon the range of energies in the primary beam which emerges from the X-ray tube.

3   Underneath the copper stepwedges is a lead sheet with holes in it. There

are ten columns of holes with ten holes to a column. The columns are grouped as five pairs, there being one pair of columns in each of the five regions of the cassette: 60 kVp, 80 kVp, 100 kVp, 120 kVp and lastly the half-value layer region. In each pair of columns, the left-hand column of holes is positioned so that each hole is beneath a copper stepwedge in an

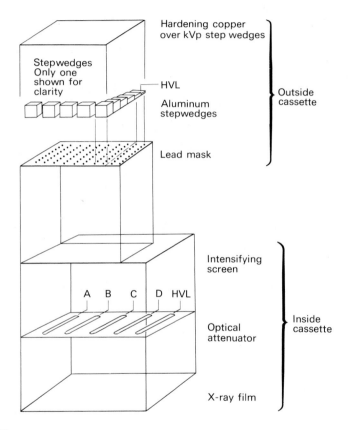

Fig. 17.17

arrangement of one step of the wedge for each hole: thus each hole is covered by a different thickness of copper. The right-hand column of holes in each pair of columns is *not* beneath a copper stepwedge. The use of the lead sheet improves the contrast of the radiographic result (seen in Fig. 17.18) by absorbing scattered radiation.

4 Beneath the lead sheet with the holes is an intensifying screen which extends through all the 5 regions of the cassette. It is a single screen, there

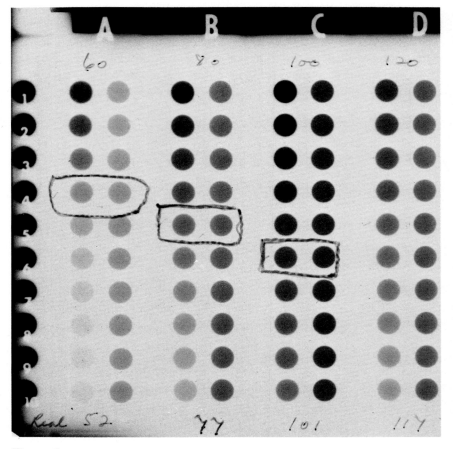

Fig. 17.18

being no other in this cassette. The use of a single screen instead of a pair eliminates the effect of possible changes in the relative speeds of different screens.

5   Beneath the intensifying screen is an optical filter which is designed to filter the light which the intensifying screen emits when it is energized by X-rays. This optical filter or attenuator is arranged in bars so that it filters the light emitted from the parts of the screen which are beneath the right-hand column of holes in each pair of columns in the lead sheet. This action of the bars of the optical filter is effectively to reduce the speed of the intensifying screen in those areas which are covered by the filtering bars.

6   The last essential in this test cassette is the film which is the detector of the radiation.

Principle of operation of the Wisconsin test cassette

We have described as a component of the test cassette a lead mask with columns of holes arranged in pairs. It will by now be realized that in each pair of columns:

1 the right-hand column of holes has the optical attenuator beneath it but no absorbing copper stepwedge above it and the circular densities which are produced as images of the holes (see Fig. 17.18) result from a combination of an unattenuated X-ray beam and an attenuated light from the screen: the attenuation of light does not vary down the column of holes for the optical filter achieves a fixed degree of attenuation.

2 the left-hand column of holes has a different thickness of copper absorber above each hole but no optical attenuator under any of the holes and the circular densities in the radiograph (see Fig. 17.18) are the result of an X-ray beam which is variously attenuated by the copper stepwedges and an unattenuated light from the screen: the copper stepwedges increase in thickness down the columns.

So for the circles of density shown in Fig. 17.18 the situation is as below.

Left-hand column of each pair of columns:

1 copper X-ray absorbers;
2 unattenuated screen;
3 circles show a density-gradient, density diminishing down the column as the thickness of the copper absorbers increases.

Right-hand column of each pair of columns:

1 no copper X-ray absorbers;
2 attenuated screen;
3 density of the circles is nearly uniform as the optical attenuation is fixed: this density should be between 0·5 and 2·0.

For a copper absorber used in conjunction with an unattenuated intensifying screen (the situation in the left-hand columns) there is a particular thickness which results in a radiographic density that is equal to the one resulting from the use of an attenuated intensifying screen used without a copper absorber (the situation in the right-hand columns). This means that there is a given thickness of copper stepwedge at which a circle of density in a left-hand column matches its immediate neighbour in the adjacent right-hand column.

Figure 17.18 shows three matching pairs of circles indicated by enclosing hand-drawn lines. It can be seen that in the 60 kVp region step 4 of the copper absorber was the thickness required to produce a match; in the 80 kVp region step 5 was the thickness that produced a match: at 100 kVp step 6 was the thickness of copper absorber needed to achieve a match.

If the attenuation of the intensifying screen is fixed (as we have seen it is in this cassette) the thickness of copper required for a match in density increases with rising kilovoltage. Furthermore, it is almost a linear function of kilovoltage when the X-ray beam has had its spectral distribution narrowed by the use of the copper sheet described earlier. So 'match thickness' can be used to measure kilovoltage and also (as it is here) to estimate the half-value layer for a beam generated at a given kilovoltage (in this case 60 kVp). Fig. 17.19 shows the two columns of circular densities in

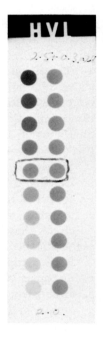

Fig. 17.19

the half-value layer region of the cassette with a matching pair enclosed in a hand-drawn line.

For the determination of half-value layer, the energy-distribution of the beam emerging from the X-ray tube must be left unchanged and the spectrum is not narrowed by passing the beam through the copper sheet. It is for this reason that the copper sheet does not extend over the region of the cassette where the half-value layer is to be measured.

Wisconsin test cassettes are each calibrated individually by the manufacturers (Radiation Measurements Inc.) against a master standard cassette. They come to the user accompanied by calibration data which allow 'match thicknesses' or step numbers to be related to kilovoltage-values and to half-values layers.

Method of use of the Wisconsin test cassette

1   When the Wisconsin test cassette is used to check a particular X-ray set for the exactness of its kilovoltage-settings, comparing actual kilovoltage-values with those indicated on the control panel, and for the estimation of half-value layer at 60 kVp, five exposures must be made: one exposure on each of the four kilovoltage regions of the cassette and one on the half-value layer region. For each exposure, the areas of the cassette which are not being used must be masked with lead and it is most important that this lead shield is adequate. At least 2 mm of lead (*not* a lead-rubber sheet) must be used.

2   The cassette is loaded with any type of X-ray film and is put on the X-ray table, placed as is any conventional cassette with its front aspect towards the X-ray tube. The long sides of the cassette should be parallel to the long anode-cathode axis of the X-ray tube. This is so that the columns of holes and the copper stepwedge absorbers lie along lines at right-angles to the anode-cathode axis of the X-ray tube: such a placing will prevent the anode heel-effect from significantly modifying the findings of the test. The X-ray tube should be centred to the long central axis of the cassette-front and will be directly over each of the five measuring regions of the cassette in its turn as the area to receive exposure.

3   Exposures are made in series over each region separately with the other regions masked with lead and with the beam-collimator so adjusted that the whole of a region is irradiated to its complete length and width.

4   When the half-value layer region is being exposed, the area next to it which is marked Identification should be included within the field: lead letters or other markers for radiographic identification placed in this panel before exposure can record data relevant to the test.

5   Before the exposures are made, the line voltage compensator of the generator should be set as precisely as possible if it is a manual control and the kilovoltage-settings each in their turn should be accurately made. If the generator of the X-ray set which is being tested does not provide the higher kilovoltages which are marked on the cassette, then those regions are not used and no exposures are made for them.

6   The 60 kVp setting on the generator must be checked as correctly providing 60 kVp before testing the half-value layer. This means that you must re-load the cassette with a second film and make the half-value layer test separately, for you cannot know the result of the test of the 60 kVp setting until you have processed the film on which it was made. Fig. 17.19 shows a radiograph taken to test the half-value layer.

7   Exposure factors which are suggested are set out below in Table 17.2.
   There are some points about these exposure factors to be noted as follows.

Table 17.2

Region of the cassette	Focus-film distance	kV setting	mA	Time in seconds
A 60 kVp	50 cm (20 inches)	60	100	1·0
B 80 kVp	100 cm (40 inches)	80	100	0·5
C 100 kVp	100 cm (40 inches)	100	100	0·12
D 120 kVp	100 cm (40 inches)	120	100	0·04
HVL	100 cm (40 inches)	60	100	0·03

(a) The milliamperage and the times should be set to give values of milliampereseconds which are as close as possible to those in the table.

(b) In the resultant radiograph (see Fig. 17.18) the density of the circles in the right-hand column of each pair (which is considered as a reference column) should be between 0·5 and 2·0. If the density is outside this range, then the cassette should be re-loaded and the test should be repeated with an increase in the milliampereseconds-values if the density is less than 0·5 and a decrease in the milliampereseconds-values if the density is more than 2·0.

(c) The milliampereseconds-values which are to be used for three-phase generators should be half those which are used with single-phase units because a three-phase generator gives a higher radiographic output for every kilovolt and milliampere used. This is a result of the rippling voltage waveform which is applied to the X-ray tube and enables it to produce useful X rays throughout the cycle of the alternating mains supply. Such a condition of operation is to be contrasted with the pulsating voltage waveform from a single phase generator in which the voltage falls from the peak kilovoltage and reaches zero on three occasions in the period of one full cycle of mains alternation.

(d) The milliampereseconds-value for the half value layer test which is undertaken at 60 kVp is much lower than that given for the test of the 60 kVp setting itself. The explanation for this lies in the copper sheet which covers the 60 kVp to 120 kVp stepwedge absorbers but does not cover the stepwedge in the half-value layer region of the cassette. The beam of radiation reaching the film in the half-value layer region has not had the range of energies of its photons narrowed by the removal of those photons which have low energy. There are therefore more photons (that is, greater intensity of radiation) reaching the film in that area of the cassette than in the other four regions of measurement.

Interpreting the results of the test

When the film has been processed, it is viewed to determine the results of the test. As can be seen in Fig. 17.18 the radiograph shows a series of circles of density arranged in columns. Across the top the letters A (60 kVp region), B (80 kVp region), C (100 kVp region), D (120 kVp region) indicate the regions of the cassette which are available for the tests of kilovoltage.

It can be seen that the circles are arranged, as would be expected from a description of the cassette, in paired columns, one pair in each region of the cassette. The right-hand column of each pair shows circles with no change of density and is considered to be the reference column: the circles of density are produced through the optical attenuator which modifies the light from the single intensifying screen in the cassette. The left-hand column in each pair shows circles of density produced through the copper stepwedges which attenuate the X-ray beam and these show a range of diminishing densities down each column.

A feature of the radiograph shown in Fig. 17.18 to the viewer's left hand is a column of circular densities labelled 1 to 10 downwards. The figures indicate the ten steps of each of the copper stepwedge absorbers which are in the cassette over the left-hand columns in the A, B, C, D and HVL regions. It is obvious from the radiograph that step 1 is the thin end and step 10 is the thick end of each copper stepwedge.

To interpret the radiograph you should take each of the pairs of columns in turn. With the aid of a densitometer, measure densities and locate in the paired columns the step where a circle in the left-hand column has a density to match that of the adjacent circle in the right-hand column. This has been done for sections A, B and C in Fig. 17.18.

It can be seen that in section A step 4 produced the matched density, in section B step 5 gave the match and in section C step 6 is the level of the circles which match. If there is no densitometer, the circles must be matched by eye and this clearly introduces subjective variables which must affect the accuracy of the result. The manufacturers of the Wisconsin test cassette say that the visual assessment is approximate at plus/minus 3 kVp: good viewing conditions and visual acuity in the assessor must be presumed.

When the match-step has been determined, a calibration curve supplied by the manufacturers is consulted. Typical samples are shown in Figs 17.20 and 17.21: in them the broken lines give the curves for three-phase generators and the solid lines are the curves for single-phase generators. On the left of the graph, locate your match-step number and then on that line proceed across the graph until there is intersection with the calibration curve appropriate to the unit which you are testing. From the point of intersection, drop a line straight down to the kVp axis (or HVL axis, if that

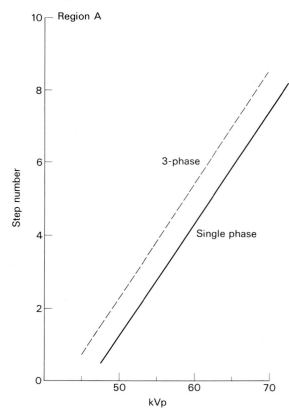

Fig. 17.20

is what you are measuring) at the foot of the graph. This determines for you the kilovoltage (or half-value layer) existing when the exposure was made.

If in any of the paired columns there is no density match, you should note the steps between which the match may be assumed to occur. It is then possible to make accurate interpolation with the aid of data supplied by the manufacturers. This interpolation involves measuring densities and applying a formula. If your assessment of density is merely visual you cannot apply a formula since you have no figures on which to calculate. In that case assume that the match-step number is at a half-way point between integral step numbers. For example, if the match appears to occur between step number 7 and step number 8, take it that the actual match-step number is 7.5 and locate that point on the step-number axes of the calibration curves which are used.

Each Wisconsin test cassette is calibrated by the manufacturers against their master cassette and comes to the user with calibration data as indicated in previous paragraphs. This information relates the step numbers at which

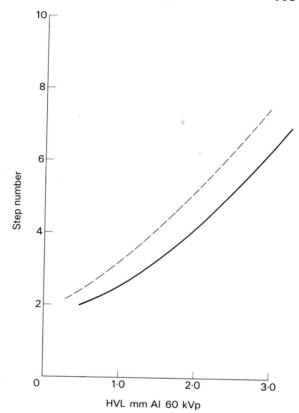

Step number

HVL mm Al 60 kVp

Fig. 17.21

matches occur to the actual kilovoltages across the X-ray tube at each of the four settings displayed on the cassette and in the fifth section to the half-value layer at 60 kVp in millimetres of aluminium.

Acceptable limits of variation

The manufacturers of the Wisconsin test cassette suggest that acceptable variations in kilovoltage from the selected values are less than 5 kVp at the 60 kVp and 80 kVp settings and less than 8 kVp at the 100 kVp and 120 kVp settings.

A half-value layer finding that is low (say, about 1·0 mm of aluminium) suggests that the added aluminium filtration which is required for the protection of patients is no longer in place. A half-value layer that is high (say, 3·0 mm of aluminium) suggests that an ageing X-ray tube is near the end of its useful life.

Testing for maintenance of kilovoltage

The controls of X-ray sets include one for the selection of kilovoltage. The settings of the selector have accompanying indications of the kilovoltages expected to be available across the X-ray tube when radiographic exposures are made. The indications may be by a pre-reading kilovolt meter or on a calibrated illuminated panel or by a digital display or other markings. Each setting of the control results in an indication of the kilovoltage which it is expected to give. All the methods of indication provide pre-exposure advice of the kilovoltage and none of them directly measures and shows the actual kilovoltage which is across the X-ray tube when the exposure is made.

The kilovoltage for an X-ray tube comes from the high tension transformer in the generator which provides the power. For this high tension transformer there is an important difference between its pre-exposure state and its condition while the exposure is taking place: this difference is that during the exposure the transformer is on load, providing power to the X-ray tube, and a load current is flowing in the transformer windings and the tube circuit. In the pre-exposure state the transformer is in a 'no load' condition and there is no load current through its windings.

When the load current flows, a voltage drop occurs on the high tension transformer. This voltage drop under load takes place because the current must flow through the ohmic resistance of the windings and some voltage is required to make it do this. This required voltage is the voltage drop under load and its magnitude is related to the load current: so it increases as the load current (which is the current through the X-ray tube) is raised.

From this it follows that any given setting of the kilovoltage selector may provide for the X-ray tube a kilovoltage which becomes lower in value for each increase in the selected milliamperes. Compensation for this effect can be arranged within the circuitry of the X-ray set: the generator is provided with an additional voltage to match the voltage drop which occurs when the load current flows. This compensation is called variously the *kilovoltage compensation*, the *milliamperage calibration* or simply the *calibration* of the generator.

If the compensating voltages actually match the voltage drops which occur, then the kilovoltage available from any given setting of the selector is maintained over the whole range of milliampere settings which is used. If the compensating voltage does not match the voltage drop that occurs at any selected milliamperes, then the kilovoltage will be lower (undercompensation) or higher (over-compensation) than it should be. A kilovoltage that is correctly maintained through all milliampere settings is essential to assure the quality of the radiographic result. The selection of appropriate kilovoltages is the most important control of contrast in the image which can be varied by the radiographer.

In monitoring the performance of an X-ray set, one of the tests to be made is to check the effectiveness of the kilovoltage compensation for the high tension generator which the controls provide. This might be done as a routine once a year and of course should be done as soon as there is any reason to suspect that the compensating voltage is not correctly matched to the voltage drops which are occurring in the range of milliamperes to be used.

Tests to be used must provide the answer to this question: is the kilovoltage available from a particular setting of the selector satisfactorily maintained when the milliamperes are raised and is it reasonably constant through the range of tube currents which is most commonly used? Undoubtedly the most precise answer to such questions is given when the kilovoltage which exists across the tube for the exposure is measured by means of a test cassette as described in the previous section. To use the Wisconsin test cassette to investigate the maintenance of kilovoltage, the procedure is as follows.

1 The test cassette, loaded with film, is placed on the X-ray table with the long sides of the cassette parallel to the anode-cathode axis of the X-ray tube.

2 Each kilovoltage region of the cassette will be exposed in turn, the rest being shielded with lead of thickness adequate to provide a screen at the highest kilovoltage to be tested (at least 2·00 mm are required). The X-ray tube is centred to each region in turn and the collimator is set so that the beam just covers completely the region in use.

3 The line voltage compensator is carefully set, together with other factors of the several exposures as indicated below and in Table 17.3.

4 A series of separate exposures is made as shown in Table 17.3. For each film the A, B, C regions of the cassette are exposed and the cassette is reloaded with fresh film for the second, third and fourth sets of 3 exposures. The end result is four radiographs, one for each of the following milliampere settings: 100, 200, 400 and 500. The suggested exposure factors are appropriate to three phase generators. The milliampereseconds should be doubled for single phase X-ray sets. It will be realized from a study of Table 17.3 that in the series of exposures 1, 4, 7 and 10 test the 60 kV setting at 100 mA, 200 mA, 400 mA and 500 mA at a constant milliampereseconds value of 100; exposures 2, 5, 8 and 11 test the 80 kV setting at the same several milliamperages with a constant milliampereseconds value of 50; exposures 3, 6, 9 and 12 test the 100 kV setting at a constant milliampereseconds value of 12 through the same range of milliamperes. The exposures can be made to cover any series of milliamperes which are commonly used

Table 17.3

Exposure number	Region of cassette	Focus-film distance (cm)	kV setting	mA setting	Time in seconds
First loading					
1	A 60kV	50	60	100	1·0
2	B 80 kV	100	80	100	0·5
3	C 100 kV	100	100	100	0·12
Second loading					
4	A 60 kV	50	60	200	0·5
5	B 80 kV	100	80	200	0·25
6	C 100 kV	100	100	200	0·06
Third loading					
7	A 60 kV	50	60	400	0·25
8	B 80 kV	100	80	400	0·125
9	C 100 kV	100	100	400	0·03
Fourth loading					
10	A 60 kV	50	60	500	0·2
11	B 80 kV	100	80	500	0·1
12	C 100 kV	100	100	500	0·024
Loading to test 120 kV if wished					
13	D 120 kV	100	120	100	0·24
14	D 120 kV	100	120	200	0·02
15	D 120 kV	100	120	400	0·01
16	D 120 kV	100	120	500	0·008

on the X-ray generator under test. The milliampereseconds values should be maintained throughout the test close to the values suggested here. Alteration in them does not affect the validity of the result, for the test cassette does not have its accuracy affected by a change in milliampereseconds. The milliampereseconds value does of course affect the density of the circles in the right-hand columns in the resultant radiographs. These reference columns should have a density which is between 0·5 and 2·0. It is relative to this density that the selection of milliampereseconds is significant.

5 The actual kilovoltage values available on the different settings can be checked by interpreting the processed radiographs as explained on p. 599. The 120 kV setting has been left out of the test described since it is not so commonly used. It could of course be included in each of the four exposure groups and suggestions are made for this at the foot of Table 17.3. However, if the X-ray set performs consistently over the range 60–100 kV, it is reasonable to assume that kilovoltage settings outside this range are also acceptably without variation.

Measurement of the focal spot of an X-ray tube

The effective size of the focal spot of an X-ray tube is important to the radiographic image. It is a factor in determining the extent in the image of the penumbra: that is, of the area of half-shadow which surrounds each structural detail in the image and contributes to unsharpness of outline. Penumbra increases in magnitude with greater focal spot area, if other conditions remain unchanged.

A manufacturer who supplies an X-ray tube makes a statement on its focal spots, assigning to each a nominal effective size: for example, a dual focus tube may have a broad focus stated to be 2·0 mm and a fine focus given as 1·0 mm. Tests of an X-ray tube's performance in the X-ray department should include one to assess the effective sizes of the focal spots, checking them against the manufacturer's statements. Such testing repeated at intervals throughout the working life of the tube allows the states of its focal spots to be monitored.

Using a pinhole camera

It is possible to produce a radiograph to show the projected focal spot of an X-ray tube by making use of the pinhole camera principle. Fig. 17.22 illustrates in simple terms how an image is formed by a pin-hole. Its

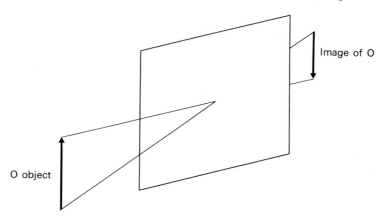

Image of O

O object

Fig. 17.22   The formation of an image by a pinhole.

production is seen to depend upon the fact that light travels in straight lines. From the triangular geometry of the system two other facts are readily apparent:

1   the further away from the pin-hole is the object O, the smaller will be its image, and conversely;

2   the ratio **object-size/image-size** is equal to the ratio **distance of object from pinhole/distance of image from pinhole**.

We can now go even further and state that if we have a system in which the object-distance (from pin-hole) is the same as the image-distance (from pin-hole) then the dimensions of the image are the same as those of the object.

X rays share with light the characteristic of travelling in straight lines and we can use a pin-pole to produce an X-ray image in a manner exactly similar to the one just depicted and described in terms of light.

In Fig. 17.23 A is the target area of an X-ray tube; it is shown as having a stationary anode for the sake of simplicity. Below the X-ray tube is a sheet

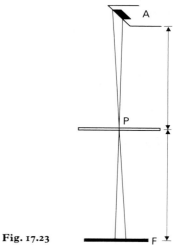

Fig. 17.23

of lead in which there is a pinhole P. Below this again is a film F and the vertical distances AP and PF are equal. From the diagram we can see that if an X-ray exposure is made the film will record an image of the apparent focal area of the tube and that this image will be a true representation of the focal spot's effective dimensions.

The drawings have depicted a pin-hole without finite size. In practice, however small we make the pin-hole, it is bound to have a finite area of its own. This influences the experimental result, for the geometry is such that the linear dimensions which we take from the radiograph are too great by twice the diameter of the pin-hole.

To be accurate in this we would need to know the diameter of the pin-hole and make the necessary deductions from the area of the image. Other physical considerations are also important and the conditions necessary for precise focal spot measurement have been studied and published (1960) by a subcommittee of the International Commission of Radiological Units and Measurements. This defined—among other matters—the diameter of the pin-hole appropriate to a certain focal spot size, the thickness and material of the diaphragm (gold-platinum alloy), the length and precise shape of the pin-hole, the type of film used for the record (dental film), the density of the image and even the strength of the illumination against which it is to be viewed. It is no simple matter, for decision by a random pin-sticking! In fact we can say that, while it is easy to obtain a picture of the effective focal area of an X-ray tube, it is very much more difficult to take correct measurements from it.

Radiographs as shown in Fig. 17.24 are easily obtained by covering the

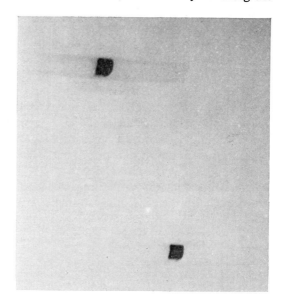

Fig. 17.24 Pinhole radiographs of effective focal areas.

portal of the X-ray tube with a piece of lead which is 2·0 mm thick and has pierced in it a small pinhole which is placed to be in the centre of the X-ray field. Through the pinhole, the radiographic exposures are made with the X-ray beam emerging through the pinhole at right angles to the film which is put on the X-ray table. The sheet of lead is at a distance from the film which is estimated to be half the distance separating the tube focus from the film.

The radiographs shown in Fig. 17.24 certainly depict the focal spots of X-ray tubes. The depictions give no better indication of the sizes than would a map drawn free-hand and without scale tell you how far you must walk in going from Birmingham to Brighton Pier.

Generally speaking, when a radiographer obtains a pin-hole radiograph of a tube in use in the department, the intention is less to discover exactly the effective size of the X-ray source than to know if the target area is in normal working condition. Distortion of the target, due to pitting of the tungsten as a result of overheating, will be seen on the radiograph of the anode because in this case X-rays are produced not from a single nearpoint source but from a number of irregular sources formed by cavities and prominences in the metal. It is not difficult either to take or to interpret such 'pictures'.

A pin-hole radiograph is sometimes employed to locate the target area accurately in the tube-shield—or rather to enable an accurate deduction to be made of the anode-film distance. (This information must be obtained with exactness for such radiographic procedures as the depth-localization of foreign bodies or even for the accurate measurement of effective focal area by radiographic tests as here described.)

For this purpose the diaphragm placed between the tube and the film must now have two pin-holes which are a known distance apart. These are represented in Fig. 17.25 by P_1 and P_2 and the images which they produce on the film respectively by F_1 and F_2. The distance P_1P_2 is physically measurable on the surface of the lead or other absorber; the distance F_1F_2 can be similarly obtained from the radiograph. Also determinable by direct measurement is the vertical height of the lead sheet above the film, indicated in the diagram by the arrow VH.

The experimental procedure is depicted in more geometric form in Fig. 17.26 but with the same diagrammatic lettering. We can see that what we

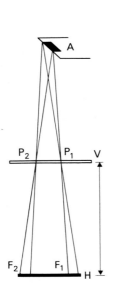

Fig. 17.25

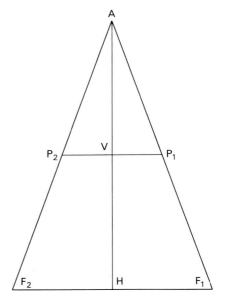

Fig. 17.26

wish to discover is the length of the line AV, since it gives the anode-film distance (AV + VH). Because the smaller and the larger triangles are similar, their side and heights have equal ratios.

Therefore we can say that,

$$\frac{AV + VH}{AV} = \frac{F_1 F_2}{P_1 P_2}$$

Except for AV, the other factors in this expression, as we have seen, are known and measurable with whatever degree of accuracy may be required. Suitable pinhole cameras can be obtained from the manufacturers and marketers of test tools. When pinhole cameras are correctly used in exact conditions, information may be obtained as to the size, shape and location of the focal spot.

Using the Wisconsin test tool

Test tools are available for convenient checks on the focal spot size alone of X-ray tubes and the choice of suitable tools allows radiographers to make such tests easily. One such tool is the Wisconsin focal spot test tool which can be used to measure the effective sizes of focal spots from a stated 0·3 mm to a stated 2·4 mm.

The tool is shown in Fig. 17.27. Its heart is a disc of plexiglass which is 7·62 cm (3 inches) in diameter and bears at its centre a test pattern in a target of heavy metal: in the checks, radiographs of this test pattern are made. The plexiglass disc incorporates a lead shield which sometimes has two small holes which are 3 cm apart: these can be used, as explained below, to locate the position of the tube focus as the X-ray source at a distance above the film. The pattern is 15·2 cm (6 inches) above the base of the tool.

Figure 17.28 is a radiograph of the test pattern. The pattern is made by slots in a radiopaque metal which reproduce in the radiograph as black bars of density where the radiation is transmitted. The white strips between the bars result from the attenuation achieved by the heavy metal in which the slots are set.

As can be seen in Fig. 17.28, there are 11 groups of bars. Fig. 17.29 is a diagram of the group numbered 1. It shows that there are 6 black bars in each group, arranged in trios which are at right angles. The 11 groups of bars become smaller in size, reduced both in length and in breadth as the serial numbers of the group rise. The spacing of the slots for the group numbered 1 is 0·84 line pairs (a black bar and a white strip) per millimetre and for the group numbered 11 the spacing is 4.76 line pairs per millimetre.

Chapter 17

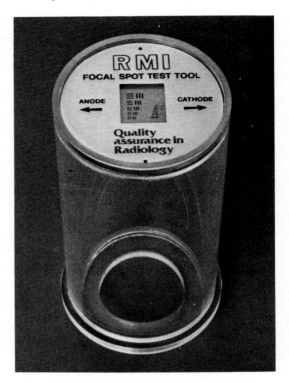

Fig. 17.27

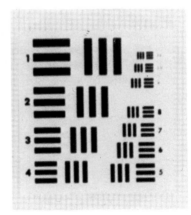

Fig. 17.28

The procedure for testing an overtable tube

The procedure for using the Wisconsin test tool to determine the effective size of the focal spot of an overtable X-ray tube is as follows.

1   Take an X-ray film held in a cassette or pack which is without intensifying

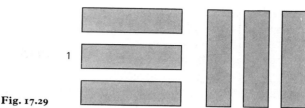

Fig. 17.29

screens: it might be, for example, a direct exposure film for the examination of extremities, a dental film for use in the occlusal plane (57 mm × 76 mm) or a film for mammography.

2 Place the film in its light-tight holder on the X-ray table, tube aspect uppermost, and put the tool directly on the film-holder. Turn the tool so that the horizontal bar groups (those are the ones nearest the identifying numbers in the test pattern) are along the anode-cathode axis of the X-ray tube. Attention to this point ensures that the orientation for the focal spot test pattern is standardized. This aids comparison among the results of tests made at different times.

3 Centre the X-ray tube with the beam at 90 degrees to the film directly over the tool and adjust the collimator so that the tool is just covered.

4 Adjust the tube height so that the focal spot to film distance is exactly 70 cm (24 inches). Since the pattern is 15·2 cm (6 inches) above the base of the tool, the focal spot to pattern distance is 54·8 cm (18 inches). This gives a magnification factor of 4/3 or 1·33.

5 On the control console, select factors at commonly used kilovoltage and milliampere settings to give about 10 mAs. Typical settings might be 80 kVp, 200 mA and 0·05 second. For uniform results, in any tests maintained over a period of time as a continuous assessment of an X-ray tube, the same settings must be used for all the tests. Focal spot size may change with kilovoltage and milliamperage. It is easy to show such a change by means of this test tool if two separate exposures are made on separate films: make one at 80 kVp, 100 mA and 0·1 second and the other at the highest tube current available from the selector with the time adjusted to give 10 mAs.

6 Make a radiographic exposure.

7 Process the film the view the result.

Interpreting the result

If they are present in the tool that you are using, look first at the images of the two small holes in the lead shield of the tool. The holes are 3 cm apart and since the magnification factor is 4/3 (i.e. 1·33) the images should be 4 cm apart. If the images of the holes as shown in the test radiograph are in fact

4 cm apart, then you know that the focal spot to film distance was in fact 70 cm: that is that the indicated setting on the tubestand is truthful.

If the image size is smaller than the expected 4 cm spacing between the black spots, then the magnification is less than 1·33. For example, an image spacing of 3·5 cm gives a magnification of 3·5/3, that is 1·1. This smaller magnification means that the 70 cm setting on the tubestand was in fact giving a focus-film distance greater than 70 cm. If the image spacing is longer than 4 cm, then the magnification is greater than 1·33: for example, a 5 cm image gives a magnification of 5/3 which is 1·6 times. This greater magnification indicates that the tube to film distance is less than the 70 cm which are set.

If the distance setting on the tubestand proves to be untruthful you must correct it empirically: that is, you must lower or raise the tube on its tubestand and make test radiographs of the tool until you find that the images of the pinholes are 4 cm apart. For future use, note at what setting on the tubestand indicator the true distance of 70 cm was obtained. The difference between this and 70 cm is the extent of the error and if it is greater than 1·4 cm at 70 cm distance then it should be corrected: 1·4 cm is a 2 per cent error on 70 cm.

With that point (or those pin points!) settled, the next step is to interpret the images of the groups of bars. This is simply done. You find the smallest group in which you can see distinct images of all six black bars in a group. Disregard those in which you see 2 or 4 bars in a group of 3 or in which you find that the bars are not separately distinguishable as clear black bars. Note the identifying number of the smallest group of 6 black bars which are clearly resolved and then from the information provided establish the largest dimension of the focal spot (see Table 17.4).

Table 17.4

Smallest group resolved	Line pairs per millimetre	Magnification = 4/3 Largest dimension of focal spot (mm)
1	0·84	2·4 mm
2	1·00	2·00 mm
3	1·19	1·8 mm
4	1·41	1·4 mm
5	1·68	1·2 mm
6	2·00	1·0 mm
7	2·38	0·8 mm
8	2·83	0·7 mm
9	3·36	0·9 mm
10	4·00	0·5 mm
11	4·76	0·4 mm

Errors may be present in this test because the sizes of the groups of bars change in separate distinct steps and not as a continuous progression of change. The error can be as large as 16 per cent.

Procedure for testing an undertable X-ray tube

The Wisconsin test tool can be used to check the effective focal spot size of an X-ray tube used in a fluoroscopic system. In describing the procedure, we are assuming a conventional arrangement in which the tube is beneath the X-ray table and the image intensifier and its recording system are above the table.

A crucial point is the distance between the focal spot of the undertable tube and the table-top. It is an important factor for the magnification in the image obtained when the test tool is radiographed. If the focus to table-top distance can be assumed to be 46 cm (18 inches), when the test tool is placed on the table with its target and bar pattern in contact with the table-top and the film at the base of the tool (see Fig. 17.30) the magnification is 4/3 as when the overtable tube is being tested. This magnification is a standard condition for the test and allows the results to be interpreted in accordance with the published tables. If the focus to table-top distance is longer than 46 cm (18 inches) the magnification becomes less and if this distance is shorter than 46 cm (18 inches) the magnification becomes greater. The procedure for the test is as follows.

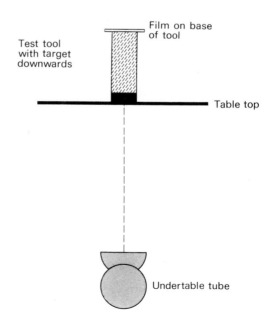

Fig. 17.30

1 Place the test tool upside down on the X-ray table. Its metal plate with the bar pattern is then in direct contact with the table-top and it should be positioned to the centre-line of the table.

2 Centre the fluoroscopic unit over the tool.

3 Adjust the diaphragms of the undertable tube until the X-ray beam just covers the face of the tool and its bar pattern.

4 Take an X-ray film held in a cassette or pack which is without intensifying screens. For example, it might be a direct exposure film for radiography of the extremities, a film to be used for mammography, a dental film for use in the occlusal plane (57 mm × 76 mm).

5 Position the film in its light-tight holder on the base of the tool. The base is now uppermost as shown in the diagram in Fig. 17.30.

6 On the control console set radiographic exposure factors for the undertable tube as follows:

80 kV   8 mAs (approximately)

For uniform results, in any tests maintained over a period of time as a continuous assessment of an X-ray tube the same settings must be used for all the tests.

7 Make the radiographic exposure

8 Process the film and view the result.

Interpreting the result

A radiograph made with the undertable tube to show an image of the test tool is interpreted as is one made with an overtable tube. You should find the smallest group of bars in which you can see distinct images of all six black bars in the group. Disregard those in which you see 2 or 4 bars in a group of 3 or in which you find that the bars are not separately distinguishable as clear black bars. Note the identifying number of the smallest group of six black bars which are resolved and then from the information provided (see Table 17.4) establish the largest dimension of the focal spot.

If the two small holes previously mentioned are present in the target of the tool, you can check whether your test conditions do in fact give the stipulated 4/3 magnification. The holes are 3 cm apart and the images should be 4 cm apart if the standard conditions have been applied: that is, with the focus of the X-ray tube 46 cm (18 inches) from the table-top, with the tool upside down on the table and with the film resting on the upturned base of the tool. If the images are more than 4 cm apart, the focus of the X-ray tube can be presumed to be closer to the table top than at a distance of 46 cm (18 inches). If the images are less than 4 cm apart, the tube focus is presumably further than 46 cm (18 inches) from the table-top. Because the bar group sizes change by discrete steps, the error in this test may be as large as 16 per cent.

Testing the light beam diaphragm

If it is suspected that the mirror in a beam delineator is out of adjustment (see Chapter 8, page 306) proof of misalignment can easily be obtained by either of the following tests.

Method 1

An empty cassette is placed open beneath the suspected X-ray tube which is then centred over one of the exposed intensifying screens. Choose the one which is at the front of the cassette. The diaphragms are adjusted to produce any appropriate field of radiation which is smaller than the area of the intensifying screen.

The delineator's lamp is then switched on and the edges of the light beam carefully outlined by means of some suitable markers; for example, a row of paper clips may be arranged along the edges of the field or—if the department possesses a tool kit—a number of Allen keys are useful implements for this purpose.

Afterwards the radiographer should withdraw from the vicinity of the X-ray table and use the footswitch to energize the X-ray tube at a fluoroscopic value of current. It is then easy to observe whether the fluorescing area on the intensifying screen coincides—or fails to coincide—with the positions of the markers. The presence, extent and direction of any misalignment are made obvious.

Method 2

This is an alternative method of making the test which avoids the use of a fluoroscopic footswitch in the event of the X-ray installation concerned not offering this facility.

In this case a loaded cassette is placed as usual beneath the X-ray tube; the latter is centred upon the cassette and the diaphragms are closed sufficiently to provide a radiation field which can be contained within the area of the film. As before, the delineator's lamp is switched on and the edges of the light field are defined with radio-opaque markers.

A radiographic exposure is then made and the film processed; the exposure should be such as to produce a visible density on the film without over-penetration of the markers. The positions of the two fields can then be compared by observation of the resultant radiograph (Fig. 17.31).

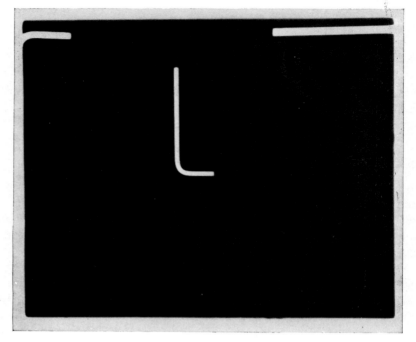

Fig. 17. 31 A light beam diaphragm which is incorrectly adjusted.

The fitting of the mirror in a light beam diaphragm is such that its position can be altered by means of a screw. It is not a difficult adjustment, although the screw is not accessible without removal of the delineator from the tubehead.

Tests to be made of tomographic equipment

Special radiographic tests may be made of tomographic equipment to check whether the system is functioning effectively to give the expected results. Answers to the following questions may be sought.

1 Is the location of the cut layer recorded in the subject at the same height above the film or depth in the subject as the control setting is said to give?

2 How thick is the layer which is sharply recorded?

3 What is the path taken by the beam during the exposure?

4 What is the overall resolution in the recorded layer?

5 Is the exposure uniform throughout the time of the tube travel?

Test tools are available which can provide answers to all these questions and we describe one later in this chapter. Not every radiographer has access to such a tool so let us first consider simple 'home-made' devices which might be used to confirm the levels and the thicknesses of tomographic layers.

It is suggested that student readers should construct their own phantoms for this purpose, using a cardboard box, a sharp pencil, a ruler scaled in centimetres and a collection of straight pins. Cardboard boxes are usually readily available in an X-ray department and an empty film box will serve this occasion very well. The experimental procedure is given below.

1   On one long edge of the box, upwards from the base, draw a vertical line—say 12 cm in length.

2   Indicate centimetre intervals on this by pushing one pin through the card at the height of the first centimetre, two pins at 2 cm, three pins at 3 cm and so in similar progression up to the full height of the line. This arrangement is shown in Fig. 17.32. The horizontal rows of pins should be

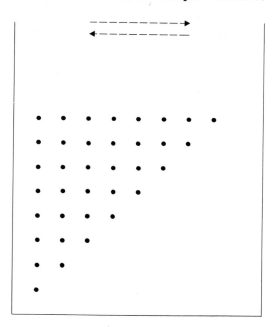

Fig. 17.32   A phantom which can be constructed from pins and a cardboard box and used for testing the accuracy of the determination of tomographic planes.

placed carefully so that they are parallel to the base of the box and to each other. It is convenient to make the horizontal spacing between the pins also 1 cm.

3   Place the assembly on the tomographic table and take a number of tomographs at any desired levels. The tube movement—if linear—should be in the direction indicated by the arrows in the sketch; that is, at right angles to the axes of the pins, in order to obtain maximum blurring of their shadows at levels above and below the selected one.

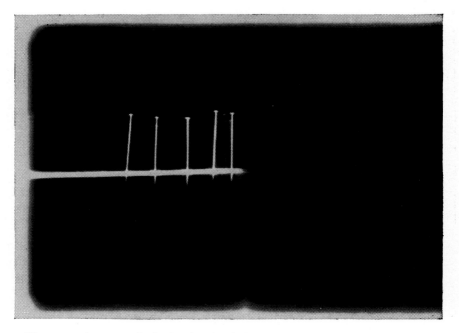

Fig. 17.33 A tomograph of a pin-phantom showing the determination of a tomographic plane.

4 Process and examine the films obtained. On any one of them, the number of pins to be seen most sharply gives the height above the table of the sectioned plane. Again, it should of course coincide with the height previously determined and selected by the operator. A radiograph obtained in this way is shown in Fig. 17.33.

A somewhat similar experiment with pins can be performed to show the thickness of the sharp layer obtained (see Chapter 13) by any given tomographic apparatus at different angles of exposure (tube swing). For this a single row of pins is constructed likewise in a box. The pins are arranged in a slanting line at vertical levels which differ by not more than 2 mm; a separation of 1 mm would be more satisfiactory but is practically so finicking a matter that we recommend it only for the slender fingered. Fig. 17.34 depicts the arrangement of the pins at different heights.

Two tomographs at least are taken, for one of which a narrow angle of exposure (25 degrees) is used and for the other a wider angle of exposure (50 degrees). When the radiographs are processed and viewed the number

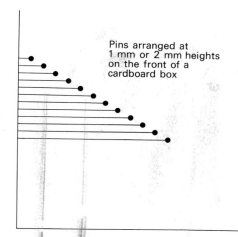

Pins arranged at
1 mm or 2 mm heights
on the front of a
cardboard box

Fig. 17.34 A pin-phantom
for determining the thickness
of any selected tomographic
layer.

of pins seen to be sharp indicates the thickness in millimetres of the section
obtained (see Fig. 17.35). In making this experiment the height of the
selected plane should be such as to cut the line of pins in the region of the
half-way mark. This will ensure that pins are 'available' for recording on
the film and avoid the possibility of the plane of interest lying partly beyond
the extremes of the line.

A tomographic test tool

An available tool for trials of tomographic equipment enables radiographs
to be made which test the following:
1 the accuracy of layer-level selection (location of the fulcrum height);
2 the thickness of the recorded layer;
3 the resolving capability of the system;
4 the trajectory of the X-ray tube and the uniformity of exposure during
its journey.

The tool about to be described comprises the following items:
1 a plastic tomographic phantom;
2 a steel plate with a small hole in its centre;
3 two sets of metal spacers, one of the sets providing a spacing of 10 cm
and the second set giving a spacing of 15 cm.

Plastic tomographic phantom

The plastic tomographic phantom is a square of sides 15 cm and it is 2·2 cm
thick. Embedded in its centre are 4 copper mesh strips which are arranged
side by side as indicated in the diagram in Fig. 17.36. Each strip is 1·2 cm

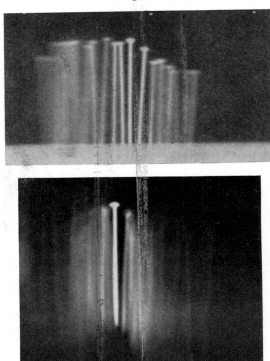

Fig. 17.35 Tomographs of a pin-phantom which show the thickness of tomographic planes.

wide and 5 cm long and their meshes are different, each strip being individual in its mesh. The four pitches of the holes are 0·8 holes/mm, 1·2 holes/mm, 1·6 holes/mm and 2·0 holes/mm. Each strip has a different pitch.

These strips serve as a test for the resolving capability of the tomographic system which is under trial. Along their length, the strips lie at an inclined plane such that each has its top edge about 12 mm or so above the base of the phantom and its lower edge about 1·0 mm or so above the base of the phantom.

Round the copper strips is a helix of lead numbers which are embedded in the plastic phantom as indicated in Figs. 17.36 and 17.37. The numbers are 1 to 12 and the helix ascends within the plastic from the numeral 1 which is 1 mm above the base to the numeral 12 which is 12 mm above the base of the phantom. It can be appreciated that each numeral is approximately at a height above the base of the tool which is shown by the digital values. These numbers are used for locating the fulcrum height and indicating the layer thickness which is obtained.

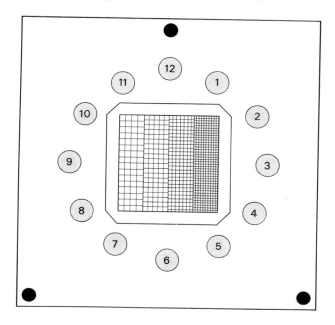

Fig. 17.36

The aperture plate

The steel plate matches the plastic phantom in its surface area, being a square of side 15 cm. It is 1 mm thick and the hole at its centre is 3·0 mm in diameter. This plate is used to show the trajectory of the X-ray tube and the uniformity of exposure during the tomographic movement.

The metal spacers

The metal spacers are rods which serve as supports or 'legs' for the phantom or the steel plate (see Fig. 17.37). One set consists of three rods in length 10 cm. The other set is three rods which are like those in the first set but are longer, being 15 cm in length.

Using the test tool

In order to use the test tool, there are certain requirements for setting up the trial as follows.

1 There should be an absorber to represent the patient and this phantom-patient is set up on the X-ray table to undergo tomographic examination. The 'patient' might be a commercially available phantom or something provided by hospital workshops: for example, a square block of aluminium

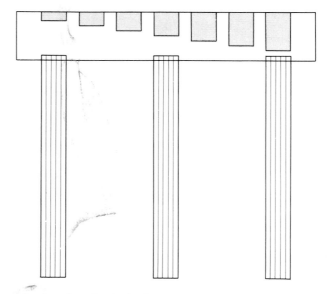

Fig. 17.37 A sketch to show the plastic phantom as seen from the side when mounted on the three 10 cm spacers.

of 2·5 cm thickness and sides 23 cm long. In our later description of the tests we call this the aluminium absorber.

2 Exposure factors should be selected to give an average density in the image which is between 0·5 and 1·2 when the plastic phantom is radiographed: and between 0·6 and 1·3 when the plate with the aperture is used. The appropriate settings for the exposure factors must be determined empirically having regard to the absorber and the equipment used. Once established, the exposure factors should be recorded.

3 The tests should be carried out in the condition which is most demanding for the equipment: that is, with the fastest sweep. After that, other conditions may be tested.

To test the location of the fulcrum layer

To test the location of the fulcrum layer by means of this test tool in conjunction with an aluminium absorber, you should proceed as follows.

1 Place the aluminium absorber on top of the tomographic table, setting it in position for tomography.

2 Screw the 10 cm spacers into the plastic phantom and set the phantom mounted on these legs over the aluminium absorber. Since it is on 10 cm legs the plastic phantom now has its base 10 cm above the aluminium absorber.

3   Measure the distance from the table to the bottom of the plastic phantom and add 7·5 mm (the level of the lead number 7). Then set the fulcrum control to that setting. In Fig. 17.38 we have assumed an aluminium absorber which is 2·5 cm thick. In this case the bottom of the plastic phantom on its 10 cm legs is

$$10 + 2\cdot5 = 12\cdot5 \text{ cm } (125 \text{ mm}) \text{ above the table top}$$
$$125 \text{ mm} + 7\cdot5 \text{ mm} = 132\cdot5 \text{ mm}$$

So here the setting for the control should be 132·5 mm (13·25 cm).

4   Operate the equipment to make a tomograph of the plastic phantom, setting the controls for a large angle of exposure and a thin layer. If it proves difficult to see the centre of the field as shown by an indicator which is a light beam, a piece of white paper placed on top of the plastic phantom makes the delineation easy.

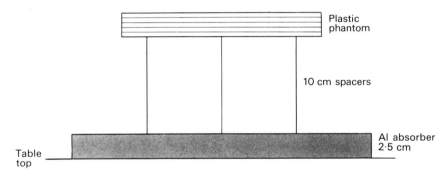

Fig. 17.38

5   Process the film and inspect the resultant radiograph. The figure 7 should be clearly seen, figures 4 and 9 should be somewhat blurred and figures 1 and 12 should be very blurred. Errors within 1 mm for pluridirectional movement and within 3 mm for linear tomographic attachments can be accepted.

To demonstrate the thickness of layer

A radiograph obtained in a test for the location of layer height can be used also if layer thickness is to be checked. The lead digits are each separated by 1 mm as they ascend successively above the table, so the number of them that is acceptably sharp indicates the layer thickness. Supposing that the digits which are acceptably sharp are 6, 7 and 8, with 5 and 9 blurred, then the layer is 2 mm thick: if the sharply recorded numerals are 5, 6, 7, 8 and 9 with 4 and 10 blurred, then the layer is 4·0 mm thick.

Overall resolution

In a tomograph made of the plastic phantom there is an image of the four strips of wire mesh which are embedded in the plastic. Satisfactory conditions can be taken as the resolution of 3 mm or more of the length of the strip which has 1·6 holes/mm as its mesh. If about 3·0 mm in length of the mesh with 2·0 holes/mm are resolved, the equipment gives excellent resolution. If the equipment cannot resolve the two coarse meshes of 1·2 holes/mm and 0·8 holes/mm, it certainly will not resolve fine structural details within a patient's anatomy and its usefulness is to be seriously questioned.

Interpretation of Figure 17.39

Figure 17.39 is a radiograph of the plastic phantom with its helix of numbers round the four wire meshes, the coarsest of which is to the viewer's left. The absorber used to make this radiograph was not a block of aluminium. It was a very simple and cheap equivalent of an aluminium absorber and was a plastic lidded box which had held 2 litres of icecream. With the icecream all eaten, the box was filled with tap water to which was added 100 ml of an iodine-constituted positive contrast agent as used for urography. This proved a satisfactory absorber and the lid accomodated the plastic phantom standing on the three 10 cm spacers as described for the test. It was set up to record in a sharp layer the figure 7 as follows: the base of the phantom was 210 mm from the table-top and this (with 7·5 mm added to it) gave 217·5 mm as the setting for the fulcrum height.

In the original radiograph which resulted, the number 12 looked to be the sharpest in outline, with 11, 10, 9, 8, 7 slightly and progressively more blurred. Numbers 6, 5, 4, 3, 2, 1 were all unaccepted as being sharp and were progressively more blurred.

These results suggest the following:
1   there is a 5·0 mm error in the stated location of the fulcrum plane since it is 12 and not 7 which is the least unsharp;
2   the layer recorded is at least about 5·0 mm thick.

Since 12 is the last numeral and is the sharpest, we cannot tell how far above 12 the zone of increasing unsharpness reaches the limit of acceptability, as we can for the figures below 12. If we assume that the sharpest figure is in the middle of the tomographic layer with the unsharpness distributed symmetrically on each side, then we would conclude that in this case the layer is about 10 mm thick. The matter could be tested further by repeating the radiograph with the fulcrum level lowered (in this case by 6·0 mm) so that the number most sharply recorded is one in the middle of the helix (say 6).

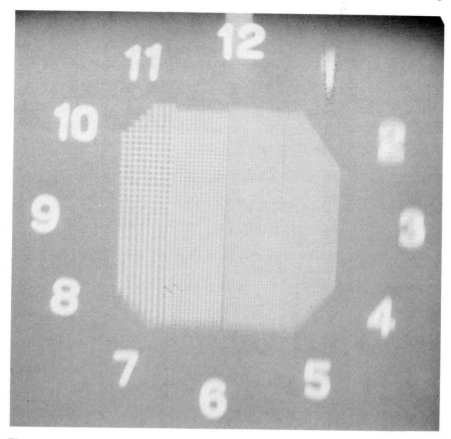

Fig. 17.39

The test of overall resolution was considered to give a satisfactory result here. The original radiograph of Fig. 17.39 shows resolved more than 3·0 mm of the mesh which has 1·6 holes/mm. The equipment used for this test was a simple device which gave linear tomography.

Trajectory and uniformity of exposure

A test to show the tube trajectory during a tomographic sweep can be made using the steel plate of this test tool. This plate has a hole in its centre which is 3·0 mm in diameter. A satisfactory test can be done if this steel plate is set directly on top of the aluminium absorber with the aperture in the centre of the absorber. The equipment is set up to make a tomograph of the plate-absorber combination, with the X-ray beam centred to the aperture. The fulcrum setting should be for a level which is some centimetres (say 5 to 10 cm) away from the level of the plate. This ensures that the image produced by the beam as it passes through the hole is spread by tomographic blurring to give an outline which is broad enough and large enough to be useful. It is not required of the outline that it should appear sharp.

Figure 17.40 is a radiograph made in this way using an elliptical movement. It can be seen that the result is an elliptical trace. Uniformity of exposure is assessed by studying the trace in a search for uneven density. The original radiograph of Fig. 17.40 appears to show four areas of greater

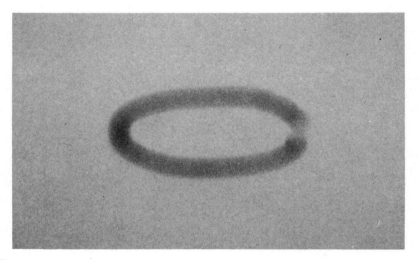

Fig. 17.40

density. Three of these are close together at the cusp of the ellipse which is on the viewer's right in the radiograph; the fourth is on the opposite cusp to the viewer's left. This disposition suggests that the incidents producing the patches of greater density occurred at the start and the end of the tube travel (right cusp) and at the point where it turned back (left cusp) to trace the opposing arc of the ellipse.

Indications of the failure of an X-ray tube

Whenever an X-ray tube is used it is subject to wearing processes to which it will ultimately succumb. Sometimes a tube may fail without any warning of which the radiographer is aware: for example, a thinned filament may fracture and exposure on the focus controlled by that filament is then impossible. The attempt to make such further exposures may increase the damage if the selected kilovoltage happens to be high, for example of the order of 90–100 kVp or more. In these circumstances the 'no-load' voltage (see Chapter 3) developed across the tube could be very high indeed and there is the possibility of fracturing the glass envelope as a result of the unduly elevated tension.

A typical sequence of events in tube failure is for the tube—maybe gradually—to lose its vacuum as the result of overheating of the anode and the liberation of occluded gases. Metal from the anode may be sprayed by electron bombardment round the sides of the tube. Whenever conduction through the tube is altered by factors like these, the milliampere meter is a good witness and this is a further reason why control consoles should include one and radiographers should read it.

Instability of the current through the X-ray tube will be reflected in a similar instability of the milliampere and milliampereseconds meters. Usually the needle is seen to swing sharply across the dial and any radiographer who sees this occur should know the probability that the tube has failed. When it happens, the urge to make a second radiographic exposure—'to see if it's real'—should be resisted. Any further investigation on these lines should be made whenever appropriate with the fluoroscopic switch, which normally energizes the tube at not more than 2–5 milliamperes. Even under abnormal conditions it will limit the current passed and may save the life of other components in the circuit, particularly the high tension rectifiers.

High tension cables

Like X-ray tubes, high tension cables sometimes fail. A breakdown of the insulation in a cable will cause high tension to track to earth, with noisy side effects—and again an abruptly swinging needle on the milliampere meter. It is not suggested that student radiographers should make any investigation of such dramatic events, though it is possible for an experienced radiographer to determine that the failure is indeed with the cable and not arising from faulty conditions in the X-ray tube.

This can be done by disconnecting both cables from the X-ray tube. They can be unscrewed quite simply at their ends and withdrawn from the cable receptables in the tube-shield. It is of obvious importance to have the mains switch 'off' when this is attempted. Furthermore immediately each cable is withdrawn from its socket, the end should be held against some metal part of the X-ray unit to discharge the residual high tension in it; a spark may often be seen or a crackle of electricity heard when this is done. It is a most important precaution and should be observed by any one who in any circumstances exposes either end of a high tension cable.

Often, after withdrawal of the cable, inspection of its tapered end and of the cable receptacle makes obvious the site of the high tension 'tracking'—both to the eye and the nose it is evident as a burned carbon pathway. An air-gap at the cable terminal is the most likely cause of high tension tracking. X-rays ionise air which thus constitutes the greatest risk to electrical insulation. To avoid such a gap, it is common practice when an engineer fits a cable to pack the cable receptacle with a suitable grease such as white vaseline.

If the break in insulation is elsewhere in the cable than at its terminal, a further test may be made.

The cables should be arranged so that their ends are not touching each other or any other conductor: they can often conveniently be placed over the back of a wooden chair. The unit is then switched on and the fluoroscopic footswitch briefly depressed. If the cables are sound, no conduction will occur and the fault may be presumed to lie with the X-ray tube. If—as is suspected—the circuit is being completed to earth via a breakdown in the cable's insulation, the erratic reading of the milliampere meter will be repeated—and no doubt the sound effects. Radiographers with sufficient confidence and experience to make this investigation should equally have enough common sense to switch off the unit and discharge the cable ends again before handing the situation over to the engineer who brings the replacement cable.

A cable may fail because one of the conductors in it is fractured. In this case the nature of the trouble may be made apparent if gentle manipulation of the cable intermittently restores the tube current. However, if this is not so, the condition may need to be distinguished from breakage of the tube filaments, since either situation presents as a failure to obtain exposure.

Again, this is a matter for the experienced radiographer, though it is not really a difficult test to make. It obviously saves an engineer's time—always expensive—and may ensure that when expert aid reaches the department the appropriate replacement is also brought. To make the differential test, the *cathode* cable is detached from the tube shield, executing the precautions previously described. It is quite easy to know which is the cathode end of the X-ray tube, since it will *not* carry the supplementary low tension cable which supplies the anode stator windings. The X-ray set is then switched on: it is most important to be certain that no one attemps to make an exposure at this or any other stage.

When the cable is withdrawn from its socket it will be found to have three pins at the end. Usually there will also be a 'key' or raised section which fits into a keyway or indexing groove in the cable receptacle, so that the cable can be put into the tube-shield only in one defined position. Fig. 17.41 is a sketch of these features but it is no substitute for reality. If they do

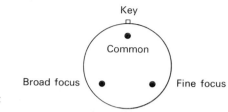

Fig. 17.41

not see them in the course of class teaching or tutorials, students may often prevail upon the good nature of an engineer who is fitting cables in the department to demonstrate the points discussed.

The three pins at the cable's termination are for connection to the filament leads; one is for the small focus, another for the large focus and the third for the common terminal of both. If the end of the cable is considered as a clock face and the cable held in one hand by its earthed sheath so that the 'key' is at the 12 o'clock position, the pin immediately underneath it is the common pin; moving clockwise, the next is for connection to the fine focus and the third is for connection to the broad focus.

Once the investigator has determined the identity of the leads, the shaft of a screwdriver with an adequately insulating (amber) handle should be laid across the appropriate pair of conductors to test in turn the supply to each filament: that is, one connection should be made between the common pin and that for the large focus, and the next between the common pin and the one for the fine focus. In each case, if the cable is sound, a spark will occur, indicating that the supply is reaching the tube—assuming the actual cable connections were tight—and that the circuit is breached in the tube filament itself. On the other hand, if a conductor is fractured at some point in its length—damage in fact occurs usually near a cable's end—then there will be an absence of any spark when the relevant pin is connected to its fellow in the trio; if the broken conductor is the common lead it will naturally affect both foci.

While the cathode cable must have three effective conductors to supply a dual-focus tube, only one conductor is necessary to carry high tension to the anode. This means that in a high tension cable of the modern 150 kVp type—which all carry three conductors—one, or even two, damaged conductors do not prevent its function if it can be transferred to supplying the anode. When an exchange of this kind is made between each of a pair of high tension cables, a record of the matter should be entered in the log book of the unit concerned. If this is not done the fact may be forgotten, or become impossible to know, should the engineer or radiographer responsible for it afterwards be unavailable. At a later similar breakdown time may be spent profitlessly—the writers have known this to occur—in switching the cables again. At this stage the purchase of a new cable has become inevitable.

Index